HEALTH OCCUPATIONS
ENTRANCE EXAMS

Fourth Edition

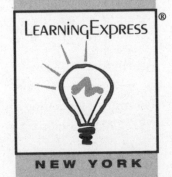

NEW YORK

Copyright © 2017 LearningExpress.

All rights reserved under International and Pan-American Copyright Conventions.
Published in the United States by LearningExpress, New York.

Cataloging-in-Publication Data is on file with the Library of Congress.

ISBN 978-1-61103-095-2

Printed in the United States of America

9 8 7 6 5 4

Fourth Edition

For more information on LearningExpress, other LearningExpress products, or bulk sales, please write to us at:
    224 West 29th Street
    3rd Floor
    New York, NY 10001

CONTRIBUTORS

Dr. Alec Durrell received his Ph.D. in chemistry from the California Institute of Technology and his B.S. in chemistry from the University of North Carolina at Chapel Hill. He is currently a postdoctoral associate at Yale University.

Mark Kalk is a member of the biology faculty at Washington University in St. Louis. He works in the University's Science Outreach program, providing classes, classroom materials, and support to local K–12 teachers. He is a frequent speaker at science education conferences and the author of several books and curriculum materials.

Cindy Phillips has been a high school mathematics teacher for the past eight years. She is currently teaching at White Plains High School in Westchester County, just north of New York City. She is also a Texas Instruments certified instructor in graphing calculator technology.

Margaret Muirhead is a writer and editor from Arlington, Massachusetts. She is a contributor for LearningExpress's *Healthcare Career Starter* and *Nursing School Entrance Exam*. She has also written about a range of health topics for the Harvard University Health Services and the University of Virginia Health System.

Ghislain Mandouma was educated in France (Orsay) and England (Imperial College), where he graduated with a B.Sc. degree in chemistry. He obtained his Ph.D. in chemistry from the City University of New York while teaching at Hunter College. After doing postdoctoral research at the University of Virginia, he joined the faculty of the department of Natural Sciences at the University of Maryland, Eastern Shore, in 2003.

Tyler Volk is associate professor of biology at New York University and codirector of the program in earth and environmental science. He is the author of the books *Gaia's Body: Toward a Physiology of Earth*; *What is Death: A Scientist Looks at the Cycle of Life*; and *Metapatterns Across Space, Time, and Mind*.

CONTENTS

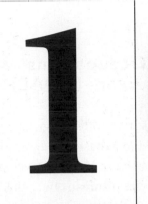

HEALTH OCCUPATIONS ENTRANCE EXAM PLANNER

CHAPTER SUMMARY

In this chapter, you will learn about what you can expect on a health occupations entrance exam, as well as how to use this book to your best advantage. You will learn tips about how to prepare for the exam and develop a study plan that meets your specific needs. After conducting a self-evaluation, you can choose from among four customized test-preparation schedules.

You have chosen this book because you want to pursue a rewarding career in healthcare. The healthcare field encompasses a wide range of exciting career choices, and the employment prospects for jobs in the next decade are excellent. Healthcare services make up the largest industry today and include occupations that are projected to be some of the fastest-growing jobs in the United States.

Healthcare occupations are composed of professionals and paraprofessionals, assistants and aides, technologists and technicians. You may be preparing for a job as a medical records technician, physical therapist, respiratory therapist, speech-language pathologist, or one of the other professions under the broad umbrella of health services.

But to begin your career, you need to get into a training program, and most likely, you will face a health occupations entrance exam. Because there is no one standard test that applies to all training programs, this book is not test-specific, but rather encompasses the core knowledge and skills you will need to pass *any* health occupations entrance exam. Developed from real tests commonly used in the field today, this book offers a study planner, valuable practice tests, and a review of the subjects tested—in short, everything you need to succeed.

Test Overview

To begin preparing for the test, you need an overview of the type of exam you are facing and some tips about how to use this book to achieve your best test score. Again, there is no single test required by all health occupations training programs. Schools have different requirements for admission, depending on the institution, your choice of study, and whether you are applying for a certification course, a one-, two-, or four-year degree, or a graduate program. Many accredited health education programs ask candidates to pass either the Health Occupations Aptitude Exam (HOAE) or the Test of Essential Academic Skills (TEAS). However, even if the school of your choice uses another exam, you will most likely need to demonstrate the essential skills covered in this book. You must show that you can communicate effectively, are able to read and understand college-level materials, and have basic math skills. You may also be asked to demonstrate that you have fundamental knowledge about biology, chemistry, natural science, anatomy, and physiology.

Contact the school of your choice immediately to find out exactly which tests you will need to pass. Many institutions offer a test guide or sample questions from the entrance exam that they use—be sure to take advantage of any information that the school provides about the test.

If you have not done so already, find out about test dates and sites in your area. The dates when the test is offered in your area may determine when you take the exam. However, if you have a choice of test dates, and if you have not already applied to take the exam, do not apply until you have conducted the self-evaluation outlined in this chapter. The results of that self-evaluation can help you decide when to take the exam.

In this chapter, you will find contact information and an overview of two common health occupations entrance exams, the HOAE and the TEAS. If you know you will need to take one of these tests, contact the following testing agencies for more information about registration, testing locations, and dates.

Health Occupations Aptitude Exam (HOAE)

Educational programs that offer degrees ranging from the associate level to a master's degree may require that applicants take the HOAE. Developed by the Psychological Services Bureau, Inc., this exam consists of five parts and takes about two-and-a-half hours to complete. The first section is divided into three subsections.

- Academic Aptitude, 75 questions
  1. Verbal
  2. Math
  3. Analytical Reasoning
- Spelling, 45 questions
- Reading Comprehension, 35 questions
- Natural Science, 60 questions
- Vocational Adjustment, 90 questions

To register for this test or learn about testing sites, contact the school of your choice or:

Psychological Services Bureau, Inc.
977 Seminole Trail PMB 317
Charlottesville, VA 22901
434-293-5865
www.psbtests.com

Test of Essential Academic Skills (ATI TEAS 6 or TEAS)

All nursing programs require the TEAS, a pre-admittance test administered through the Assessment Technologies Institute (ATI) Nursing Education. This three-and-a-half-hour test measures your ability in four general academic areas—your knowledge of English language and usage, your reading skills, your understanding of science, and your ability to solve math problems. The test includes 170 questions, 20 of which are not scored, over four academic sections:

- English Language and Usage
- Reading
- Science
- Mathematics

When you are ready to register for the TEAS, you can do so on the official ATI website, which offers a select number of institutions offering the test.

www.atitesting.com/ctccteas/

If your school is not featured on the site, contact the school directly to learn how to register for the TEAS.

How to Use This Book

This book contains three practice exams (in Chapters 3, 10, and 11) that include the same types of questions as the health occupations entrance exam that you will face. You may be tempted to start right in with a practice exam—but before you do, read on in this chapter. You will learn how to use the first practice exam as a self-evaluation to diagnose your strengths and the areas in which you need more preparation. This chapter will also show you how to customize your study plan so that you can achieve a top score.

In Chapter 2, "LearningExpress Test Preparation System," you will learn strategies to manage your study time as well as practical test-taking tips, such as how to pace yourself during the exam, when to guess, and how to combat test anxiety. Be sure to review the helpful strategies in this chapter before you begin the self-evaluation process.

Chapters 4–9 cover the subject areas found on most health occupations entrance exams: Verbal Ability, Reading Comprehension, Math, Biology, Chemistry, and General Science. Each of these chapters will provide an overview of the kinds of questions you will encounter on the exam and how to tackle them. And you will find practice questions throughout—so you can hone your test-taking skills while you review each topic.

Self-Evaluation

Your first step is to evaluate your level of preparedness. Begin by taking the practice test in Chapter 3 to highlight the areas in which you are strongest and those in which you need more work. You do not have to time yourself—just make sure you have allotted enough time (approximately four hours) so that you can complete the test in one sitting. When you have finished, score your exam using the answer key at the end. Then match your percentages on each section with the following analysis.

SECTION SCORE	ANALYSIS
under 50%	You need concentrated work in this area. Your best bet is to take an additional course. If that is not possible, contact your school's guidance or academic counseling office to arrange for a tutor. Turn to the chapter of this book pertaining to this section of the test only after you have taken a review course or spent at least two months in tutoring; at that point, you will be ready to get maximum benefit from the tips and practice questions in the chapter.
51–70%	This area may not be your strong suit, which is why you should not only work through the relevant chapter of this book, but also use the additional resources listed at the end of that chapter. You might want to find a tutor or form a study group with other students preparing for a health occupations entrance exam.
71–85%	You can probably get all the additional help you need from the chapter of this book pertaining to this section of the test—unless science falls into this category, in which case you should also refer to a biology, chemistry, natural science, or anatomy and physiology textbook.
over 85%	Congratulations! You do not need a lot of work in this area. Turn to the relevant chapter of this book to pick up vital tips and practice that can give you extra points in this area.

Most people do better on some sections of the exam than on others, but most also find that the variation is within a certain range; that is, it is rare to score under 50% in one section and over 90% in another. If you are one of those rare types, do not worry; it just shows you where most of your preparation time should go.

But if you are more typical, where your section scores tend to cluster on the chart should tell you something about when you should take the exam (if you have a choice) and how much time you will have to put in to prepare. If your scores cluster in the "under 50%" category, you should really consider postponing taking the exam until you have had some time for serious study. If your scores tend to be in the middle ranges, then you can go ahead and take the exam, but you should plan to put aside a fair amount of time for study between now and exam day. And if most or all of your scores are in the "over 85%" category, you can still benefit from the practice tests and review chapters in this book—your study time will most likely ensure a high score on the entrance exam.

Planning for Success

There are four customized schedules on the following pages, based on the amount of time you have before the exam. If you are the kind of person who needs deadlines and assignments to motivate you for a project, here they are. If you prefer to design your own study timeline, use the suggested schedules here to help you create an effective plan.

Be sure to research the content of the specific entrance test you will be taking in order to adapt the given schedules for your exam. For example, if you are taking the TEAS, you may plan to skip the verbal chapter, since only the HOAE features spelling questions.

In constructing your plan, you should take into account how much work you need to do. If your scores on the first practice exam were not what you hoped, you should take some of the steps from Schedule A and get them into Schedule D somehow, even if you do have only two weeks before the exam.

Similarly, your scores on the practice exam should help determine how much time you have to spend each week. If you scored low, you might need to devote several hours a day to test preparation. If you scored high, a few hours a week will probably be enough.

Even more important than making a plan is making a commitment. You cannot get ready overnight for a health occupations entrance exam. Set aside some time every day—every other day, if your scores were high and you have months until the exam—for study and practice. An hour every day or every other day will do you much more good than a day or two of cramming right before the exam.

Schedule A: Six Months to Exam

You have taken the first practice test in Chapter 3 and know that you have at least six months in which to build on your strengths and improve in areas where you are weak. Do not put off your preparation. In six months, five hours a week can make a significant difference in your score.

- **Exam minus 6 months:** Pick the one section in which your percentage score on the practice exam was lowest to concentrate on this month. Read the relevant chapter from among Chapters 4–9 and work through the exercises. Use the additional resources listed in that chapter. When you get to that chapter in the following plan, review it.
- **Exam minus 5 months:** Read Chapter 5, "Reading Comprehension," and work through the exercises. Practice reading textbooks and professional journal articles about healthcare, and quiz yourself on each chapter or article you read. Read Chapter 9, "General Science Review," using your reading comprehension skills. Find other people who are preparing for the exam and form a study group.

- **Exam minus 4 months:** Read Chapter 7, "Biology Review," and work through the sample questions. Use the resources listed at the end of the chapter for a comprehensive review. All this reading is a good time to practice your reading comprehension skills, too.
- **Exam minus 3 months:** Read Chapter 8, "Chemistry Review," and work through the exercises. Use the resources listed at the end of the chapter, or your old textbooks, to review topics you are shaky on.
- **Exam minus 2 months:** Read Chapter 6, "Math Review," and work through the exercises. Give yourself additional practice by making up your own test questions in the areas that give you the most trouble.
- **Exam minus 4 weeks:** Read Chapter 4, "Verbal Ability," and work through the exercises. Use at least one additional resource listed here.
- **Exam minus 2 weeks:** Take the practice exam in Chapter 10. Use your scores to help you decide your focus for this week. Go back to the relevant chapters, and get the help of a teacher or your study group.
- **Exam minus 1 week:** Review the first two sample tests, especially the answer explanations. Then, take the practice exam in Chapter 11 for extra practice. As you study this week, concentrate on your strongest areas and decide not to let any areas where you still feel uncertain bother you. Go to bed early every night this week so you can be at your best by test time.
- **Exam minus 1 day:** Relax. Do something unrelated to your health occupations entrance exam. Eat a healthy meal and go to bed at your new early bedtime.

Schedule B: Three to Six Months to Exam

If you have three to six months until the exam, you have just enough time to prepare, as long as you put in at least seven or eight hours a week. This schedule assumes you have four months; stretch it out or compress it if you have more or less time.

- **Exam minus 4 months:** Read Chapter 5, "Reading Comprehension," and work through the exercises. Practice your reading comprehension skills as you work through Chapter 9, "General Science Review," and the resources listed at the end of that chapter. Find other people who are preparing for the exam and form a study group.
- **Exam minus 3 months:** Read Chapters 7 and 8, "Biology Review" and "Chemistry Review," and work through the exercises. Use the resources listed at the end of the chapters, or your old textbooks, to review topics you're shaky on.
- **Exam minus 2 months:** Read Chapter 6, "Math Review," and work through the exercises. Give yourself additional practice by making up your own test questions in the areas that give you the most trouble.
- **Exam minus 4 weeks:** Read Chapter 4, "Verbal Ability," and work through the exercises. Use at least one of the additional resources listed there.
- **Exam minus 2 weeks:** Take the practice test in Chapter 10. Use your scores to help you decide where to concentrate your efforts this week. Go back to the relevant chapters, and get help from a teacher or your study group.
- **Exam minus 1 week:** Review the first two sample tests, especially the answer explanations. Read over the test-taking strategies in Chapter 2. Then, take the sample test in Chapter 11 for extra practice. Choose the one area in which your scores are lowest to review this week. Go to bed early every night this week so you can be at your peak by test time.
- **Exam minus 1 day:** Relax. Do something unrelated to your health occupations entrance exam. Eat a healthy meal and go to bed at your new early bedtime.

Schedule C: One to Three Months to Exam

If you have one to three months until the exam, you still have time to get ready, but you should plan to put in 10 hours a week. This schedule is built around a two-month time frame. If you have only one month, spend a couple of extra hours a week so you can get all the steps in. If you have three months, include some of the steps from Schedule B.

- **Exam minus 8 weeks:** Read Chapter 5, "Reading Comprehension," and work through the exercises. Use your reading comprehension skills as you review Chapter 9, "General Science Review."
- **Exam minus 6 weeks:** Read Chapters 7 and 8, "Biology Review" and "Chemistry Review," and work through the exercises. Use the resources listed at the end of the chapters, or your old textbooks, to review topics you're shaky on.
- **Exam minus 4 weeks:** Read Chapter 6, "Math Review," and work through the exercises.
- **Exam minus 2 weeks:** Read Chapter 4, "Verbal Ability," and work through the exercises.
- **Exam minus 1 week:** Take the practice test in Chapter 10. Use your scores to help you decide where to concentrate your efforts this week. Go back to the relevant chapters, and get the help of a teacher or friend. Go to bed early every night this week so you can be at your peak by test time.
- **Exam minus 4 days:** Take the practice exam in Chapter 11 for extra practice.
- **Exam minus 1 day:** Relax. Do something unrelated to your health occupations entrance exam. Eat a healthy meal and go to bed at your new early bedtime.

Schedule D: Two to Four Weeks to Exam

If you have three weeks or less before the test, you really have your work cut out for you. Carve half an hour out of your day, every day, for studying. This schedule assumes you have the whole three weeks to prepare; if you have less time, you will have to compress the schedule accordingly.

- **Exam minus 14 days:** Read Chapter 5, "Reading Comprehension," and work through the exercises. Use your reading comprehension skills as you review Chapter 9, "General Science Review." Work through the exercises in that chapter.
- **Exam minus 12 days:** Read Chapters 7 and 8, "Biology Review" and "Chemistry Review," and work through the exercises. Use the resources listed at the end of the chapters, or your old textbooks, to review topics you're shaky on.
- **Exam minus 10 days:** Read Chapter 6, "Math Review," and work through the exercises.
- **Exam minus 8 days:** Read Chapter 4, "Verbal Ability," and work through the exercises. Go to bed early every night this week so you can be at your peak by test time.
- **Exam minus 6 days:** Take the practice test in Chapter 10. Choose one or two areas to review until the day before the exam, based on your scores. Go back to the relevant instructional chapters, and get the help of a teacher or friend.
- **Exam minus 4 days:** Take the practice exam in Chapter 11 for extra practice.
- **Exam minus 1 day:** Relax. Do something unrelated to your health occupations entrance exam. Eat a healthy meal and go to bed at your new early bedtime.

Score Your Best

The final step in your study plan is to plan to succeed on exam day. Preparation is the key to building your confidence and giving you the edge you will need to do your best on the exam. If you use this book to customize and follow a study plan, learn the secrets of test success, study the kinds of questions on the exam, and take the practice tests, you *will* score your best—because you will be prepared.

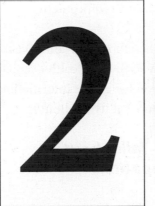

THE LEARNINGEXPRESS TEST PREPARATION SYSTEM

CHAPTER SUMMARY
Taking a health occupations entrance exam can be tough, and your career in healthcare depends on your passing the exam. The LearningExpress Test Preparation System, developed exclusively for LearningExpress by leading test experts, gives you the discipline and attitude you need to succeed.

Taking the health occupations entrance exam can be challenging, and preparing yourself for the test will take work. Your future career in healthcare depends on passing the test, but there are all sorts of pitfalls that can keep you from doing your best on this all-important exam. Here are some of the obstacles that can stand in the way of your success:

- being unfamiliar with the format of the exam
- being paralyzed by test anxiety
- leaving your preparation to the last minute
- not preparing at all!
- not knowing vital test-taking skills: how to pace yourself through the exam, how to use the process of elimination, and when to guess
- not being in your best mental and physical shape
- arriving late at the test site, having to work on an empty stomach, or shivering through the exam because the room is cold

What's the common denominator in all these test-taking pitfalls? One word: control. Who's in control, you or the exam?

Now the good news: The LearningExpress Test Preparation System puts you in control. In just nine easy-to-follow steps, you will learn everything you need to know to make sure that you are in charge of your preparation and your performance on the exam. Other test takers may let the test get the better of them; other test takers may be unprepared or out of shape—but not you. You will have taken all the steps you need to take to get a high score on the health occupations entrance exam.

Here's how the LearningExpress Test Preparation System works: Nine easy steps lead you through everything you need to know and do to get ready to master your exam. Each of the following steps includes both reading about the step and one or more activities. It is important that you do the activities along with the reading, or you won't be getting the full benefit of the system.

Step 1. Get Information
Step 2. Conquer Test Anxiety
Step 3. Make a Plan
Step 4. Learn to Manage Your Time
Step 5. Learn to Use the Process of Elimination
Step 6. Know When to Guess
Step 7. Reach Your Peak Performance Zone
Step 8. Get Your Act Together
Step 9. Do It!

If you have several hours, you can work through the whole LearningExpress Test Preparation System in one sitting. Otherwise, you can break it up and do just one or two steps a day for the next several days. It is up to you—remember, you are in control.

Step 1: Get Information

Activities: Read Chapter 1, "Health Occupations Entrance Exam Planner," and use the suggestions there to find out about your requirements.

Knowledge is power. Therefore, first, you have to find out everything you can about the health occupations entrance exam. Once you have your information, the next steps will show you what to do about it.

Part A: Straight Talk about the Health Occupations Entrance Exam

Why do you have to take this exam, anyway? Because an increasing number of people, particularly elderly people, need to be cared for. And, since more and more people need these services, there is growing concern about the quality of care the patients get. One way to try to ensure quality of care is to test the people who give that care to find out if they have been well trained. And that's why your state, your schools, or the agency you want to work for may require you to take a written exam.

It is important for you to remember that your score on the written exam does not determine how smart you are or even whether you will make a good healthcare professional. There are all kinds of things a written exam like this can't test: whether you are likely to show up late or call in sick a lot, whether you can be patient with a trying client, or whether you can be trusted with confidential information about people's health. Those kinds of things are hard to evaluate on a written exam. Meanwhile, it is easy to evaluate whether you can correctly answer questions about your job duties.

This is not to say that correctly answering the questions on the written exam is not important! The knowledge tested on the exam is knowledge you will need to do your job, and your ability to enter the profession you have trained for depends on your passing this exam. And that's why you are here—to achieve control over the exam.

Part B: What's on the Test

If you haven't already done so, stop here and read Chapter 1 of this book, which gives you an overview of the written exam. Later, you will have the opportunity to take the sample practice exams in Chapters 3, 10, and 11.

Step 2: Conquer Test Anxiety

Activity: Take the Test Anxiety Quiz on page 12.

Having complete information about the exam is the first step in getting control of the exam. Next, you have to overcome one of the biggest obstacles to test success: test anxiety. Test anxiety can not only impair your performance on the exam itself; it can even keep you from preparing! In this step, you will learn stress management techniques that will help you succeed on your exam. Learn these strategies now, and practice them as you complete the exams in this book so that they will be second nature to you by exam day.

Combating Test Anxiety

The first thing you need to know is that a little test anxiety is a good thing. Everyone gets nervous before a big exam—and if that nervousness motivates you to prepare thoroughly, so much the better. Many well-known people throughout history have experienced anxiety or nervousness—from performers such as actor Sir Laurence Olivier and singer Aretha Franklin to writers such as Charlotte Brontë and Alfred Lord Tennyson. In fact, anxiety probably gave them a little extra edge—just the kind of edge you need to do well, whether on a stage or in an examination room.

Stop here and complete the Test Anxiety Quiz on the next page to find out whether your level of test anxiety is something you should worry about.

Stress Management before the Test

If you feel your level of anxiety getting the best of you in the weeks before the test, here is what you need to do to bring the level down again:

- **Get prepared.** There's nothing like knowing what to expect and being prepared for it to put you in control of test anxiety. That's why you are reading this book. Use it faithfully, and remind yourself that you are better prepared than most of the people taking the test.

- **Practice self-confidence.** A positive attitude is a great way to combat test anxiety. This is no time to be humble or shy. Stand in front of the mirror and say to your reflection, "I'm prepared. I'm full of self-confidence. I'm going to ace this test. I know I can do it." If you hear it often enough, you will come to believe it.

- **Fight negative messages.** Every time someone starts telling you how hard the exam is or how it is almost impossible to get a high score, start telling them your self-confidence messages above. If the someone with the negative messages is you, telling yourself *You don't do well on exams* or *You just can't do this*, don't listen.

- **Visualize.** Imagine yourself reporting for duty on your first day as a healthcare professional. Think of yourself helping patients and making them more comfortable. Imagine coming home with your first paycheck. Visualizing success can help make it happen—and it reminds you of why you are working so hard to pass the exam.

You need to worry about test anxiety only if it is extreme enough to impair your performance. The following questionnaire will provide a diagnosis of your level of test anxiety. In the blank before each statement, write the number that most accurately describes your experience.

0 = Never
1 = Once or twice
2 = Sometimes
3 = Often

_____ I have gotten so nervous before an exam that I put down the books and did not study for it.

_____ I have experienced disabling physical symptoms such as vomiting and severe headaches because I was nervous about an exam.

_____ I have simply not shown up for an exam because I was afraid to take it.

_____ I have experienced dizziness and disorientation while taking an exam.

_____ I have had trouble filling in the little circles because my hands were shaking too hard.

_____ I have failed an exam because I was too nervous to complete it.

_____ **Total: Add up the numbers in the blanks above.**

Your Test Stress Score

Here are the steps you should take, depending on your score. If you scored:

- **Below 3:** Your level of test anxiety is nothing to worry about; it is probably just enough to give you that little extra edge.
- **Between 3 and 6:** Your test anxiety may be enough to impair your performance, and you should practice the stress management techniques in this section to try to bring your test anxiety down to manageable levels.
- **Above 6:** Your level of test anxiety is a serious concern. In addition to practicing the stress management techniques listed in this section, you may want to seek additional, personal help. Call your local high school or community college and ask for the academic counselor. Tell the counselor that you have a level of test anxiety that sometimes keeps you from being able to take the exam. The counselor may be willing to help you or may suggest someone else you should talk to.

- **Exercise.** Physical activity helps calm down your body and focus your mind. Besides, being in good physical shape can actually help you do well on the exam. Go for a run, lift weights, go swimming—and do it regularly.

Stress Management on Test Day

There are several ways you can bring down your level of test anxiety on test day. They will work best if you practice them in the weeks before the test, so you know which ones work best for you.

- **Deep breathing.** Take a deep breath while you count to five. Hold it for a count of one, then let it out for a count of five. Repeat several times.
- **Move your body.** Try rolling your head in a circle. Rotate your shoulders. Shake your hands from the wrist. Many people find these movements very relaxing.
- **Visualize again.** Think of the place where you are most relaxed: lying on the beach in the sun, walking through the park, or whatever makes you feel good. Now close your eyes and imagine you are actually there. If you practice in advance, you will find that you only need a few seconds of this exercise to experience a significant increase in your sense of well-being.

When anxiety threatens to overwhelm you right there during the exam, there are still things you can do to manage the stress level.

- **Repeat your self-confidence messages.** You should have them memorized by now. Say them quietly to yourself, and believe them!
- **Visualize one more time.** This time, visualize yourself moving smoothly and quickly through the test answering every question correctly and finishing just before time is up. Like most visualization techniques, this one works best if you have practiced it ahead of time.

- **Find an easy question.** Skim over the test until you find an easy question, and answer it. Getting even one circle filled in gets you into the test-taking groove.
- **Take a mental break.** Everyone loses concentration once in a while during a long test. It is normal, so you shouldn't worry about it. Instead, accept what has happened. Say to yourself, "Hey, I lost it there for a minute. My brain is taking a break." Put down your pencil, close your eyes, and do some deep breathing for a few seconds. Then you will be ready to go back to work.

Try these techniques ahead of time, and see which ones work best for you!

Step 3: Make a Plan

Activity: Construct a study plan.

One of the most important things you can do to get control of yourself and your exam is to make a study plan. Too many people fail to prepare simply because they fail to plan. Spending hours poring over sample test questions the day before the exam not only raises your level of test anxiety, but it also will not replace careful preparation and practice over time.

Don't fall into the cram trap. Take control of your preparation time by mapping out a study schedule. On pages 5–7 are four sample schedules, based on the amount of time you have before you take the written exam. If you are the kind of person who needs deadlines and assignments to motivate you for a project, here they are. If you are the kind of person who doesn't like to follow other people's plans, you can use the suggested schedules to construct your own.

Even more important than making a plan is making a commitment. You can't review everything you learned in your healthcare courses in one night. You need to set aside some time every day for study and practice. Try for at least 20 minutes a day. Twenty minutes daily will do you much more good than two hours on Saturday—divide your test preparation into smaller pieces of the larger work. In addition, making study notes, creating visual aids, and memorizing can be quite useful as you prepare. Each time you begin to study, quickly review your last lesson. This act will help you retain all you have learned and help you assess if you are studying effectively. You may realize you are not remembering some of the material you studied earlier. Approximately one week before your exam, try to determine the areas that are still most difficult for you.

Don't put off your study until the day before the exam. Start now. A few minutes a day, with half an hour or more on weekends, can make a big difference in your score.

Learning Styles

Each of us absorbs information differently. Whichever way works best for you is called your dominant learning method. If someone asks you to help them construct a bookcase they just bought, which may be in many pieces, how do you begin? Do you need to read the directions and see the diagram? Would you rather hear someone read the directions to you—telling you which part connects to another? Or do you draw your own diagram?

The three main learning methods are visual, auditory, and kinesthetic. Determining which type of learner you are will help you create tools for studying.

1. **Visual learners** need to see the information in the form of maps, pictures, text, words, or mathematical equations. Outlining notes and important points in colorful highlighters and taking note of diagrams and pictures may be key in helping you study.
2. **Auditory learners** retain information when they can hear directions, the spelling of a word, a math theorem, or a poem. Repeating information aloud or listening to a recording of your notes may help. Many auditory learners also find working in study groups or having someone quiz them is beneficial.

3. **Kinesthetic learners** must *do!* They need to draw diagrams, write directions, and so on. Rewriting notes on index cards or making margin notes in your textbooks also helps kinesthetic learners to retain information.

Mnemonics

Mnemonics are memory tricks that help you remember what you need to know. The three basic principles in the use of mnemonics are imagination, association, and location. Acronyms (words created from the first letters in a series of words) are common mnemonics. One acronym you may already know is **HOMES**, for the names of the Great Lakes (**H**uron, **O**ntario, **M**ichigan, **E**rie, and **S**uperior). **ROY G. BIV** reminds people of the colors in the spectrum (**R**ed, **O**range, **Y**ellow, **G**reen, **B**lue, **I**ndigo, and **V**iolet). Depending on the type of learner you are, mnemonics can also be colorful or vivid images, stories, word associations, or catchy rhymes such as "Thirty days hath September . . ." created in your mind. Any type of learner, whether visual, auditory, or kinesthetic, can use mnemonics to help the brain store and interpret information.

Step 4: Learn to Manage Your Time

Activities: Practice these strategies as you take the sample tests in this book.

Steps 4, 5, and 6 of the LearningExpress Test Preparation System put you in charge of your exam by showing you test-taking strategies that work. Practice these strategies as you take the sample tests in this book, and then you will be ready to use them on test day.

First, you will take control of your time on the exam. Most health occupations entrance exams have a time limit, which may give you more than enough time to complete all the questions—or may not. It is a terrible feeling to hear the examiner say, "Five minutes left," when you are only three-quarters of the way through the test. Here are some tips to keep that from happening to you.

- **Follow directions.** If the directions are given orally, listen to them. If they are written on the exam booklet, read them carefully. Ask questions before the exam begins if there's anything you don't understand. If you are allowed to write in your exam booklet, write down the beginning time and the ending time of the exam.
- **Pace yourself.** Glance at your watch every few minutes, and compare the time to how far you have gotten in the test. When one-quarter of the time has elapsed, you should be one-quarter of the way through the test, and so on. If you are falling behind, pick up the pace a bit.
- **Keep moving.** Don't spend too much time on one question. If you don't know the answer, skip the question and move on. Circle the number of the question in your test booklet in case you have time to come back to it later.
- **Keep track of your place on the answer sheet.** If you skip a question, make sure that you also skip the question on the answer sheet. Check yourself every five to ten questions to make sure that the number of the question still corresponds with the number on the answer sheet.
- **Don't rush.** Though you should keep moving, rushing won't help. Try to keep calm and work methodically and quickly.

Step 5: Learn to Use the Process of Elimination

Activity: Complete worksheet on Using the Process of Elimination (see pages 17–18).

After time management, your next most important tool for taking control of your exam is using the process of elimination wisely. It is standard test-taking wisdom that you should always read all the answer choices before choosing your answer. This helps you find the right answer by eliminating wrong answer choices. And, sure enough, that standard wisdom applies to your health occupations entrance exam, too.

Let's say you are facing a question like this:

Which of the following lists of signs and symptoms indicates a possible heart attack?
a. headache, dizziness, nausea, confusion
b. dull chest pain, sudden sweating, difficulty breathing
c. wheezing, labored breathing, chest pain
d. difficulty breathing, high fever, rapid pulse

You should always use the process of elimination on a question like this, even if the right answer jumps out at you. Sometimes, the answer that jumps out isn't right after all. Let's assume, for the purpose of this exercise, that you are a little rusty on your signs and symptoms of a heart attack, so you need to use a little intuition to make up for what you don't remember. Proceed through the answer choices in order.

- **Start with choice a.** This one is pretty easy to eliminate; none of these signs and symptoms is likely to indicate a heart attack. Mark an **X** next to choice **a** so you never have to look at it again.
- **On to choice b.** "Dull chest pain" looks good, though if you are not up on your cardiac signs and symptoms you might wonder if it should be "acute chest pain" instead. "Sudden sweating" and "difficulty breathing"? Check. And that's what you write next to choice **b**—a check mark, meaning "good answer, I might use this one."
- **Choice c is a possibility.** Maybe you don't really expect "wheezing" in a heart attack victim, but you know "chest pain" is right, and let's say you are not sure whether "labored breathing" is a sign of cardiac difficulty. Put a question mark next to choice **c**, meaning "well, maybe."

- **Choice d is also a possibility.** "Difficulty breathing" is a good sign of a heart attack. But wait a minute. "High fever"? Not really. "Rapid pulse"? Well, maybe. This doesn't really sound like a heart attack, and you have already got a better answer picked out in choice **b**. If you are feeling sure of yourself, put an **X** next to this one. If you want to be careful, put a question mark. Now your question looks like this:

Which of the following lists of signs and symptoms indicates a possible heart attack?
X **a.** headache, dizziness, nausea, confusion
✓ **b.** dull chest pain, sudden sweating, difficulty breathing
? **c.** wheezing, labored breathing, chest pain
? **d.** difficulty breathing, high fever, rapid pulse

You have just one check mark for a good answer. If you are pressed for time, you should simply mark choice **b** on your answer sheet. If you have got the time to be extra careful, you could compare your check-mark answer to your question-mark answers to make sure that it is better.

It is good to have a system for marking good, bad, and maybe answers. We recommend this one:

X = bad
✓ = good
? = maybe

If you don't like these marks, devise your own system. Just make sure you do it long before test day—while you are working through the practice exams in this book—so you won't have to worry about it during the test.

Key Words

Often, identifying key words in a question will help you in the process of elimination. Words such as *always, never, all, only, must,* and *will* often make statements incorrect. Here is an example of an incorrect statement:

When a nursing assistant is preparing to ambulate a client, making sure the client is wearing proper footwear will always prevent them from falling.

The word *always* in this statement makes it incorrect. Nursing assistants must also take other measures, in addition to providing proper footwear, when ambulating a resident, such as proper body mechanics and providing support to the client.

Words like *usually, may, sometimes,* and *most* may make a statement correct. Here is an example of a correct statement:

Clients of healthcare facilities and hospitals may need help with tasks such as being fed and bathed.

The word *may* makes this statement correct. There are clients in facilities who may be too ill or weak to perform daily tasks such as feeding and bathing themselves.

Even when you think you are absolutely clueless about a question, you can often use the process of elimination to get rid of at least one answer choice. If so, you are better prepared to make an educated guess, as you will see in Step 6. More often, you can eliminate answers until you have only two possible answers. Then you are in a strong position to guess.

Try using your powers of elimination on the questions in the following worksheet, Using the Process of Elimination. The questions are not about healthcare work; they are just designed to show you how the process of elimination works. The answer explanations for this worksheet show one possible way you might use the process to arrive at the right answer.

Step 6: Know When to Guess

Activity: Complete worksheet on Your Guessing Ability (see pages 18–19).

Armed with the process of elimination, you are ready to take control of one of the big questions in test tak-

Use the process of elimination to answer the following questions.

1. Ilsa is as old as Meghan will be in five years. The difference between Ed's age and Meghan's age is twice the difference between Ilsa's age and Meghan's age. Ed is 29. How old is Ilsa?
   a. 4
   b. 10
   c. 19
   d. 24

2. "All drivers of commercial vehicles must carry a valid commercial driver's license whenever operating a commercial vehicle." According to this sentence, which of the following people need NOT carry a commercial driver's license?
   a. a truck driver idling his engine while waiting to be directed to a loading dock
   b. a bus operator backing her bus out of the way of another bus in the bus lot
   c. a taxi driver driving his personal car to the grocery store
   d. a limousine driver taking the limousine to her home after dropping off her last passenger of the evening

3. Smoking tobacco has been linked to
   a. increased risk of stroke and heart attack.
   b. all forms of respiratory disease.
   c. increasing mortality rates over the past ten years.
   d. juvenile delinquency.

4. Which of the following words is spelled correctly?
   a. incorrigible
   b. outragous
   c. domestickated
   d. understandible

Answers

Here are the answers, as well as some suggestions as to how you might have used the process of elimination to find them.

1. **d.** You should have eliminated choice **a** off the bat. Ilsa can't be four years old if Meghan is going to be Ilsa's age in five years. The best way to eliminate other answer choices is to try plugging them in to the information given in the problem. For instance, for choice **b**, if Ilsa is 10, then Meghan must be 5. The difference in their ages is 5. The difference between Ed's age, 29, and Meghan's age, 5, is 24. Is 24 two times 5? No. Then choice **b** is wrong. You could eliminate choice **c** in the same way and be left with choice **d**.

2. **c.** Note the word *not* in the question, and go through the answers one by one. Is the truck driver in choice **a** "operating a commercial vehicle"? Yes, idling counts as "operating," so he needs to have a commercial driver's license. Likewise, the bus operator in choice **b** is operating a commercial vehicle; the question doesn't say the operator has to be on the street. The limo driver in choice **d** is operating a commercial vehicle, even if it doesn't have a passenger in it. However, the cabbie in choice **c** is not operating a commercial vehicle, but his own private car.

3. a. You could eliminate choice **b** simply because of the presence of the word *all*. Such absolutes hardly ever appear in correct answer choices. Choice **c** looks attractive until you think a little about what you know—aren't fewer people smoking these days, rather than more? So how could smoking be responsible for a higher mortality rate? (If you didn't know that mortality rate means the rate at which people die, you might keep this choice as a possibility, but you would still be able to eliminate two answers and have only two to choose from.) And choice **d** is not logical, so you could eliminate that one, too. You are left with the correct answer, choice **a**.

4. a. How you used the process of elimination here depends on which words you recognized as being spelled incorrectly. If you knew that the correct spellings were *outrageous*, *domesticated*, and *understandable*, then you were home free. Surely you knew that at least one of those words was wrong.

YOUR GUESSING ABILITY

The following are 10 really hard questions. You are not supposed to know the answers. Rather, this is an assessment of your ability to guess when you don't have a clue. Read each question carefully, just as if you did expect to answer it. If you have any knowledge of the subject, use that knowledge to help you eliminate wrong answer choices.

1. September 7 is Independence Day in
   a. India.
   b. Costa Rica.
   c. Brazil.
   d. Australia.

2. Which of the following is the formula for determining the momentum of an object?
   a. $p = MV$
   b. $F = ma$
   c. $P = IV$
   d. $E = mc^2$

3. Because of the expansion of the universe, the stars and other celestial bodies are all moving away from each other. This phenomenon is known as
   a. Newton's first law.
   b. the big bang.
   c. gravitational collapse.
   d. Hubble flow.

4. American author Gertrude Stein was born in
   a. 1713.
   b. 1830.
   c. 1874.
   d. 1901.

5. Which of the following is NOT one of the Five Classics attributed to Confucius?
   a. the *I Ching*
   b. the *Book of Holiness*
   c. the *Spring and Autumn Annals*
   d. the *Book of History*

6. The religious and philosophical doctrine that holds that the universe is constantly in a struggle between good and evil is known as
   a. Pelagianism.
   b. Manichaeanism.
   c. neo-Hegelianism.
   d. Epicureanism.

7. The third Chief Justice of the U.S. Supreme Court was

   a. John Blair.

   b. William Cushing.

   c. James Wilson.

   d. John Jay.

8. Which of the following is the poisonous portion of a daffodil?

   a. the bulb

   b. the leaves

   c. the stem

   d. the flowers

9. The winner of the Masters golf tournament in 1953 was

   a. Sam Snead.

   b. Cary Middlecoff.

   c. Arnold Palmer.

   d. Ben Hogan.

10. The state with the highest per capita personal income in 1980 was

   a. Alaska.

   b. Connecticut.

   c. New York.

   d. Texas.

Answers

Check your answers against the following correct answers.

1. c.

2. a.

3. d.

4. c.

5. b.

6. b.

7. b.

8. a.

9. d.

10. a.

How Did You Do?

You may have simply gotten lucky and actually known the answer to one or two questions. In addition, your guessing was probably more successful if you were able to use the process of elimination on any of the questions. Maybe you didn't know who the third Chief Justice was (question 7), but you knew that John Jay was the first. In that case, you would have eliminated choice **d** and therefore improved your odds of guessing right from one in four to one in three.

According to probability, you should get two and a half answers correct, so getting either two or three right would be average. If you got four or more right, you may be a really terrific guesser. If you got one or none right, you may be a really bad guesser.

Keep in mind, though, that this is only a small sample. You should continue to keep track of your guessing ability as you work through the sample questions in this book. Circle the numbers of questions you guess on as you make your guess; or, if you don't have time while you take the practice tests, go back afterward and try to remember which questions you guessed at. Remember, on a test with four answer choices, your chance of guessing correctly is one in four. So keep a separate "guessing" score for each exam. How many questions did you guess on? How many did you get right? If the number you got right is at least one-fourth of the number of questions you guessed on, you are at least an average guesser—maybe better—and you should always go ahead and guess on the real exam. If the number you got right is significantly lower than one-fourth of the number you guessed on, you would be safe in guessing anyway, but maybe you would feel more comfortable if you guessed only selectively, when you can eliminate a wrong answer or at least have a good feeling about one of the answer choices.

Even if you are a play-it-safe person with lousy intuition, you are still safe guessing every time.

ing: Should I guess? The answer is *Yes*. Some exams have what's called a "guessing penalty," in which a fraction of your wrong answers is subtracted from your right answers—but health occupations entrance exams don't tend to work like that. The number of questions you answer correctly yields your raw score. So you have nothing to lose and everything to gain by guessing.

The more complicated answer to the question "Should I guess?" depends on you—your personality and your "guessing intuition." There are two things you need to know about yourself before you go into the exam:

Are you a risk taker?
Are you a good guesser?

You will have to decide about your risk-taking quotient on your own. To find out if you are a good guesser, complete the *Your Guessing Ability* worksheet on pages 18–19.

Step 7: Reach Your Peak Performance Zone

Activity: Complete the Physical Preparation Checklist on page 21.

To get ready for a challenge like a big exam, you have to take control of your physical, as well as your mental, state. Exercise, proper diet, and rest in the weeks prior to the test will ensure that your body works with, rather than against, your mind—both on test day and during your preparation.

Exercise

If you don't already have a regular exercise program going, it's a great idea to start one in the time during which you are preparing for an exam. And if you are already keeping fit—or trying to get that way—don't let the pressure of preparing for an exam fool you into quitting now. Exercise helps reduce stress by pumping

feel-good hormones, called endorphins, into your system. It also increases the oxygen supply throughout your body, including your brain, so you will be at peak performance on test day.

A half hour of vigorous activity—enough to raise a sweat—every day should be your aim. If you are really pressed for time, every other day is okay. Choose an activity you like and get out there and do it. Jogging with a friend always makes the time go faster, as does listening to music.

But don't overdo it. You don't want to exhaust yourself. Moderation is the key.

Diet

First, cut out the junk. Go easy on caffeine and nicotine, and eliminate alcohol from your system at least two weeks before the exam. What your body needs for peak performance is simply a balanced diet. Eat plenty of fruits and vegetables, along with protein and complex carbohydrates. Foods that are high in lecithin (an amino acid), such as fish and beans, are especially good "brain foods."

The night before the exam, you might "carbo-load" the way athletes do before a contest. Eat a big plate of spaghetti, rice and beans, or whatever your favorite carbohydrate is.

Rest

You probably know how much sleep you need every night to be at your best, even if you don't always get it. Make sure you do get that much sleep, though, for at least a week before the exam. Moderation is important here, too. Extra sleep will just make you groggy.

If you are not a morning person and your exam will be given in the morning, you should reset your internal clock so that your body doesn't think you are taking an exam at 3 A.M. You have to start this process well before the exam. The way it works is to get up half an hour earlier each morning, and then go to bed half an hour earlier that night. Don't try it the other way around; you will just toss and turn if you go to bed early without having gotten up early. The next morn-

PHYSICAL PREPARATION CHECKLIST

For the week before the exam, write down (1) what physical exercise you engaged in and for how long and (2) what you ate for each meal. Remember, you are trying for at least half an hour of exercise every other day (preferably every day) and a balanced diet that is light on junk food.

Exam minus 7 days

Exercise: _____ for _____ minutes

Breakfast: _____

Lunch: _____

Dinner: _____

Snacks: _____

Exam minus 6 days

Exercise: _____ for _____ minutes

Breakfast: _____

Lunch: _____

Dinner: _____

Snacks: _____

Exam minus 5 days

Exercise: _____ for _____ minutes

Breakfast: _____

Lunch: _____

Dinner: _____

Snacks: _____

Exam minus 4 days

Exercise: _____ for _____ minutes

Breakfast: _____

Lunch: _____

Dinner: _____

Snacks: _____

Exam minus 3 days

Exercise: _____ for _____ minutes

Breakfast: _____

Lunch: _____

Dinner: _____

Snacks: _____

Exam minus 2 days

Exercise: _____ for _____ minutes

Breakfast: _____

Lunch: _____

Dinner: _____

Snacks: _____

Exam minus 1 day

Exercise: _____ for _____ minutes

Breakfast: _____

Lunch: _____

Dinner: _____

Snacks: _____

ing, get up another half an hour earlier, and so on. How long you will have to do this depends on how late you are used to getting up.

Step 8: Get Your Act Together

Activity: Complete Final Preparations worksheet on page 23.

You are in control of your mind and body; you are in charge of test anxiety, your preparation, and your test-taking strategies. Now it is time to take charge of external factors, like the testing site and the materials you need to take the exam.

Find Out Where the Test Is and Make a Trial Run

The testing agency or your healthcare course instructor will notify you when and where your exam is being held. Do you know how to get to the testing site? Do you know how long it will take to get there? If not, make a trial run, preferably on the same day of the week at the same time of day. Make note, on the worksheet Final Preparations on page 23, of the amount of time it will take you to get to the exam site. Plan on arriving at least 10–15 minutes early so you can get the lay of the land, use the bathroom, and calm down. Then figure out how early you will have to get up that morning, and make sure you get up that early every day for a week before the exam.

Gather Your Materials

The night before the exam, lay out the clothes you will wear and the materials you have to bring with you to the exam. Plan on dressing in layers; you won't have any control over the temperature of the examination room. Have a sweater or jacket you can take off if it is warm. Use the checklist on the worksheet Final Prep-

arations on the following page to help you pull together what you will need.

Don't Skip Breakfast

Even if you don't usually eat breakfast, do so on exam morning. A cup of coffee doesn't count. Don't eat doughnuts or other sweet foods, either. A sugar high will leave you with a sugar low in the middle of the exam. A mix of protein and carbohydrates is best: Cereal with milk and just a little sugar, or eggs with toast, will do your body a world of good.

Step 9: Do It!

Activity: Ace the health occupations entrance exam!

Fast forward to exam day. You are ready. You made a study plan and followed through. You practiced your test-taking strategies while working through this book. You are in control of your physical, mental, and emotional states. You know when and where to show up and what to bring with you. In other words, you are better prepared than most of the other people taking the health occupations entrance exam with you. You are psyched.

Just one more thing . . . When you are done with the exam, you deserve a reward. Plan a celebration. Call up your friends and plan a party, or have a nice dinner for two—whatever your heart desires. Give yourself something to look forward to.

And then do it. Go into the exam, full of confidence, armed with test-taking strategies you have practiced until they are second nature. You are in control of yourself, your environment, and your performance on the exam. You are ready to succeed. So do it. Go in there and ace the exam. And look forward to your future career as a healthcare professional!

Getting to the Exam Site

Location of exam site: _____

Date: _____

Departure time: _____

Do I know how to get to the exam site?   Yes _____   No _____   (If no, make a trial run.)

Time it will take to get to exam site _____

Things to Lay Out the Night Before

Clothes I will wear   _____

Sweater/jacket   _____

Watch   _____

Photo ID   _____

Four #2 pencils   _____

Other Things to Bring/Remember

_____   _____

_____   _____

_____   _____

_____   _____

▶ PRACTICE EXAM I

CHAPTER SUMMARY

This is the first of three practice exams in this book based on actual health occupations entrance exams commonly used in the field today. Use this test to see how you would do if you had to take the test today.

The practice test in this chapter is modeled after real entrance exams required by health education programs. Like many health occupations entrance exams, the practice test measures your skills, abilities, and knowledge of six core subjects: Verbal Ability, Reading Comprehension, Math, General Science, Biology, and Chemistry. It uses a multiple-choice format, with four answer choices, **a–d**. The types of questions in the practice test reflect the kinds of test questions you will likely encounter on your entrance exam. For example, the section on Quantitative Ability includes analytical reasoning questions and the Verbal Ability section features spelling questions, two types of questions that are part of the current HOAE.

The practice test is divided into six sections, covering the six main topics outlined above. In the actual test, each section will be timed separately, with the whole test taking from about two and a half to three hours. Here, you do not have to worry about timing—just try to relax and do your best. Remember, the goal of the practice test is to familiarize yourself with the test format and types of questions and to highlight the areas where you need to concentrate your study and preparation. Make sure that you have scheduled enough time to complete the test without major interruptions, taking only short breaks between sections.

On the following pages, you will find an answer sheet. Use this sheet to mark your answers, filling in the ovals that correspond with your answer choices. Each question has only one correct answer, so do not fill in more than one oval per item. The answer key is located on page 65, so be sure to review the answer explanations carefully after you have finished. Instructions on how to score your exam follow the answer key.

Section 1: Verbal Ability

1. ⓐ ⓑ ⓒ ⓓ
2. ⓐ ⓑ ⓒ ⓓ
3. ⓐ ⓑ ⓒ ⓓ
4. ⓐ ⓑ ⓒ ⓓ
5. ⓐ ⓑ ⓒ ⓓ
6. ⓐ ⓑ ⓒ ⓓ
7. ⓐ ⓑ ⓒ ⓓ
8. ⓐ ⓑ ⓒ ⓓ
9. ⓐ ⓑ ⓒ ⓓ
10. ⓐ ⓑ ⓒ ⓓ
11. ⓐ ⓑ ⓒ ⓓ
12. ⓐ ⓑ ⓒ ⓓ
13. ⓐ ⓑ ⓒ ⓓ
14. ⓐ ⓑ ⓒ ⓓ
15. ⓐ ⓑ ⓒ ⓓ
16. ⓐ ⓑ ⓒ ⓓ
17. ⓐ ⓑ ⓒ ⓓ

18. ⓐ ⓑ ⓒ ⓓ
19. ⓐ ⓑ ⓒ ⓓ
20. ⓐ ⓑ ⓒ ⓓ
21. ⓐ ⓑ ⓒ ⓓ
22. ⓐ ⓑ ⓒ ⓓ
23. ⓐ ⓑ ⓒ ⓓ
24. ⓐ ⓑ ⓒ ⓓ
25. ⓐ ⓑ ⓒ ⓓ
26. ⓐ ⓑ ⓒ ⓓ
27. ⓐ ⓑ ⓒ ⓓ
28. ⓐ ⓑ ⓒ ⓓ
29. ⓐ ⓑ ⓒ ⓓ
30. ⓐ ⓑ ⓒ ⓓ
31. ⓐ ⓑ ⓒ ⓓ
32. ⓐ ⓑ ⓒ ⓓ
33. ⓐ ⓑ ⓒ ⓓ
34. ⓐ ⓑ ⓒ ⓓ

35. ⓐ ⓑ ⓒ ⓓ
36. ⓐ ⓑ ⓒ ⓓ
37. ⓐ ⓑ ⓒ ⓓ
38. ⓐ ⓑ ⓒ ⓓ
39. ⓐ ⓑ ⓒ ⓓ
40. ⓐ ⓑ ⓒ ⓓ
41. ⓐ ⓑ ⓒ ⓓ
42. ⓐ ⓑ ⓒ ⓓ
43. ⓐ ⓑ ⓒ ⓓ
44. ⓐ ⓑ ⓒ ⓓ
45. ⓐ ⓑ ⓒ ⓓ
46. ⓐ ⓑ ⓒ ⓓ
47. ⓐ ⓑ ⓒ ⓓ
48. ⓐ ⓑ ⓒ ⓓ
49. ⓐ ⓑ ⓒ ⓓ
50. ⓐ ⓑ ⓒ ⓓ

Section 2: Reading Comprehension

1. ⓐ ⓑ ⓒ ⓓ
2. ⓐ ⓑ ⓒ ⓓ
3. ⓐ ⓑ ⓒ ⓓ
4. ⓐ ⓑ ⓒ ⓓ
5. ⓐ ⓑ ⓒ ⓓ
6. ⓐ ⓑ ⓒ ⓓ
7. ⓐ ⓑ ⓒ ⓓ
8. ⓐ ⓑ ⓒ ⓓ
9. ⓐ ⓑ ⓒ ⓓ
10. ⓐ ⓑ ⓒ ⓓ
11. ⓐ ⓑ ⓒ ⓓ
12. ⓐ ⓑ ⓒ ⓓ
13. ⓐ ⓑ ⓒ ⓓ
14. ⓐ ⓑ ⓒ ⓓ
15. ⓐ ⓑ ⓒ ⓓ
16. ⓐ ⓑ ⓒ ⓓ
17. ⓐ ⓑ ⓒ ⓓ

18. ⓐ ⓑ ⓒ ⓓ
19. ⓐ ⓑ ⓒ ⓓ
20. ⓐ ⓑ ⓒ ⓓ
21. ⓐ ⓑ ⓒ ⓓ
22. ⓐ ⓑ ⓒ ⓓ
23. ⓐ ⓑ ⓒ ⓓ
24. ⓐ ⓑ ⓒ ⓓ
25. ⓐ ⓑ ⓒ ⓓ
26. ⓐ ⓑ ⓒ ⓓ
27. ⓐ ⓑ ⓒ ⓓ
28. ⓐ ⓑ ⓒ ⓓ
29. ⓐ ⓑ ⓒ ⓓ
30. ⓐ ⓑ ⓒ ⓓ
31. ⓐ ⓑ ⓒ ⓓ
32. ⓐ ⓑ ⓒ ⓓ
33. ⓐ ⓑ ⓒ ⓓ
34. ⓐ ⓑ ⓒ ⓓ

35. ⓐ ⓑ ⓒ ⓓ
36. ⓐ ⓑ ⓒ ⓓ
37. ⓐ ⓑ ⓒ ⓓ
38. ⓐ ⓑ ⓒ ⓓ
39. ⓐ ⓑ ⓒ ⓓ
40. ⓐ ⓑ ⓒ ⓓ
41. ⓐ ⓑ ⓒ ⓓ
42. ⓐ ⓑ ⓒ ⓓ
43. ⓐ ⓑ ⓒ ⓓ
44. ⓐ ⓑ ⓒ ⓓ
45. ⓐ ⓑ ⓒ ⓓ

Section 3: Math

1.	ⓐ	ⓑ	ⓒ	ⓓ	18.	ⓐ	ⓑ	ⓒ	ⓓ	35.	ⓐ	ⓑ	ⓒ	ⓓ
2.	ⓐ	ⓑ	ⓒ	ⓓ	19.	ⓐ	ⓑ	ⓒ	ⓓ	36.	ⓐ	ⓑ	ⓒ	ⓓ
3.	ⓐ	ⓑ	ⓒ	ⓓ	20.	ⓐ	ⓑ	ⓒ	ⓓ	37.	ⓐ	ⓑ	ⓒ	ⓓ
4.	ⓐ	ⓑ	ⓒ	ⓓ	21.	ⓐ	ⓑ	ⓒ	ⓓ	38.	ⓐ	ⓑ	ⓒ	ⓓ
5.	ⓐ	ⓑ	ⓒ	ⓓ	22.	ⓐ	ⓑ	ⓒ	ⓓ	39.	ⓐ	ⓑ	ⓒ	ⓓ
6.	ⓐ	ⓑ	ⓒ	ⓓ	23.	ⓐ	ⓑ	ⓒ	ⓓ	40.	ⓐ	ⓑ	ⓒ	ⓓ
7.	ⓐ	ⓑ	ⓒ	ⓓ	24.	ⓐ	ⓑ	ⓒ	ⓓ	41.	ⓐ	ⓑ	ⓒ	ⓓ
8.	ⓐ	ⓑ	ⓒ	ⓓ	25.	ⓐ	ⓑ	ⓒ	ⓓ	42.	ⓐ	ⓑ	ⓒ	ⓓ
9.	ⓐ	ⓑ	ⓒ	ⓓ	26.	ⓐ	ⓑ	ⓒ	ⓓ	43.	ⓐ	ⓑ	ⓒ	ⓓ
10.	ⓐ	ⓑ	ⓒ	ⓓ	27.	ⓐ	ⓑ	ⓒ	ⓓ	44.	ⓐ	ⓑ	ⓒ	ⓓ
11.	ⓐ	ⓑ	ⓒ	ⓓ	28.	ⓐ	ⓑ	ⓒ	ⓓ	45.	ⓐ	ⓑ	ⓒ	ⓓ
12.	ⓐ	ⓑ	ⓒ	ⓓ	29.	ⓐ	ⓑ	ⓒ	ⓓ	46.	ⓐ	ⓑ	ⓒ	ⓓ
13.	ⓐ	ⓑ	ⓒ	ⓓ	30.	ⓐ	ⓑ	ⓒ	ⓓ	47.	ⓐ	ⓑ	ⓒ	ⓓ
14.	ⓐ	ⓑ	ⓒ	ⓓ	31.	ⓐ	ⓑ	ⓒ	ⓓ	48.	ⓐ	ⓑ	ⓒ	ⓓ
15.	ⓐ	ⓑ	ⓒ	ⓓ	32.	ⓐ	ⓑ	ⓒ	ⓓ	49.	ⓐ	ⓑ	ⓒ	ⓓ
16.	ⓐ	ⓑ	ⓒ	ⓓ	33.	ⓐ	ⓑ	ⓒ	ⓓ	50.	ⓐ	ⓑ	ⓒ	ⓓ
17.	ⓐ	ⓑ	ⓒ	ⓓ	34.	ⓐ	ⓑ	ⓒ	ⓓ					

Section 4: General Science

1.	ⓐ	ⓑ	ⓒ	ⓓ	18.	ⓐ	ⓑ	ⓒ	ⓓ	35.	ⓐ	ⓑ	ⓒ	ⓓ
2.	ⓐ	ⓑ	ⓒ	ⓓ	19.	ⓐ	ⓑ	ⓒ	ⓓ	36.	ⓐ	ⓑ	ⓒ	ⓓ
3.	ⓐ	ⓑ	ⓒ	ⓓ	20.	ⓐ	ⓑ	ⓒ	ⓓ	37.	ⓐ	ⓑ	ⓒ	ⓓ
4.	ⓐ	ⓑ	ⓒ	ⓓ	21.	ⓐ	ⓑ	ⓒ	ⓓ	38.	ⓐ	ⓑ	ⓒ	ⓓ
5.	ⓐ	ⓑ	ⓒ	ⓓ	22.	ⓐ	ⓑ	ⓒ	ⓓ	39.	ⓐ	ⓑ	ⓒ	ⓓ
6.	ⓐ	ⓑ	ⓒ	ⓓ	23.	ⓐ	ⓑ	ⓒ	ⓓ	40.	ⓐ	ⓑ	ⓒ	ⓓ
7.	ⓐ	ⓑ	ⓒ	ⓓ	24.	ⓐ	ⓑ	ⓒ	ⓓ	41.	ⓐ	ⓑ	ⓒ	ⓓ
8.	ⓐ	ⓑ	ⓒ	ⓓ	25.	ⓐ	ⓑ	ⓒ	ⓓ	42.	ⓐ	ⓑ	ⓒ	ⓓ
9.	ⓐ	ⓑ	ⓒ	ⓓ	26.	ⓐ	ⓑ	ⓒ	ⓓ	43.	ⓐ	ⓑ	ⓒ	ⓓ
10.	ⓐ	ⓑ	ⓒ	ⓓ	27.	ⓐ	ⓑ	ⓒ	ⓓ	44.	ⓐ	ⓑ	ⓒ	ⓓ
11.	ⓐ	ⓑ	ⓒ	ⓓ	28.	ⓐ	ⓑ	ⓒ	ⓓ	45.	ⓐ	ⓑ	ⓒ	ⓓ
12.	ⓐ	ⓑ	ⓒ	ⓓ	29.	ⓐ	ⓑ	ⓒ	ⓓ	46.	ⓐ	ⓑ	ⓒ	ⓓ
13.	ⓐ	ⓑ	ⓒ	ⓓ	30.	ⓐ	ⓑ	ⓒ	ⓓ	47.	ⓐ	ⓑ	ⓒ	ⓓ
14.	ⓐ	ⓑ	ⓒ	ⓓ	31.	ⓐ	ⓑ	ⓒ	ⓓ	48.	ⓐ	ⓑ	ⓒ	ⓓ
15.	ⓐ	ⓑ	ⓒ	ⓓ	32.	ⓐ	ⓑ	ⓒ	ⓓ	49.	ⓐ	ⓑ	ⓒ	ⓓ
16.	ⓐ	ⓑ	ⓒ	ⓓ	33.	ⓐ	ⓑ	ⓒ	ⓓ	50.	ⓐ	ⓑ	ⓒ	ⓓ
17.	ⓐ	ⓑ	ⓒ	ⓓ	34.	ⓐ	ⓑ	ⓒ	ⓓ					

Section 5: Biology

	a	b	c	d			a	b	c	d			a	b	c	d
1.	ⓐ	ⓑ	ⓒ	ⓓ	18.	ⓐ	ⓑ	ⓒ	ⓓ	35.	ⓐ	ⓑ	ⓒ	ⓓ
2.	ⓐ	ⓑ	ⓒ	ⓓ	19.	ⓐ	ⓑ	ⓒ	ⓓ	36.	ⓐ	ⓑ	ⓒ	ⓓ
3.	ⓐ	ⓑ	ⓒ	ⓓ	20.	ⓐ	ⓑ	ⓒ	ⓓ	37.	ⓐ	ⓑ	ⓒ	ⓓ
4.	ⓐ	ⓑ	ⓒ	ⓓ	21.	ⓐ	ⓑ	ⓒ	ⓓ	38.	ⓐ	ⓑ	ⓒ	ⓓ
5.	ⓐ	ⓑ	ⓒ	ⓓ	22.	ⓐ	ⓑ	ⓒ	ⓓ	39.	ⓐ	ⓑ	ⓒ	ⓓ
6.	ⓐ	ⓑ	ⓒ	ⓓ	23.	ⓐ	ⓑ	ⓒ	ⓓ	40.	ⓐ	ⓑ	ⓒ	ⓓ
7.	ⓐ	ⓑ	ⓒ	ⓓ	24.	ⓐ	ⓑ	ⓒ	ⓓ	41.	ⓐ	ⓑ	ⓒ	ⓓ
8.	ⓐ	ⓑ	ⓒ	ⓓ	25.	ⓐ	ⓑ	ⓒ	ⓓ	42.	ⓐ	ⓑ	ⓒ	ⓓ
9.	ⓐ	ⓑ	ⓒ	ⓓ	26.	ⓐ	ⓑ	ⓒ	ⓓ	43.	ⓐ	ⓑ	ⓒ	ⓓ
10.	ⓐ	ⓑ	ⓒ	ⓓ	27.	ⓐ	ⓑ	ⓒ	ⓓ	44.	ⓐ	ⓑ	ⓒ	ⓓ
11.	ⓐ	ⓑ	ⓒ	ⓓ	28.	ⓐ	ⓑ	ⓒ	ⓓ	45.	ⓐ	ⓑ	ⓒ	ⓓ
12.	ⓐ	ⓑ	ⓒ	ⓓ	29.	ⓐ	ⓑ	ⓒ	ⓓ	46.	ⓐ	ⓑ	ⓒ	ⓓ
13.	ⓐ	ⓑ	ⓒ	ⓓ	30.	ⓐ	ⓑ	ⓒ	ⓓ	47.	ⓐ	ⓑ	ⓒ	ⓓ
14.	ⓐ	ⓑ	ⓒ	ⓓ	31.	ⓐ	ⓑ	ⓒ	ⓓ	48.	ⓐ	ⓑ	ⓒ	ⓓ
15.	ⓐ	ⓑ	ⓒ	ⓓ	32.	ⓐ	ⓑ	ⓒ	ⓓ	49.	ⓐ	ⓑ	ⓒ	ⓓ
16.	ⓐ	ⓑ	ⓒ	ⓓ	33.	ⓐ	ⓑ	ⓒ	ⓓ	50.	ⓐ	ⓑ	ⓒ	ⓓ
17.	ⓐ	ⓑ	ⓒ	ⓓ	34.	ⓐ	ⓑ	ⓒ	ⓓ					

Section 6: Chemistry

	a	b	c	d			a	b	c	d			a	b	c	d
1.	ⓐ	ⓑ	ⓒ	ⓓ	18.	ⓐ	ⓑ	ⓒ	ⓓ	35.	ⓐ	ⓑ	ⓒ	ⓓ
2.	ⓐ	ⓑ	ⓒ	ⓓ	19.	ⓐ	ⓑ	ⓒ	ⓓ	36.	ⓐ	ⓑ	ⓒ	ⓓ
3.	ⓐ	ⓑ	ⓒ	ⓓ	20.	ⓐ	ⓑ	ⓒ	ⓓ	37.	ⓐ	ⓑ	ⓒ	ⓓ
4.	ⓐ	ⓑ	ⓒ	ⓓ	21.	ⓐ	ⓑ	ⓒ	ⓓ	38.	ⓐ	ⓑ	ⓒ	ⓓ
5.	ⓐ	ⓑ	ⓒ	ⓓ	22.	ⓐ	ⓑ	ⓒ	ⓓ	39.	ⓐ	ⓑ	ⓒ	ⓓ
6.	ⓐ	ⓑ	ⓒ	ⓓ	23.	ⓐ	ⓑ	ⓒ	ⓓ	40.	ⓐ	ⓑ	ⓒ	ⓓ
7.	ⓐ	ⓑ	ⓒ	ⓓ	24.	ⓐ	ⓑ	ⓒ	ⓓ	41.	ⓐ	ⓑ	ⓒ	ⓓ
8.	ⓐ	ⓑ	ⓒ	ⓓ	25.	ⓐ	ⓑ	ⓒ	ⓓ	42.	ⓐ	ⓑ	ⓒ	ⓓ
9.	ⓐ	ⓑ	ⓒ	ⓓ	26.	ⓐ	ⓑ	ⓒ	ⓓ	43.	ⓐ	ⓑ	ⓒ	ⓓ
10.	ⓐ	ⓑ	ⓒ	ⓓ	27.	ⓐ	ⓑ	ⓒ	ⓓ	44.	ⓐ	ⓑ	ⓒ	ⓓ
11.	ⓐ	ⓑ	ⓒ	ⓓ	28.	ⓐ	ⓑ	ⓒ	ⓓ	45.	ⓐ	ⓑ	ⓒ	ⓓ
12.	ⓐ	ⓑ	ⓒ	ⓓ	29.	ⓐ	ⓑ	ⓒ	ⓓ	46.	ⓐ	ⓑ	ⓒ	ⓓ
13.	ⓐ	ⓑ	ⓒ	ⓓ	30.	ⓐ	ⓑ	ⓒ	ⓓ	47.	ⓐ	ⓑ	ⓒ	ⓓ
14.	ⓐ	ⓑ	ⓒ	ⓓ	31.	ⓐ	ⓑ	ⓒ	ⓓ	48.	ⓐ	ⓑ	ⓒ	ⓓ
15.	ⓐ	ⓑ	ⓒ	ⓓ	32.	ⓐ	ⓑ	ⓒ	ⓓ	49.	ⓐ	ⓑ	ⓒ	ⓓ
16.	ⓐ	ⓑ	ⓒ	ⓓ	33.	ⓐ	ⓑ	ⓒ	ⓓ	50.	ⓐ	ⓑ	ⓒ	ⓓ
17.	ⓐ	ⓑ	ⓒ	ⓓ	34.	ⓐ	ⓑ	ⓒ	ⓓ					

Section 1: Verbal Ability

Find the correctly spelled word in the following lists.

1. a. pathetically
b. pathatically
c. pathetickly

2. a. beleif
b. bilief
c. belief

3. a. camaflage
b. camouflaj
c. camouflage

4. a. breach
b. breche
c. braech

5. a. percieved
b. preceived
c. perceived

6. a. shriveled
b. shrivvelled
c. shrivelled

7. a. sittuation
b. situation
c. situashun

8. a. apparently
b. apparrentely
c. apperantly

9. a. obssession
b. obsessian
c. obsession

10. a. jeoperdy
b. jepardy
c. jeopardy

11. a. magnifisint
b. magnifisent
c. magnificent

12. a. geraitrics
b. geriatrics
c. gereatrics

13. a. elicitt
b. ellicit
c. illicit

14. a. inquiry
b. inquirry
c. enquirry

15. a. terminated
b. termenated
d. termanated

16. a. persecution
b. pursecution
c. presecution

17. a. peculior
b. peculiar
c. peculliar

18. a. psycology
b. psychology
c. psychollogy

19. a. license
b. lisence
c. lycence

20. a. concise
b. concize
c. consise

21. a. nieghbor
b. neighbor
c. niehbor

22. a. stabilize
b. stablize
c. stableize

23. a. rexamining
b. reexammining
c. reexamining

24. a. aspirations
b. asparations
c. aspirrations

25. a. excercise
b. exercise
c. exersize

26. a. artificial
b. artifishal
c. artaficial

27. a. hindrance
b. hindrence
c. hindranse

28. a. testamony
b. testimonie
c. testimony

29. a. adiction
b. addictione
c. addiction

30. a. thorough
b. thorogh
c. thurugh

31. a. quantity
b. quantitie
c. quantety

32. a. imitiate
b. imitat
c. imitate

33. a. contradect
b. contradict
c. contredict

34. a. reversil
b. reversal
c. reversale

35. a. foregn
b. forein
c. foreign

36. a. ravenous
b. ravenas
c. ravenus

37. a. phenomenal
b. phenomenil
c. phenomenul

38. a. temprature
b. temperature
c. temperatur

39. a. auditoriam
b. auditorium
c. auditoreum

40. a. circumfrence
    b. circumferance
    c. circumference

41. a. worrees
    b. worries
    c. worrys

42. a. finalaty
    b. finality
    c. finalitie

43. a. religious
    b. religiouse
    c. religius

44. a. coliseum
    b. coliseam
    c. colaseum

45. a. delinquant
    b. delinquent
    c. delinquente

46. a. forcast
    b. forecaste
    c. forecast

47. a. righteous
    b. righteus
    c. righteos

48. a. sincerely
    b. sincerly
    c. sincereley

49. a. hospise
    b. hospice
    c. hospace

50. a. resparation
    b. respiration
    c. respiratione

Section 2:
Reading Comprehension

Read each passage and answer the questions based on the information in the text. You have 45 minutes to complete this section.

Asthma is no longer considered a condition with isolated, acute episodes of bronchospasm. Rather, asthma is now understood to be a chronic inflammatory disorder of the airways—that is, inflammation makes the airways chronically sensitive. When these hyper-responsive airways are irritated, air flow is limited, and attacks of coughing, wheezing, chest tightness, and difficulty in breathing occur.

Asthma involves complex interactions among inflammatory cells, mediators, and the cells and tissues in the airways. The interactions result in airflow limitation from acute bronchoconstriction, swelling of the airway wall, increased mucus secretion, and airway remodeling. The inflammation also causes an increase in airway responsiveness. During an asthma attack, the patient attempts to compensate by breathing at a higher lung volume in order to keep the air flowing through the constricted airways; the greater the airway limitation, the higher the lung volume must be to keep airways open. The morphologic changes that occur in asthma include bronchial infiltration by inflammatory cells. Key effector cells in the inflammatory response are the mast cells, lymphocytes, and eosinophils. Mast cells and eosinophils are also significant participants in allergic responses, hence the similarities between allergic reactions and asthma attacks. Other changes include mucus plugging of the airways, interstitial edema, and microvascular leakage. Destruction of bronchial epithelium and thickening of the subbasement membrane are also characteristic. In addition, there may be hypertrophy and hyperplasia of airway smooth muscle, increase in goblet cell number, and enlargement of submucous glands.

Although causes of the initial tendency toward inflammation in the airways of patients with asthma are not yet certain, to date the strongest identified risk factor is atopy. This inherited familial tendency to have allergic reactions includes increased sensitivity to allergens that are risk factors for developing asthma. Some of these allergens include domestic dust mites, animals with fur, cockroaches, pollens, and molds. Additionally, asthma may be triggered by viral respiratory infections, especially in children. By avoiding these allergens and triggers, a person with asthma lowers the risk of irritating sensitive airways. A few avoidance techniques include keeping the home clean and well ventilated, using an air conditioner in the summer months when pollen and mold counts are high, and getting an annual influenza vaccination. Of course, asthma sufferers should avoid tobacco smoke altogether. Cigar, cigarette, and pipe smoke are triggers whether the patient smokes or breathes in the smoke from others. Smoke increases the risk of allergic sensitization in children and increases the severity of symptoms in children who already have asthma. Many of the risk factors for developing asthma may also provoke asthma attacks, and people with asthma may have one or more triggers, which vary among individuals. The risk can be further reduced by taking medications that decrease airway inflammation. Most exacerbations can be prevented by the combination of avoiding triggers and taking anti-inflammatory medications. An exception is physical activity, which is a common trigger of exacerbations in asthma patients. However, asthma patients should not necessarily avoid all physical exertion, because some types of activity have been proven

to reduce symptoms. Rather, they should work with a doctor to design a proper training regimen including the use of medication.

In order to diagnose asthma, a healthcare professional must appreciate the underlying disorder that leads to asthma symptoms and understand how to recognize the condition through information gathered from the patient's history, physical examination, measurements of lung function, and allergic status. Because asthma symptoms vary throughout the day, the respiratory system may appear normal during physical examination. Clinical signs are more likely to be present when a patient is experiencing symptoms; however, the absence of symptoms at the time of the examination does not exclude the diagnosis of asthma.

1. What is the name for the familial inclination to have hypersensitivity to certain allergens?
   a. interstitial edema
   b. hyperplasia
   c. hypertrophy
   d. atopy

2. Why does a person suffering from an asthma attack attempt to inhale more air?
   a. to prevent the loss of consciousness
   b. to keep air flowing through shrunken air passageways
   c. to prevent hyperplasia
   d. to compensate for weakened mast cells, lymphocytes, and eosinophils

3. From the passage you can infer that asthma is
   a. a relatively new disease.
   b. a degenerating, life-threatening disorder.
   c. a health problem that has been around for some time.
   d. a digestive condition.

4. Which of the following describes the word *chronic* as it is used in the first paragraph of the passage?
   a. isolated
   b. acute
   c. recurring
   d. hyper

5. During an allergy attack, the bronchial epithelium might be
   a. destroyed.
   b. thickened.
   c. enlarged.
   d. increased.

6. Which of the following triggers is mentioned as possibly reducing the symptoms of asthma in some patients?
   a. using a fan instead of an air conditioner
   b. second-hand cigarette smoke
   c. a family pet
   d. physical activity

7. Why might a patient with asthma have an apparently normal respiratory system during an examination by a doctor?
   a. Asthma symptoms come and go throughout the day.
   b. Severe asthma occurs only after strenuous physical exertion.
   c. Doctors' offices are usually smoke-free and very clean.
   d. The pollen and mold count may be low that day.

8. Which of the following contribute significantly to the similarities between allergic reactions and asthma attacks?
   a. mast cells and lymphocytes
   b. eosinophils and mast cells
   c. mast cells and epithelia
   d. lymphocytes and eosinophils

9. One cause of an asthma attack is
   a. infections.
   b. swelling.
   c. secretion.
   d. hyperventilating.

Spina bifida is a defect of the spinal column that occurs during the first 28 days after fertilization of a human ovum. The broad definition of spina bifida is the condition in which the bones of the spinal column surrounding the spinal cord do not close properly, and the cord or spinal fluid bulges through a section of the lower back. Any portion of the spinal cord outside the vertebrae is undeveloped or damaged and will inevitably cause paralysis and incontinence. However, there is a minor and a major form of this condition. The symptom of the mild form, called spina bifida *occulata* ("hidden"), is a small gap in the spine covered by a dimple in the skin. This condition can be so mild that some people who have spina bifida occulata may never even know they have it.

In contrast, the more disabling form, called spina bifida *aperta*, is what most people refer to as spina bifida. On rare occasions, spina bifida aperta results in a small but noticeable sac called a *meningocele* forming on the fetus's back. The meningocele may be repaired after birth in a major surgical procedure. Afterward, the patient may suffer little or no muscle paralysis. However, in 90% of all spina bifida aperta cases, a portion of the undeveloped spinal cord itself protrudes through the spine and forms a sac. This so-called *myelocele* (or *meningomyelocele*) is visible on the baby's back. The location of the myelocele determines how severely disabled the child will be. In general, the higher it is on the spinal column, the more paralysis is possible. Doctors must repair any opening of the spine shortly after birth or the child will die. Other major surgeries often follow in the child's first years.

Depending on the severity of their condition, children with spina bifida have varying degrees of paralysis and incontinence. About 85% of them develop *hydrocephalus*, an accumulation of cerebrospinal fluid surrounding the brain. This fluid must be drained to the abdomen or blood stream with a surgically implanted tube. Some children with spina bifida develop foot and knee deformities caused by an interruption of spinal nerve circuits. Many patients require leg braces, crutches, and other devices to help them walk. They may have learning disabilities, and about 30% of these children have slight to severe mental retardation. Other results of this condition are chronic bladder infections and kidney problems, which require lifelong medical attention. Despite their need for medical attention, children with spina bifida can learn to care for many of their own needs. While once all of these children died, with proper medical treatment, between 85% and 90% of them now live to adulthood.

10. Spina bifida is a defect of the spinal column that occurs during
   a. the middle of the third trimester.
   b. the first 28 days after fertilization.
   c. the second trimester.
   d. delivery of the child.

11. Repairing the meningocele could prevent the patient from suffering
   a. spina bifida.
   b. paralysis.
   c. incontinence.
   d. deformity.

12. Which of the following describes the word *procedure* as it is used in the second paragraph of the passage?
   a. system
   b. rule
   c. process
   d. formula

13. Which of the following is the term for a pool of cerebrospinal fluid in the area around the brain?
   a. catheterization
   b. spina bifida
   c. hydrocephalus
   d. meningomyelocele

14. A sign of spina bifida occulata is
   a. a small gap in the spine covered by a dimple.
   b. total paralysis.
   c. severe mental retardation.
   d. inability to move the fingers.

15. The conclusion of this passage could best be summarized by which of the following statements?
   a. All pregnant women should have their fetuses tested for spina bifida.
   b. Infants with spina bifida are smaller than other infants.
   c. Spina bifida is a birth defect that kills millions of innocent children each year.
   d. People who have spina bifida may lead productive lives with proper medical attention.

Medical waste has been a growing concern because of recent incidents of public exposure to discarded blood vials, needles (sharps), empty prescription bottles, and syringes. Medical waste can typically include general refuse, human blood and blood products, cultures and stocks of infectious agents, laboratory animal carcasses, contaminated bedding material, and pathological wastes.

Wastes are collected by gravity chutes, carts, or pneumatic tubes. Chutes are limited to vertical transport, and there is some risk of exhausting contaminants into hallways if a door is left open during use. Another disadvantage of gravity chutes is that the waste container may get jammed while dropping, or broken upon hitting the bottom. Carts are primarily for horizontal transport of bagged or containerized wastes. The main risk here is that bags may be broken or torn during transport, potentially exposing the worker to the wastes. Using automated carts can reduce the potential for exposure. Pneumatic tubes offer the best performance for waste transport in a large facility. Advantages include high-speed movement, movement in any direction, and minimal intermediate storage of untreated wastes. However, some objects cannot be conveyed pneumatically.

Off-site disposal of regulated medical wastes remains a viable option for smaller hospitals (those with fewer than 150 beds). Some preliminary on-site processing, such as compaction or hydropulping, may be necessary prior to sending the waste off-site. Compaction reduces the total volume of solid wastes, often reducing transportation and disposal costs, but does not change the hazardous characteristics of the waste. However, compaction may not be economical if transportation and disposal costs are based on weight rather than volume.

Hydropulping involves grounding the waste in the presence of an oxidizing fluid, such as hypochlorite solution. The liquid is separated from the pulp and discharged directly into the sewer unless local limits require additional pretreatment prior to discharge. The pulp can often be disposed of at a landfill. One advantage is that waste can be rendered innocuous and reduced in size within the same system. Disadvantages are the added operating burden, difficulty of controlling fugitive emission, and the difficulty of conducting microbiological tests to determine whether all organic matters and infectious organisms from the waste have been destroyed.

On-site disposal is a feasible alternative for hospitals generating two tons or more per day of total solid waste. Common treatment techniques include steam sterilization and incineration. Although other options are available, incineration is currently the preferred method for on-site treatment of hospital waste.

Steam sterilization is limited in the types of medical waste it can treat, but is appropriate for laboratory cultures and substances contaminated with infectious organisms. The waste is subjected to steam in a sealed, pressurized chamber. The liquid that may form is drained off to the sewer or sent for processing. The unit is then reopened after a vapor release to the atmosphere, and the solid waste is taken out for further processing or disposal. One advantage of steam sterilization is that it has been used for many years in hospitals to sterilize instruments and containers and to treat small quantities of waste. However, since sterilization does not change the appearance of the waste, there could be a problem in gaining acceptance of the waste for landfilling.

A properly designed, maintained, and operated incinerator achieves a relatively high level of organism destruction. Incineration reduces the weight and volume of the waste as much as 95% and is especially appropriate for pathological wastes and sharps. The most common incineration system for medical waste is the controlled-air type. The principal advantage of this type of incinerator is low particulate emissions. Rotary kiln and grate-type units have been used, but use of grate-type units has been discontinued due to high air emissions. The rotary kiln also puts out high emissions, and the costs have been prohibitive for smaller units.

16. One disadvantage of the compaction method of waste disposal is that it
  a. cannot reduce transportation costs.
  b. reduces the volume of solid waste material.
  c. does not allow hospitals to confirm that organic matter has been eliminated.
  d. does not reduce the weight of solid waste material.

17. For hospitals that dispose of waste on their own premises, the optimum treatment method is
  a. incineration.
  b. compaction.
  c. sterilization.
  d. hydropulping.

18. Which of the following could be safely disposed of in a landfill but might not be accepted by landfill facilities?
  a. hydropulped material
  b. sterilized waste
  c. incinerated waste
  d. laboratory cultures

19. Carting away medical waste can create a risk for
  a. hospital patients.
  b. medical professionals.
  c. maintenance workers.
  d. waste removal workers.

20. Two effective methods for treating waste caused by infectious matter are
  a. steam sterilization and incineration.
  b. hydropulping and steam sterilization.
  c. incineration and compaction.
  d. hydropulping and incineration.

21. Hospitals can minimize employee contact with dangerous waste by switching from
  a. a manual cart to a gravity chute.
  b. an automated cart to a hydropulping machine.
  c. a gravity chute to a manual cart.
  d. a manual cart to an automated cart.

22. The process that both transforms waste from hazardous to harmless and diminishes waste volume is
  a. sterilization.
  b. hydropulping.
  c. oxidizing.
  d. compacting.

23. Hospitals would have a better chance of getting landfills to accept steam sterilized waste if they could change the waste's
  a. toxicity.
  b. quantity.
  c. odor.
  d. appearance.

24. The use of on-site grate-type units has been discontinued because of
  a. budgetary constraints.
  b. high air emissions.
  c. local community ordinances.
  d. lack of availability.

The immune system is equal in complexity to the combined intricacies of the brain and nervous system. The success of the immune system in defending the body relies on a dynamic regulatory-communications network consisting of millions and millions of cells. Organized into sets and subsets, these cells pass information back and forth like clouds of bees swarming around a hive. The result is a sensitive system of checks and balances, which produces an immune response that is prompt, appropriate, effective, and self-limiting.

At the heart of the immune system is the ability to distinguish between *self* and *nonself*. When immune defenders encounter cells or organisms carrying foreign or nonself molecules, the immune troops move quickly to eliminate the intruders. Virtually every body cell carries distinctive molecules that identify it as self. The body's immune defenses do not normally attack tissues that carry a self marker. Rather, immune cells and other body cells coexist peaceably in a state known as self-tolerance. When a normally functioning immune system attacks a nonself molecule, the system has the ability to "remember" the specifics of the foreign body. Upon subsequent encounters with the same species of molecules, the immune system reacts accordingly. With the possible exception of antibodies passed during lactation, this so-called immune system memory is not inherited. Despite the occurrence of a virus in your family, your immune system must "learn" from experience with the many millions of distinctive nonself molecules in the sea of microbes in which we live. Learning entails producing the appropriate molecules and cells to match up with and counteract each nonself invader.

Any substance capable of triggering an immune response is called an *antigen*. Antigens are not to be confused with *allergens*, which are most often harmless substances (such as ragweed pollen or cat hair) that provoke the immune system to set off the inappropriate and harmful response known as *allergy*. An antigen can be a virus, a bacterium, a fungus, a parasite, or even a portion or product of one of these organisms. Tissues or cells from another individual (except an identical twin, whose cells carry identical self markers) also act as antigens; because the immune system recognizes transplanted tissues as foreign, it rejects them. The body will even reject nourishing proteins unless they are first broken down by the digestive system into their primary, non-antigenic building blocks. An antigen announces its foreignness by means of intricate and characteristic shapes called *epitopes*, which protrude from its surface. Most antigens, even the simplest microbes, carry several different kinds of epitopes on their surface; some may even carry several hundred. Some epitopes will be more effective than others at stimulating an immune response. Only in abnormal situations does the immune system wrongly identify self as nonself and execute a misdirected immune attack. The result can be a so-called autoimmune disease such as rheumatoid arthritis or systemic lupus erythematosus. The painful side effects of these diseases are caused by a person's immune system actually attacking itself.

25. The surfaces of antigens have been known to carry
   a. fungi.
   b. epitopes.
   c. allergens.
   d. bacterium.

26. The immune cells and other cells in the body coexist peaceably in a state known as
   a. equilibrium.
   b. self-tolerance.
   c. harmony.
   d. tolerance.

27. What is the specific term used in the passage for the substance capable of triggering an inappropriate or harmful immune response to a harmless substance such as ragweed pollen?
a. antigen
b. microbe
c. allergen
d. autoimmune disease

28. How do the cells in the immune system recognize an antigen as "foreign" or "nonself"?
a. through an allergic response
b. through blood type
c. through fine hairs protruding from the antigen surface
d. through characteristic shapes on the antigen surface

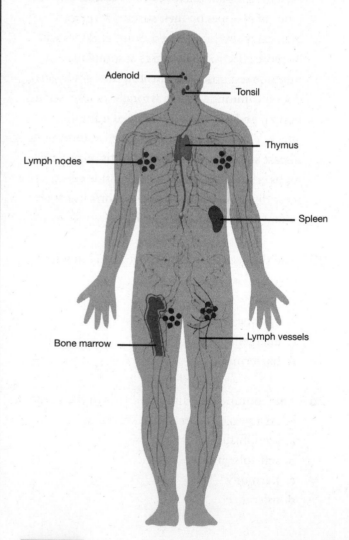

Adenoid
Tonsil
Lymph nodes
Thymus
Spleen
Bone marrow
Lymph vessels

29. A component of the immune system located in the torso is the
a. spleen.
b. pancreas.
c. tonsil.
d. adenoid.

30. Which of the following best expresses the main idea of this passage?
a. The basic function of the immune system is to distinguish between self and nonself.
b. An antigen is any substance that triggers an immune response.
c. One of the immune system's primary functions is the allergic response.
d. The human body presents an opportune habitat for microbes.

31. Rheumatoid arthritis presents an abnormal situation in which
a. antibodies were passed during lactation.
b. the immune system actually attacks itself.
c. nourishing proteins are broken down by the digestive system.
d. the immune system sets off a response known as an allergy.

Sometimes your protective immune system can suddenly become your worst enemy. When that happens, rogue killer cells may attack organs or tissues that are essential to your survival. In recent years, scientists have identified this scenario, known as an *autoimmune attack*, as the cause of many diseases whose origins previously were unknown. Psoriasis is among the latest to be included in this category.

Psoriasis is a skin disease that in severe cases disfigures patients' bodies and makes their lives miserable. Affected areas of the skin— often spreading out from elbows and knees—are red and inflamed and may be covered by silvery scales. It has long been known that many psoriasis patients belong to families that have a history of the disease, and in these psoriasis-prone families certain genetic markers, known as HLA antigens, are inherited more often than in the general population. However, until recently, it was not known whether psoriasis was primarily an immune disease or an epidermal skin disease.

Data existed that suggested immune system involvement. In studies of psoriatic skin, investigators detected immune cells, known as *T cells*, that have surface receptors for interleukin-2 (IL-2), a cellular hormone that is an important mediator of immune reactions. What wasn't clear from the studies was whether the immune contribution was a secondary phenomenon. To distinguish between the roles of the scaling, non-immune epidermal skin cells, called *keratinocytes*, and the immune cells, scientists used an experimental drug that eliminated specific T cells. They reasoned that if the absence of these cells improved the patients' psoriasis, immune cells, not epidermal skin cells, were probably the main culprit in causing the disease.

Since only T cells that are activated to participate in immune reactions carry the IL-2 receptor, selective removal of these cells did not endanger all T cells in the body. Scientists theorize that in psoriasis there is an as-yet undefined antigen that the T cells react to in an autoimmune fashion. Those reactive cells proliferate and express the IL-2 receptor.

To target and kill the activated T cells, scientists use a molecule manufactured by fusing IL-2 and diphtheria toxin. The innocuous IL-2 part of the fusion molecule binds to T cells that have IL-2 receptors and thereby delivers its poisonous partner to the target. After binding, the fusion molecule enters the cells and the diphtheria toxin blocks their protein-synthesizing machinery, killing the cells.

Scientists tested the experimental drug in ten patients who had severe psoriasis. The patients were admitted to a research center where they received the drug in five daily intravenous doses. Subsequently they were assessed as outpatients for 23 days. After this, they received an additional round of five intravenous doses of the drug followed by another 23-day assessment period. Four of the patients showed striking clinical improvement, four had moderate improvement, and two had minimal improvement after two cycles of treatment with the drug. Among the improvements were, most significantly, thinning of the psoriatic areas, reduced keratinocyte proliferation, and reduced inflammation with fewer T cells in the epidermis.

These studies suggest that the molecule is likely to be effective, but scientists caution there is a long way to go before claiming that this drug is safe and widely effective. The low doses are reasonably well tolerated, and studies have revealed that at least some cases of psoriasis are caused by a defective immune system. There is no data that refute the hypothesis that the disease is immune-mediated. Scientists point out, however, that the response was mixed since not all patients responded to the drug.

Scientists are continuing their studies with higher doses of the IL-2/diphtheria toxin drug to see if a higher proportion of the patients may respond. Because psoriasis is a uniquely human disease, it cannot be studied in animal models, an approach that allows experimental studies of many other diseases.

32. Psoriasis is a kind of
   a. deformity.
   b. skin cancer.
   c. autoimmune attack.
   d. immune reaction.

33. One reason researchers used an experimental drug was to
  a. gauge the impact of missing immune cells on psoriasis patients.
  b. identify epidermal skin cells as the cause of psoriasis.
  c. trace the genetic history of psoriasis.
  d. rule out autoimmune attacks as a cause of psoriasis.

34. People in psoriasis-prone families inherit which of the following more often than those in the general population?
  a. genetic markers known as anti-Rh antibodies
  b. genetic markers known as HLA antigens
  c. the CD103 antigen
  d. a surface receptor known as H1V1

35. The passage does not suggest that psoriasis can cause
  a. inflammations.
  b. scales.
  c. paralysis.
  d. disfigurement.

36. The impact of the experimental drug was extraordinary
  a. for over half the patients.
  b. because epidermal skin cells multiplied.
  c. for fewer than half the patients.
  d. because the drug received universal acceptance.

37. IL-2 receptors are transported by
  a. undefined antigens.
  b. cellular hormones.
  c. activated T cells.
  d. epidermal cells.

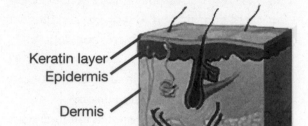

Normal skin

Keratin layer
Epidermis
Dermis
Subcutaneous layer

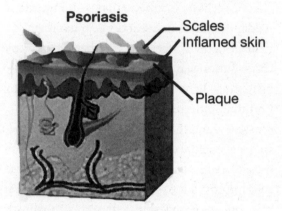

Psoriasis
Scales
Inflamed skin
Plaque

38. The keratin layer of someone suffering from psoriasis contains
  a. dermis.
  b. plaque.
  c. hormones.
  d. diphtheria.

39. The main idea of the passage is that scientists
  a. are closer than before to comprehending the causes of psoriasis.
  b. can now prove psoriasis is a genetic disease.
  c. can rule out epidermal cells as the cause of psoriasis.
  d. are closer to discrediting an immune-related cause of psoriasis.

40. Psoriasis is
  a. a uniquely human disease.
  b. an autoimmune disease.
  c. a sometimes disfiguring skin disease.
  d. all of the above

Genetic engineering, more formally known as recombinant DNA technology, allows scientists to cut segments of DNA from one type of organism and combine them with the genes of a second organism. In this way, relatively simple organisms such as bacteria or yeast, or even mammalian cells in culture, can be induced to make quantities of human proteins, including interferons or interleukins. This technology has enabled scientists to grow tobacco plants that produce monoclonal antibodies, and goats that secrete a clot-dissolving heart attack drug, *tissue plasminogen activator* (TPA), in their milk.

Another facet of recombinant DNA technology involves gene therapy. The goal of this therapy is to replace defective genes, or to endow a cell with new capabilities. In 1989, the feasibility and safety of gene transfer was demonstrated when *tumor-infiltrating lymphocytes* (TILs) were extracted from a patient, equipped with a marker gene (so they could be tracked and monitored), and then reinjected into patients with advanced cancer. To deliver the gene into the TIL, the scientists used a virus, exploiting its natural tendency to invade cells. Before being used as a vector, the virus was altered so that it could not reproduce or cause disease. This experiment demonstrated that gene-modified cells could survive for long periods in the bloodstream and in tumor deposits without harm to the patient.

The earliest attempts to use genes therapeutically focused on a form of *severe combined immunodeficiency disease* (SCID), which is caused by the lack of an enzyme due to a single abnormal gene. The gene for this enzyme—*adenosine deaminase* (ADA)—is delivered into the patient's T cells by a modified retrovirus. When the virus splices its genes into those of the T cells, it simultaneously introduces the gene for the missing enzyme. After the treated T cells begin to produce the missing enzyme, they are injected back into the patient.

Gene therapy is now being used with some cancer patients. TILs reinforced with a gene for the anti-tumor cytokine known as *tumor necrosis factor* (TNF) have been administered to patients with advanced melanoma, a deadly form of skin cancer. Plans are under way to engineer a cancer "vaccine" designed to improve anti-cancer immune responses by taking small bits of tumor from patients with cancer, outfitting the tumor cells with genes for immune-cell-activating cytokines such as IL-2, and reinjecting these gene-modified tumors into the patient. While the thought of reintroducing a cancerous tumor into a patient seems somewhat frightening, the enhanced immune response triggered by this technique may help prevent the recurrence of cancer.

41. The fourth paragraph is chiefly concerned with the use of gene therapy to combat
   a. necrosis.
   b. cancer.
   c. cytokine.
   d. melanoma.

42. Recombinant DNA technology can lead to heart attack drugs to be produced by
   a. yeast.
   b. bacteria.
   c. tobacco plants.
   d. goats.

43. Why might cancer patients be leery of the prospect of a cancer "vaccine"?
   a. Vaccine recipients will be reinjected with cancerous material.
   b. The vaccine is derived from the tobacco plant.
   c. The safety of genetic transfer has not yet been proven.
   d. Genetic material from the vector could invade the vaccine recipient's bloodstream.

44. Tumor-infiltrating lymphocytes reinforced with tumor necrosis factor have been used to treat
   a. heart attacks.
   b. melanoma.
   c. SCID.
   d. blood diseases.

45. Adenosine deaminase (ADA) is transferred into the T cells of a patient via which of the following?
   a. marker gene
   b. TIL
   c. interferon
   d. modified retrovirus

Section 3: Math

Use scratch paper if needed to answer the following 50 questions. You have 45 minutes to complete this section.

1. 292 × 50 is equal to
   a. 14,600.
   b. 14,500.
   c. 10,500.
   d. 1,450.

2. What is $\frac{5}{8}$ of 600?
   a. 75
   b. 375
   c. 400
   d. 225

3. Reduce $\frac{52}{117}$ to lowest terms.
   a. $\frac{1}{2}$
   b. $\frac{25}{49}$
   c. $\frac{4}{9}$
   d. $\frac{15}{17}$

4. Which value of x makes the number sentence $x - 14 = 53$ true?
   a. $x = 89$
   b. $x = 29$
   c. $x = 37$
   d. $x = 67$

5. $\frac{-\frac{1}{4}}{-\frac{1}{8}}$ is equal to
   a. 2.
   b. $\frac{1}{2}$.
   c. $-\frac{1}{2}$.
   d. –2.

6. About how many liters of water will a 5-gallon container hold? (1 liter = 1.06 quarts)
   a. 5
   b. 11
   c. 20
   d. 21

7. What is another way to write 20,706?
   a. 200 + 70 + 6
   b. 2,000 + 700 + 6
   c. 20,000 + 70 + 6
   d. 20,000 + 700 + 6

8. If $\frac{x}{54} = \frac{2}{9}$, then x is
   a. 6.
   b. 12.
   c. 18.
   d. 108.

9. Which of the following is divisible by 6 and 7?
   a. 63
   b. 74
   c. 84
   d. 96

10. Which is equivalent to 0.0004?
    a. 4×10^4
    b. 4×10^{-4}
    c. 0.4×10^3
    d. 40×10^{-2}

11. What is the value of $44 + 18 \div 6 - 9$?
    a. −1
    b. 8
    c. 38
    d. 33

12. The perimeter of a rectangle is 148 feet. Its two longest sides add up to 86 feet. What is the length of each of its two shortest sides?
    a. 31 ft.
    b. 42 ft.
    c. 62 ft.
    d. 74 ft.

13. The cost of a list of supplies for a hospital ward is as follows: $19.98, $52.20, $12.64, and $7.79. What is the total cost?
    a. $91.30
    b. $92.61
    c. $93.60
    d. $93.61

14. If jogging for one mile uses 150 calories and brisk walking for one mile uses 100 calories, a jogger has to go how many times as far as a walker to use the same number of calories?
    a. $\frac{1}{2}$
    b. $\frac{2}{3}$
    c. $\frac{3}{2}$
    d. 2

15. A dosage of a certain medication is 12 cc per 100 pounds. What is the dosage for a patient who weighs 175 pounds?
    a. 15 cc
    b. 18 cc
    c. 21 cc
    d. 24 cc

16. A gram of fat contains 9 calories. An 1,800-calorie diet allows no more than 20% of calories from fat. How many grams of fat are allowed in that diet?
    a. 40 g
    b. 90 g
    c. 200 g
    d. 360 g

17. How much water must be added to 1 liter of a 5% saline solution to get a 2% saline solution?
  a. 1 liter
  b. 1.5 liters
  c. 2 liters
  d. 2.5 liters

18. A 15 cc dosage must be increased by 20%. What is the new dosage?
  a. 17 cc
  b. 18 cc
  c. 30 cc
  d. 35 cc

19. What is the volume of the liquid in this cylinder?

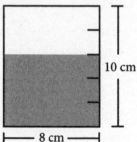

  a. 64π cm^3
  b. 80π cm^3
  c. 96π cm^3
  d. 160π cm^3

20. The following figure contains both a circle and a square. What is the area of the entire shaded figure?

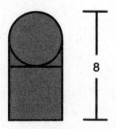

  a. $16 + 4\pi$
  b. $16 + 16\pi$
  c. $24 + 2\pi$
  d. $24 + 4\pi$

21. In the following figure, angle *POS* measures 90°. What is the measure of angle *ROQ*?

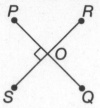

  a. 45°
  b. 90°
  c. 180°
  d. 270°

22. A line intersects two parallel lines in the following figure. If angle *P* measures 40°, what is the measure of angle *Q*?

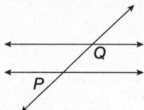

  a. 50°
  b. 60°
  c. 80°
  d. 140°

23. A nurse is paid $33.55 per hour. She works 22.75 hours during one week. How much total pay will she receive for the week?
  a. $726.00
  b. $7,632.65
  c. $627.26
  d. $763.26

24. Of 9,125 patients treated in a certain emergency room in one year, 72% were male. Among the males, three out of five were under the age of 25. How many of the emergency room patients were males age 25 or older?
  a. 2,628
  b. 3,942
  c. 5,475
  d. 6,570

25. 62.5% is equal to

a. $\frac{1}{16}$.

b. $\frac{5}{8}$.

c. $6\frac{1}{4}$.

d. $6\frac{2}{5}$.

26. $\frac{7}{40}$ is equal to

a. 0.0175.

b. 0.175.

c. 1.75.

d. 17.5.

27. A certain water pollutant is unsafe at a level over 20 ppm (parts per million). A city's water supply now contains 50 ppm of this pollutant. What percentage improvement will make the water safe?

a. 30%

b. 40%

c. 50%

d. 60%

28. In half of migraine sufferers, a certain drug reduces the number of migraines by 50%. What percentage of all migraines can be eliminated by this drug?

a. 25%

b. 50%

c. 75%

d. 100%

29. Nationwide, in one year, there were about 21,500 fire-related injuries associated with furniture. Of these, 11,350 were caused by smoking materials. About what percent of the fire-related injuries were smoking-related?

a. 47%

b. 49%

c. 51%

d. 53%

30. 0.63×0.42 is equal to

a. 26.46.

b. 2.646.

c. 0.2646.

d. 0.02646.

31. Which of the following numbers is the smallest?

a. 0.45

b. 2^{-2}

c. $\frac{2}{5}$

d. $\frac{3}{9}$

32. $3\frac{9}{16} - 1\frac{7}{8}$ is equal to

a. $1\frac{11}{16}$.

b. $2\frac{1}{8}$.

c. $2\frac{1}{4}$.

d. $2\frac{5}{16}$.

33. If the average woman burns 8.2 calories per minute while riding a bicycle, how many calories will she burn if she rides for 35 minutes?

a. 286

b. 287

c. 387

d. 980

34. The basal metabolic rate (BMR) is the rate at which our body uses calories. The BMR for a man in his twenties is about 1,700 calories per day. If 204 of those calories should come from protein, about what percentage of this man's diet should be protein?

a. 1.2%

b. 8.3%

c. 12%

d. 16%

35. One lap on a particular outdoor track measures a quarter of a mile around. To run a total of $3\frac{1}{2}$ miles, how many complete laps must a person finish?
a. 7
b. 10
c. 13
d. 14

36. Down syndrome occurs in about one in 1,500 children when the mothers are in their twenties. About what percentage of all children born to mothers in their twenties are likely to have Down syndrome?
a. 0.0067%
b. 0.067%
c. 0.67%
d. 6.7%

37. If a population of yeast cells grows from 10 to 320 in a period of five hours, what is the rate of growth?
a. It doubles its numbers every hour.
b. It triples its numbers every hour.
c. It doubles its numbers every two hours.
d. It triples its numbers every two hours.

38. Which value of x will make this number sentence true? $x + 25 \leq 13$
a. −12
b. −11
c. 12
d. 38

39. How many faces does a cube have?
a. 4
b. 6
c. 8
d. 12

40. What is the length of a rectangle if its width is 9 ft. and its area is 117 sq. ft.?
a. 1.3 ft.
b. 10.5 ft.
c. 12 ft.
d. 13 ft.

41. The cost of a patient's X-ray is $830. The insurance company pays 85% of the cost and the patient pays the remaining amount. How much does the patient pay for the X-ray?
a. $15.00
b. $124.50
c. $664.00
d. $705.50

42. $2\frac{1}{4} + 4\frac{5}{8} + \frac{1}{2}$ is equal to
a. $6\frac{7}{8}$.
b. $7\frac{1}{4}$.
c. $7\frac{3}{8}$.
d. $7\frac{3}{4}$.

43. What percentage of 600 is 750?
a. 80%
b. 85%
c. 110%
d. 125%

44. What is the value of $d = rt$ if $r = 65$ and $t = 12$?
a. 780
b. 715
c. 650
d. 845

45. What is another way to write 0.32×10^3?
a. 3.2
b. 32
c. 320
d. 3,200

46. In the following figure, triangle *QRS* is a right triangle. If angle *S* measures 37°, what is the measure of angle *Q*?

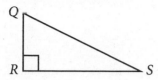

   a. 63°
   b. 37°
   c. 53°
   d. 180°

47. 3.6 − 1.89 is equal to
   a. 1.47.
   b. 1.53.
   c. 1.71.
   d. 2.42.

48. If a particular woman's resting heartbeat is 72 beats per minute and she is at rest for six and a half hours, about how many times will her heart beat during that period of time?
   a. 4,320
   b. 4,680
   c. 28,080
   d. 43,200

49. The number of red blood corpuscles in one cubic millimeter is about 5 million, and the number of white blood corpuscles in one cubic millimeter is about 8,000. What, then, is the ratio of white blood corpuscles to red blood corpuscles?
   a. 1:625
   b. 1:40
   c. 4:10
   d. 5:1,250

50. $\frac{5}{12} - \frac{3}{8}$ is equal to
   a. $\frac{1}{10}$.
   b. $\frac{1}{24}$.
   c. $\frac{5}{48}$.
   d. $\frac{19}{24}$.

Section 4: General Science

This section will test your accumulated knowledge in general science.

1. Which of the following is NOT one of the four fundamental forces of the universe?
   a. gravity
   b. electromagnetism
   c. pressure
   d. weak nuclear force

2. This Dutchman charmed Europe with his letters that contained drawings depicting the extraordinary details visible under the high-power microscopes he built himself.
   a. Isaac Newton
   b. Baron von Humboldt
   c. Antonie van Leeuwenhoek
   d. Benedict Spinoza

3. When studying the orbit of the planet Mars, he discovered the law that planets move around the Sun in ellipses.
   a. Kepler
   b. Galileo
   c. Newton
   d. Copernicus

4. Sixteenth-century astronomer Nicolaus Copernicus stirred up controversy, now referred to as the "Copernican Revolution," with his book *On the Revolutions of the Heavenly Spheres*. What did Copernicus propose that was so revolutionary for the time?
  a. All the planets revolved around the Sun.
  b. The Sun and planets revolved around Earth.
  c. The planets revolved around the Sun, and the Sun in turn revolved around Earth.
  d. Earth revolved around the Sun, and the planets in turn revolved around Earth.

5. He was the Austrian monk who spent years in scientific isolation while he bred pea plants and studied the results, which we now know as heredity.
  a. Rutherford
  b. Darwin
  c. Mendel
  d. Watson

6. A mass extinction occurred at the end of which geologic period?
  a. Cambrian
  b. Jurassic
  c. Permian
  d. Silurian

7. What did Galileo do?
  a. first split light into its colors
  b. first used the x- and y-axes
  c. first realized the antiquity of Earth
  d. first observed the moons of Jupiter

8. If you want to test the effect of a new malaria vaccine, the group of people who receive shots that contain no vaccine is called the
  a. control group.
  b. experiment group.
  c. fake group.
  d. zero group.

9. How many milligrams are in one gram?
  a. 10
  b. 100
  c. 1,000
  d. 10,000

10. The biggest concepts in science are called
  a. predictions.
  b. theories.
  c. experiments.
  d. hypotheses.

11. Doing science in a Popperian manner means
  a. selecting only data that fits your hypothesis.
  b. actively seeking experiments that will falsify your hypothesis.
  c. creating data that goes with hypothetical explanations.
  d. wanting your experiments to work.

12. Which of the following is not a flavor of quark?
  a. up
  b. middle
  c. strange
  d. charm

13. What year was the first successful landing of a U.S. rover on Mars?
  a. 1969
  b. 1957
  c. 1997
  d. 2011

14. Reductionism in science refers to what?
  a. rejecting holism as unessential
  b. making the hypothesis small enough to fit the facts
  c. creating an alternative pattern that uses previous ideas
  d. explaining behaviors in terms of interacting parts

15. In an XY graph comparing time versus distance, time is the
   a. dependent variable and located on the *x*-axis.
   b. dependent variable and located on the *y*-axis.
   c. independent variable and located on the *x*-axis.
   d. independent variable and located on the *y*-axis.

16. The typical human hair is about 50 micrometers in diameter. That means it is 50 _____ of a meter.
   a. billionths
   b. thousandths
   c. parts
   d. millionths

17. Humans are putting about 6 billion tons of carbon into the atmosphere each year in the form of carbon dioxide. Which of the following is another way of expressing this number?
   a. 6 megatons
   b. 6 kilotons
   c. 6 petatons
   d. 6 gigatons

18. Which of the following is the standard metric unit of energy?
   a. joule
   b. mole
   c. watt
   d. ampere

19. What exponent or power of 10 would you use to express how many meters are in a kilometer?
   a. 10^5
   b. 10^3
   c. 10^4
   d. 10^2

20. The presence of life is responsible for the relatively high concentration of which gas in Earth's atmosphere?
   a. carbon dioxide
   b. hydrogen
   c. methane
   d. oxygen

21. The nanosecond is one _____ of one second.
   a. thousandth
   b. millionth
   c. billionth
   d. trillionth

22. How many milliliters (mL) are there in a 1-liter (L) soda bottle?
   a. 0.001
   b. 0.01
   c. 100
   d. 1,000

23. Satellites have measured differences in this quantity, which came into existence before the formation of galaxies and shows that inhomogeneities existed in the early universe—in other words, that the universe was "lumpy." What is the quantity?
   a. radiation temperature
   b. black hole wavelength
   c. electron density
   d. galaxy patterns

24. Based on current scientific observations, most cosmologists are in agreement that the universe is
   a. contracting.
   b. expanding.
   c. static.
   d. oscillating.

25. Put in order the following events, from earliest (closest in time to the Big Bang) to latest (closest in time to today): electrons become stable around atomic nuclei (E); stable combinations of protons and neutrons (S); near annihilation of matter and antimatter (N); protogalaxies start to form (P).
   a. N-S-E-P
   b. E-S-N-P
   c. P-E-S-N
   d. S-E-P-N

26. In the electromagnetic spectrum, infrared wavelengths are slightly longer than those of visible red, and ultraviolet wavelengths are slightly shorter than visible blue. If an absorption spectrum from a calcium atom here on Earth has a characteristic pattern in the red wavelengths, looking at calcium in the absorption spectrum of a distant galaxy will show the same characteristic pattern toward the
   a. ultraviolet.
   b. blue.
   c. red (the same).
   d. infrared.

27. Of the following elements, which is formed last in the stages of nuclear fusion inside stars?
   a. hydrogen
   b. helium
   c. carbon
   d. oxygen

28. Which events or processes disperse elements born in the internal nuclear fires of stars, making those elements available for subsequent formations of new stars and planets?
   a. supernovas
   b. expanding universe
   c. fusion reactions
   d. red shift

29. The innovation that allowed the human population to first grow above 10 million was
   a. fire.
   b. hunting.
   c. agriculture.
   d. industrial technology.

30. Which element in the universe (including inside our Sun) is both primordial (meaning some of it was made shortly after the Big Bang, before any stars formed) and made inside stars during fusion reactions?
   a. carbon
   b. hydrogen
   c. helium
   d. iron

31. Which increases in density as the universe ages?
   a. energy
   b. microwave radiation
   c. hydrogen
   d. carbon

32. The planet nearest to Earth is
   a. Venus.
   b. Jupiter.
   c. Neptune.
   d. Saturn.

33. Astronomers sometimes make units that fit the large scales of space and time. Consider the time interval from today back to the formation of Earth (in other words, Earth's condensation from the gas cloud that also formed the Sun). For just this question, call this amount of time one Earth Formation Unit (1 EFU). About how many EFUs from today must you go back in time to reach the Big Bang?
   a. 1 EFU
   b. 3 EFUs
   c. 8 EFUs
   d. 15 EFUs

34. Our best dates for the origin of the solar system come from
    a. rocks found on the Moon.
    b. the oldest rocks on Earth.
    c. meteorites.
    d. gases in the Sun.

35. Which planet does not have a well-developed atmosphere because of its small size?
    a. Neptune
    b. Mars
    c. Venus
    d. Mercury

36. Humans are currently in space on the
    a. Mir space station.
    b. International Space Station.
    c. Mars rover.
    d. Apollo capsule.

37. Which of the following is considered a dwarf planet?
    a. Mercury
    b. Eris
    c. Oort
    d. Dysnomia

38. Which body in our solar system has very good evidence for the presence, at one time in the past, for liquid water?
    a. Moon
    b. Mars
    c. Venus
    d. Mercury

39. In 2006, the International Astronomical Union voted to reclassify Pluto from a planet to a(n)
    a. dwarf planet.
    b. asteroid.
    c. moon.
    d. Oort cloud.

40. We know there is matter that cannot be seen by any means available to us, including the different wavelengths of the electromagnetic spectrum. Yet we know this so-called "dark matter" exists. How?
    a. Black holes have consumed much of the matter that once existed.
    b. At the origin of the universe was a large amount of antimatter that became hidden.
    c. Einstein's equation shows us the equivalence of energy that could also be considered matter.
    d. The spins of galaxies cannot be explained by the amount of known, ordinary matter.

41. Today, we know fairly well the composition of the universe, in terms of types of matter (or types of energy that can be put into amounts of equivalent matter, using Einstein's equation $E = mc^2$). What percentage of the universe is dark energy?
    a. 98%
    b. 73%
    c. 23%
    d. 4%

42. One element crucial to life is carbon, which forms about 40% of our body's dry weight. If planets had formed around the very earliest stars in the universe, why would it have been unlikely for life to start on those earliest planets?
    a. Carbon is made slowly as the expanding energy of the Big Bang is converted to matter.
    b. Carbon leaks into our universe through black holes.
    c. Carbon is made by fusion reactions in stars.
    d. Carbon is made by the fission of oxygen.

43. The geographical region of the ocean that meets the deep ocean floor is the
   a. continental alluvium.
   b. continental abyss.
   c. continental slope.
   d. continental shelf.

44. What word in ancient Greek meant indivisible?
   a. atom
   b. molecule
   c. ion
   d. isotope

45. The radioactive isotope of carbon is
   a. carbon-11.
   b. carbon-12.
   c. carbon-13.
   d. carbon-14.

46. If positively charged and negatively charged particles are considered "opposites," which pair of atomic particles would be "opposite"?
   a. protons and neutrons
   b. neutrons and electrons
   c. electrons and protons
   d. neutrons and quarks

47. Parts of the atomic nucleus are sometimes collectively called *nucleons*. Nucleons are therefore
   a. protons and mesons.
   b. electrons and neutrons.
   c. mesons and electrons.
   d. neutrons and protons.

48. In measuring electricity, the unit for resistance is the
   a. volt.
   b. ohm.
   c. amp.
   d. watt.

49. Electromagnetism is the force that
   a. causes the interaction between electrically charged particles.
   b. binds protons and neutrons together to form the nucleus of an atom.
   c. is responsible for the radioactive decay of subatomic particles.
   d. causes dispersed matter to coalesce.

50. What is 10^{-12} meters?
   a. a picometer
   b. a nanometer
   c. a micrometer
   d. a femtometer

Section 5: Biology

There are 50 questions in this section. You have 45 minutes to complete this section.

1. Which of the following is NOT a pyrimidine base of nucleic acids?
   a. thymine
   b. cytosine
   c. uracil
   d. guanine

2. In primates, what is the epithelial lining of the uterus?
   a. fimbria
   b. cervix
   c. myometrium
   d. endometrium

3. What is the clinical term for abnormal tissue growth?
   a. atrophy
   b. karyolysis
   c. dysplasia
   d. thrombosis

4. Which of the following is an example of genetic engineering?
   a. gene deletion
   b. genetic screening
   c. selective breeding
   d. pedigree analysis

5. What is the protein coat that encloses the genome of a virus?
   a. cell wall
   b. myelin sheath
   c. envelope
   d. capsid

6. An organism with two different alleles for a trait is
   a. homozygous for that trait.
   b. heterozygous for that trait.
   c. phenotypic for that trait.
   d. genotypic for that trait.

7. Which of the following organelles are found in plants, but NOT in animals or bacteria?
   a. mitochondria
   b. chloroplasts
   c. nucleus
   d. cell wall

8. Which of the following scientists is known as the founder of modern genetics?
   a. Johannes Kepler
   b. Sir Charles Lyell
   c. Gregor Mendel
   d. Robert Hooke

9. Which of the following is an air- or fluid-filled space in the cytoplasm of a living cell?
   a. a vacuum
   b. a vacuole
   c. a centriole
   d. a centrosome

10. Which of the following hormones is a peptide?
   a. insulin
   b. adrenaline
   c. testosterone
   d. thyroxine

11. These organelles generate the majority of ATP in eukaryotic cells.
   a. mitochondria
   b. chloroplasts
   c. ribosomes
   d. lysosomes

12. Which of the following lists the phases of mitosis in the correct order?
   a. prophase, metaphase, anaphase, telophase
   b. prophase, anaphase, telophase, metaphase
   c. metaphase, prophase, anaphase, telophase
   d. telophase, metaphase, anaphase, prophase

13. A reproductive cell, or gamete, is a unique kind of cell because it
   a. is a haploid cell.
   b. is a diploid cell.
   c. does not contain protein.
   d. is much smaller than other cells.

14. The function of the lysosome is to
   a. contain the cell's genetic material.
   b. combine amino acids into proteins.
   c. break down waste material in the cell.
   d. generate ATP.

15. During which stage of meiosis I does crossing over occur?
   a. prophase
   b. metaphase
   c. anaphase
   d. telophase

16. A part of what type of cell is shown in the following figure?

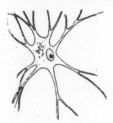

    a. a blood cell
    b. a fat cell
    c. a muscle cell
    d. a nerve cell

17. Hepatitis is an inflammation of the
    a. joints.
    b. lungs.
    c. liver.
    d. large intestine.

18. The process of cellular reproduction in bacteria is known as
    a. mitosis.
    b. meiosis.
    c. telophase.
    d. binary fission.

19. The principal function of blood platelets is to
    a. help clot blood.
    b. carry oxygen.
    c. produce antibodies.
    d. phagocytize bacteria.

20. The two or more related genes that control a trait are known as
    a. chromosomes.
    b. chromatids.
    c. phenotypes.
    d. alleles.

21. Bacteria can undergo genetic recombination through
    a. binary fission.
    b. translation.
    c. transformation.
    d. meiosis.

22. The term *mutation* refers to
    a. a change in one or more genes.
    b. rapidly multiplying cells.
    c. a bacterial infection.
    d. a change in the organism's metabolic rate.

23. The complementary RNA sequence for CATTGAA is
    a. GTAACTT.
    b. TGCCTGG.
    c. GUAACUU.
    d. ACGGTCC.

24. In some flowers, the alleles for red and white produce pink flowers in heterozygotes. This phenomenon is called
    a. the genotypic ratio.
    b. the law of independent assortment.
    c. incomplete metamorphosis.
    d. incomplete dominance.

25. The term *biological catalyst* most closely describes
    a. RNA.
    b. DNA.
    c. a mitochondrion.
    d. an enzyme.

26. Which of the following is NOT a member of the class of fungi?
    a. common bread mold
    b. mushrooms
    c. kelp
    d. yeast

27. Which plasma protein plays the greatest role in maintaining the osmotic pressure of blood?
a. fibrinogen
b. albumin
c. prothrombin
d. gamma globulins

28. Initial classification of a bacterium is based on its
a. size.
b. shape.
c. color.
d. ability to cause disease.

29. Which of the following is NOT caused by a virus?
a. polio
b. rabies
c. malaria
d. cold sores (herpes simplex)

30. Bacteria and viruses can both have genomes made up of
a. single-stranded DNA.
b. double-stranded DNA.
c. single-stranded RNA.
d. double-stranded RNA.

31. The process of a complementary strand of RNA being made from a sequence of DNA is known as
a. transcription.
b. translation.
c. mitosis.
d. replication.

32. The broadest classification of plants is whether they are
a. vascular or nonvascular.
b. angiosperms or gymnosperms.
c. monocots or dicots.
d. seedless or seeded.

33. The structure formed by the union of male and female gametes is the
a. zoospore.
b. zygote.
c. ova.
d. oocyte.

34. The metabolic pathway for the degradation of glucose into pyruvate to produce ATP is known as
a. glycolysis.
b. gluconeogenesis.
c. the Calvin cycle.
d. the Krebs cycle.

35. During strenuous exercise, a build-up of what substance may cause muscle cramps?
a. lactic acid
b. lactose
c. adrenaline
d. serotonin

36. Which of the following organs functions to absorb water and create feces from undigested food?
a. small intestine
b. liver
c. large intestine
d. stomach

37. During a latent period in muscle tissue, what is released from the sarcoplasmic reticulum?
- **a.** calcium
- **b.** sodium
- **c.** lactic acid
- **d.** acetylcholine

38. Beriberi is caused by a deficit of which vitamin?
- **a.** vitamin B_1
- **b.** vitamin C
- **c.** vitamin E
- **d.** vitamin D

39. This molecule is responsible for the green color of leaves.
- **a.** deoxyribonucleic acid
- **b.** adenosine triphosphate
- **c.** chlorophyll
- **d.** glucose

40. Which of the following is NOT characteristic of anaphylaxis?
- **a.** circulatory shock
- **b.** bronchospasm
- **c.** hives
- **d.** hypertension

41. What is the generic term for any substance which blocks ONLY the sensory perception of pain?
- **a.** analgesic
- **b.** general anesthetic
- **c.** local anesthetic
- **d.** acetylcholine

42. Which of the following is NOT an amino acid?
- **a.** tyrosine
- **b.** tryptophan
- **c.** thymine
- **d.** threonine

43. Which organelle of a bacterium plays the greatest role in movement of the bacterium?
- **a.** flagella
- **b.** ribosomes
- **c.** cytoplasm
- **d.** cell wall

44. "Energy cannot be destroyed; it can only be transformed" is a statement of what physical law?
- **a.** first law of thermodynamics
- **b.** second law of thermodynamics
- **c.** law of entropy
- **d.** law of constant composition

45. In complementary base pairing, cytosine pairs only with
- **a.** adenine.
- **b.** guanine.
- **c.** thymine.
- **d.** uracil.

46. The primary component of alcoholic beverages that acts as a central nervous system (CNS) depressant is
- **a.** isopropyl alcohol.
- **b.** methanol.
- **c.** methionine.
- **d.** ethanol.

47. Primary structure refers to a protein's
- **a.** amino acid sequence.
- **b.** α-helices and β-sheets.
- **c.** shape.
- **d.** active site.

48. A benign tumor usually caused by a *papillomavirus* is a
- **a.** wart.
- **b.** sarcoma.
- **c.** adenoma.
- **d.** cold sore.

49. What is the light-sensitive pigment found in the vertebrate retina?

   a. cytochrome

   b. hemoglobin

   c. rhodopsin

   d. melanin

50. What is another term for excessively high blood pressure?

   a. cardiomyopathy

   b. hypertension

   c. hypoglycemia

   d. hemophilia

Section 6: Chemistry

There are 50 questions in this section. You have 45 minutes to complete this section. Use the periodic table on this page when necessary to help you answer the following questions.

1 IA								9 VIIIB									18 VIIIA
1 **H** 1.00794	2 IIA											13 IIIA	14 IVA	15 VA	16 VIA	17 VIIA	2 **He** 4.002602
3 **Li** 6.941	4 **Be** 9.012182											5 **B** 10.811	6 **C** 12.0107	7 **N** 14.00674	8 **O** 15.9994	9 **F** 8.9984032	10 **Ne** 20.1797
11 **Na** 22.989770	12 **Mg** 24.3050	3 IIIB	4 IVB	5 VB	6 VIB	7 VIIB	8	VIIIB	10	11 IB	12 IIB	13 **Al** 26.981538	14 **Si** 28.0855	15 **P** 30.973761	16 **S** 32.066	17 **Cl** 35.4527	18 **Ar** 39.948
19 **K** 39.0983	20 **Ca** 40.078	21 **Sc** 44.955910	22 **Ti** 47.867	23 **V** 50.9415	24 **Cr** 51.9961	25 **Mn** 54.938049	26 **Fe** 55.845	27 **Co** 58.933200	28 **Ni** 58.6934	29 **Cu** 63.546	30 **Zn** 65.39	31 **Ga** 69.723	32 **Ge** 72.61	33 **As** 74.92160	34 **Se** 78.96	35 **Br** 79.904	36 **Kr** 83.80
37 **Rb** 85.4678	38 **Sr** 87.62	39 **Y** 88.90585	40 **Zr** 91.224	41 **Nb** 92.90638	42 **Mo** 95.94	43 **Tc** (98)	44 **Ru** 101.07	45 **Rh** 102.90550	46 **Pd** 106.42	47 **Ag** 107.8682	48 **Cd** 112.411	49 **In** 114.818	50 **Sn** 118.710	51 **Sb** 121.760	52 **Te** 127.60	53 **I** 126.90447	54 **Xe** 131.29
55 **Cs** 132.90545	56 **Ba** 137.327	57 **La*** 138.9055	72 **Hf** 178.49	73 **Ta** 180.9479	74 **W** 183.84	75 **Re** 186.207	76 **Os** 190.23	77 **Ir** 192.217	78 **Pt** 195.078	79 **Au** 196.96655	80 **Hg** 200.59	81 **Tl** 204.3833	82 **Pb** 207.2	83 **Bi** 208.98038	84 **Po** (209)	85 **At** (210)	86 **Rn** (222)
87 **Fr** (223)	88 **Ra** (226)	89 **Ac**** (227)	104 **Rf** (265)	105 **Db** (268)	106 **Sg** (271)	107 **Bh** (270)	108 **Hs** (277)	109 **Mt** (276)	110 **Ds** (281)	111 **Rg** (280)	112 **Cn** (285)	113 **Nh** (286)	114 **Fl** (289)	115 **Mc** (289)	116 **Lv** (293)	117 **Ts** (294)	118 **Og** (294)

* Lanthanide series	58 **Ce** 140.116	59 **Pr** 140.90765	60 **Nd** 144.24	61 **Pm** (145)	62 **Sm** 150.36	63 **Eu** 151.964	64 **Gd** 157.25	65 **Tb** 158.92534	66 **Dy** 162.50	67 **Ho** 164.93032	68 **Er** 167.26	69 **Tm** 168.93421	70 **Yb** 173.04	71 **Lu** 174.967
** Actinide series	90 **Th** 232.0381	91 **Pa** 231.03588	92 **U** 238.0289	93 **Np** (237)	94 **Pu** (244)	95 **Am** (243)	96 **Cm** (247)	97 **Bk** (247)	98 **Cf** (251)	99 **Es** (252)	100 **Fm** (257)	101 **Md** (258)	102 **No** (259)	103 **Lr** (262)

1. Which of the following substances has a pH closest to 7?

   a. ammonia

   b. blood

   c. lemon juice

   d. vinegar

2. In the equilibrium reaction $AgCl_{(s)} \rightleftharpoons$ $Ag^+_{(aq)} + Cl^-_{(aq)}$ that occurs when silver chloride is added to water, what happens when more chloride ions are added to the solution?
   a. less AgCl dissolves
   b. less AgCl forms
   c. more Ag^+ ions form
   d. more Cl^- ions form

3. Which of the following groups is common to the majority of amino acids?
   a. CH_3
   b. H_2O
   c. NH_2
   d. SO_4^{-2}

4. When amino acids polymerize to make a protein, which of the following is produced as a byproduct?
   a. H_2O
   b. H_2
   c. O_2
   d. CO_2

5. The α-helices and β-sheets in a protein make up its
   a. primary structure.
   b. secondary structure.
   c. tertiary structure.
   d. quaternary structure.

6. ^{35}Cl has 17 protons. How many neutrons does it have?
   a. 17
   b. 18
   c. 35
   d. 52

7. By which of the following mechanisms does a catalyst operate?
   a. It decreases the activation energy barrier for a reaction.
   b. It serves as a reactant and is consumed.
   c. It increases the temperature of a reaction.
   d. It increases the concentration of reactants.

8. If an atom has a mass number of 40 and an atomic number of 18, how many neutrons does it contain?
   a. 18
   b. 22
   c. 40
   d. 58

9. Which is the best Lewis structure for acetone, $CH_3C(O)CH_3$?
   a.

$$H-\underset{\underset{H}{|}}{\overset{\overset{H}{|}}{C}}-\ddot{C}=\ddot{O}-\underset{\underset{H}{|}}{\overset{\overset{H}{|}}{C}}-H$$

   b.

$$H-\underset{\underset{H}{|}}{\overset{\overset{H}{|}}{C}}-\ddot{C}-\ddot{O}-\underset{\underset{H}{|}}{\overset{\overset{H}{|}}{C}}-H$$

   c.

$$H-\underset{\underset{H}{|}}{\overset{\overset{H}{|}}{C}}-\overset{\overset{:O:}{||}}{C}-\underset{\underset{H}{|}}{\overset{\overset{H}{|}}{C}}-H$$

   d.

$$H-\underset{\underset{H}{|}}{\overset{\overset{H}{|}}{C}}-\overset{\overset{:\ddot{O}:}{|}}{C}-\underset{\underset{H}{|}}{\overset{\overset{H}{|}}{C}}-H$$

10. Which of the following represents *t*-butyl?

a. $CH_3 - CH_2 - CH_2 - CH_3$

b.
$$CH_3$$
$$|$$
$$CH_3 - C - CH_3$$
$$|$$
$$CH_3$$

c. $CH_3 - CH_2 - CH_3$

d.
$$H$$
$$|$$
$$CH_3 - C - CH_3$$
$$|$$
$$CH_3$$

11. O^{-2} has how many electrons?

a. 6
b. 8
c. 10
d. 18

12. Which of the following groups on the periodic table is most likely to form negative ions?

a. alkali metals
b. alkaline earth metals
c. halogens
d. noble gases

13. Which of the following is the correct, balanced equation for the combustion of propane?

a. $C_3H_{8(g)} + 5O_{2(g)} + N_{2(g)} \rightarrow 3CO_{2(g)} + 2NO_{2(g)} + 4H_{2(g)}$

b. $C_3H_8(g) + 5O_{2(g)} \rightarrow 3CO_{2(g)} + 4H_2O_{(g)}$

c. $C_3H_{8(g)} + 6O_{2(g)} + 2H_{2(g)} \rightarrow 3CO_{2(g)} + 6H_2O_{(g)}$

d. $C_3H_{8(g)} + O_{2(g)} + 4H_2O_{(g)} \rightarrow 3CO_{2(g)} + 6H_{2(g)}$

14. What is the electron configuration of a Cl^- ion?

a. $[Ne]3s^23p^5$
b. $[Ne]3s^2p^63d^1$
c. $[Ne]3s^23p^4$
d. $[Ne]3s^23p^6$

15. Which of the following is the hybridization of the carbon atom in methane, CH_4?

a. sp
b. sp^2
c. sp^3
d. sp^4

16. Which of the following electron configurations is NOT possible?

a. $1s^22s^1$
b. $1s^22s^4$
c. $1s^22s^22p^2$
d. $1s^22s^22p^6$

17. When a liquid is at its boiling point, the vapor pressure of the liquid

a. is less than the external pressure on the liquid.
b. is equal to the external pressure on the liquid.
c. is greater than the external pressure on the liquid.
d. can be either less or greater than the external pressure on the liquid.

18. What is the oxidation state of iron in Fe_2O_3?

a. 0
b. +2
c. +3
d. +6

19. Which of the following is the empirical formula for ethylene glycol, $C_2H_6O_2$?

a. CH_3O
b. $C_2H_6O_2$
c. $C_4H_{12}O_4$
d. CH_2

20. What is the most likely oxidation state of Mg?
   a. +2
   b. +1
   c. 0
   d. –6

21. Which of the following is the chemical symbol for the species that has 16 protons, 17 neutrons, and 18 electrons?

   a. $^{33}_{16}S$

   b. $^{33}_{17}Cl$

   c. $^{35}_{17}Cl$

   d. $^{33}_{16}S^{2-}$

22. Which of the following equations correctly describes the reaction between $SO_{3(g)}$ and $KOH_{(aq)}$?
   a. $4SO_{3(g)} + 4KOH_{(aq)} \rightarrow 2H_2SO_{4(aq)} + 4K_{(s)} + O_{2(g)}$
   b. $SO_{3(g)} + 2KOH_{(aq)} \rightarrow K_2SO_{4(aq)} + H_2O_{(1)}$
   c. $2SO_3 + 4KOH_{(aq)} \rightarrow 2K_2SO_{3(aq)} + 2H_2O_{(1)} + O_{2(g)}$
   d. No reaction occurs.

23. Which of the following is a Lewis acid, but not a Bronsted acid?
   a. HCl
   b. H_2SO_4
   c. CH_4
   d. $AlCl_3$

24. Butane, C_4H_{10}, combusts to form CO_2 and H_2O. Which of the following is the balanced chemical equation that describes this reaction?
   a. $C_4H_{10} + O_2 \rightarrow CO_2 + H_2O$
   b. $C_4H_{10} + 7O_2 + H_2 \rightarrow 4CO_2 + 6H_2O$
   c. $C_4H_{10} + 7O_2 \rightarrow 4CO_2 + 5H_2O$
   d. $2C_4H_{10} + 13O_2 \rightarrow 8CO_2 + 10H_2O$

25. One liter of solution is made by dissolving 29.2 g of NaCl in water. What is the molarity of the solution?
   a. 0.5 M
   b. 2.0 M
   c. 1.3 M
   d. 0.82 M

26. Which of the following is an ether?
   a. $CH_3CH_2OCH_2CH_3$
   b. CH_3CH_2COOH
   c. $CH_3CH_2NH_2$
   d. $CH_3CH=CHCH_3$

27. Which of the following is the oxidation number of sulfur in the compound sodium thiosulfate, $Na_2S_2O_3$?
   a. +1
   b. –1
   c. +2
   d. –2

28. Two liters of air at a pressure of 2 atm are condensed to 0.5 liters. If the temperature is constant, what is the new pressure?
   a. 16 atm
   b. 8 atm
   c. 2 atm
   d. 0.5 atm

29. The composition of dry air consists of approximately 78% nitrogen, N_2, and 21% oxygen, O_2. If the air pressure of a 5-liter sample of dry air is 800 torr, what is the approximate partial pressure of oxygen?
   a. 620 torr
   b. 720 torr
   c. 210 torr
   d. 170 torr

30. In an experiment, 0.5 grams of copper was reacted with 100 mL of a 0.5 M HCl solution. The reaction was then repeated using 0.5 grams of copper and 100 mL of a 0.1 M HCl solution. Compared to the first reaction, the second reaction
   a. would proceed at a slower rate.
   b. would proceed at a faster rate.
   c. would proceed at the same rate.
   d. would not proceed.

31. The electronic configuration $1s^2 2s^2 2p^6 3s^2 3p^3$ describes which atom?
   a. N
   b. Ne
   c. Ar
   d. P

32. If a gas is heated at a constant volume, the pressure
   a. increases, because molecules collide with walls more slowly.
   b. increases, because molecules collide with walls more quickly.
   c. decreases, because molecules collide with walls more slowly.
   d. decreases, because molecules collide with walls more quickly.

33. How much heat is required to raise the temperature of 100 grams of water from 25°C (near room temperature) to 100°C (its boiling point)? The specific heat of water is approximately 4.2 J per g·K.
   a. 3.2×10^4 J
   b. 32 J
   c. 4.2×10^4 J
   d. 76 J

34. Which temperature is equivalent to 100°C?
   a. −273.15 K
   b. 0 K
   c. 273.15 K
   d. 373.15 K

35. Primary intermolecular interactions between a K cation and H_2O molecules are
   a. hydrogen bonds.
   b. dipole-dipole interactions.
   c. ion-dipole interactions.
   d. London forces.

36. In a chemical reaction, there is a single reactant and two products. Which type of reaction must have occurred?
   a. combination
   b. decomposition
   c. double displacement
   d. single displacement

Answer questions 37 and 38 based on the following phase diagram for a compound.

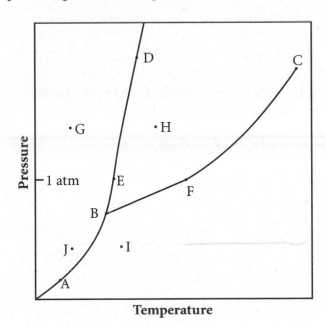

37. At which point is the compound a solid?
  a. F
  b. G
  c. H
  d. I

38. Sublimation occurs when moving from
  a. G to H.
  b. I to J.
  c. J to I.
  d. I to H.

39. Which of following is the balanced equation for the reaction between NH_3 and O_2?
  a. $4NH_3 + 5O_2 \rightarrow 4NO + 6H_2O$
  b. $2NH_3 + 3O_2 \rightarrow 2NO + 3H_2O$
  c. $2NH_3 + 2O_2 \rightarrow NO_2 + 3H_2O$
  d. $NH_3 + O_2 \rightarrow N_2O + 3H_2O$

40. In the reaction $4Al + 3O_2 \rightarrow 2Al_2O_3$, how many grams of O_2 are needed to completely react with 1.5 moles of Al?
  a. 24 g
  b. 36 g
  c. 48 g
  d. 60 g

41. What is the equilibrium constant K_c for the following equation?

$$2SO_{2(g)} + O_{2(g)} \rightleftharpoons 2SO_{3(g)}$$

  a. $K_c = \dfrac{[SO_3]}{[SO_2][O_2]}$
  b. $K_c = \dfrac{[SO_2][O_2]}{[SO_3]}$
  c. $K_c = \dfrac{[SO_2]^2[O_2]}{[SO_3]^2}$
  d. $K_c = \dfrac{[SO_3]^2}{[SO_2]^2[O_2]}$

42. What is the pH of a solution with $[OH^-] = 1 \times 10^{-8}$?
  a. 4
  b. 6
  c. 8
  d. 14

43. Which of the following has the highest electronegativity?
  a. S
  b. Se
  c. Cl
  d. Br

44. How many moles of 0.2 M HCl are needed to titrate 100 ml of 0.4 M NaOH?

$$HCl_{(aq)} + NaOH_{(aq)} \rightarrow NaCl_{(aq)} + H_2O_{(1)}$$

  a. 0.2 mol
  b. 0.1 mol
  c. 0.04 mol
  d. 0.02 mol

45. Which of the following is an example of an ionic crystal?
  a. LiF
  b. SiO_2
  c. CO_2
  d. $C_{12}H_{22}O_{11}$

46. Which of the following would have to happen to a neutral chlorine atom for it to have the same stable configuration as argon?
  a. lose one electron
  b. gain one electron
  c. lose two electrons
  d. gain two electrons

47. Electronegativity increases on the periodic table traveling
   a. down and to the left.
   b. down and to the right.
   c. up and to the left.
   d. up and to the right.

48. When 100 mL of 0.1 M $Pb(NO_3)_2$ and 100 mL of 0.1 M $BaCl_2$ are mixed, 1.67 g of $PbCl_2$ form. What is the percent yield of this reaction?
   a. 100%
   b. 60%
   c. 40%
   d. 10%

49. What is the empirical formula for glucose, $C_6H_{12}O_6$?
   a. CH_2O
   b. CHO
   c. $C_3H_4O_3$
   d. $[CH_2O]_6$

50. Which of the following is the molecular weight of calcium chloride ($CaCl_2$)?
   a. 75.53 g/mol
   b. 110.98 g/mol
   c. 115.61 g/mol
   d. 151.06 g/mol

Answers

Section 1: Verbal Ability
1. a. pathetically
2. c. belief
3. c. camouflage
4. a. breach
5. c. perceived
6. a. shriveled
7. b. situation
8. a. apparently
9. c. obsession
10. c. jeopardy
11. c. magnificent
12. b. geriatrics
13. c. illicit
14. a. inquiry
15. a. terminated
16. a. persecution
17. b. peculiar
18. b. psychology
19. a. license
20. a. concise
21. b. neighbor
22. a. stabilize
23. c. reexamining
24. a. aspirations
25. b. exercise
26. a. artificial
27. a. hindrance
28. c. testimony
29. c. addiction
30. a. thorough
31. a. quantity
32. c. imitate
33. b. contradict
34. b. reversal
35. c. foreign
36. a. ravenous
37. a. phenomenal
38. b. temperature

39. b. auditorium
40. c. circumference
41. b. worries
42. b. finality
43. a. religious
44. a. coliseum
45. b. delinquent
46. c. forecast
47. a. righteous
48. a. sincerely
49. b. hospice
50. b. respiration

Section 2: Reading Comprehension

1. d. Many asthma sufferers have an inherited tendency to have allergies, referred to as *atopy* in the third paragraph.

2. b. The second paragraph explains that during an attack, the asthmatic will compensate for constricted airways by breathing a greater volume of air.

3. c. The first sentence begins "Asthma is no longer . . . ," indicating that asthma is not a new disease and that it has been around for some time.

4. c. The first paragraph indicates that asthma was once *considered a condition with isolated, acute episodes of bronchospasm*, but it *is now understood to be a chronic* disorder. Since these sentences show that *chronic* has the opposite meaning of *isolated*, choice **c** is the best answer.

5. a. According to the second paragraph of the passage, *destruction of bronchial epithelium* can occur during asthma.

6. d. The third paragraph discusses triggers in detail. Only physical activity is listed as a possible symptom reducer.

7. a. Since asthma symptoms vary throughout the day, relying on the presence of an attack or even just on the presence of a respiratory ailment to diagnose asthma is flawed logic.

8. b. The second paragraph states that mast cells, lymphocytes, and eosinophils are all key to an asthma attack, but also clarifies that only mast cells and eosinophils account for the similarity between asthma attacks and allergic responses. Epithelia are body tissues and are not mentioned in the passage.

9. a. The passage only mentions viral respiratory infections as a trigger for asthma, so they are a cause of asthma, not an effect of the disorder. Choices **b** and **c** are mentioned as effects of asthma.

10. b. During the first 28 days after fertilization is correct, as stated in the first sentence of the passage, long before the second or third trimester or delivery.

11. b. According to the second paragraph, *the meningocele may be repaired after birth in a major surgical procedure. Afterward, the patient may suffer little or no muscle paralysis.* While the other answer choices could be correct, there is no direct evidence in the passage to support any of them.

12. c. The second paragraph refers to the removal of a meningocele by a medical procedure. Although each answer choice is a synonym of *procedure*, the only one that would make sense if used in place of the word in this context is *process*.

13. c. Hydrocephalus is the correct term and is given in the final paragraph of the passage.

14. a. The first paragraph states that a small gap covered by a dimple is a sign of the mild form of spina bifida (spina bifida occulata). The text also explains that this form may be so mild that some people never know they have it, so the other answer choices would not apply.

15. d. The passage concludes with the thought that although spina bifida is a serious condition, sufferers may lead productive lives. The other options are never stated or are false.

16. d. See the last sentence of the third paragraph. Compaction may well reduce transportation costs (choice **a**) according to the third paragraph. That it reduces the volume of waste (choice **b**) is an advantage, not a disadvantage. Compaction is not designed to eliminate organic matter, so confirming that it has been eliminated (choice **c**) is not an issue.

17. a. See the last sentence of the fifth paragraph, which states that *incineration is . . . the preferred method for on-site treatment.*

18. b. See the last sentence of the sixth paragraph, which points out that steam sterilization does not change the appearance of the waste, thus perhaps raising questions at a landfill.

19. d. According to the second paragraph of the passage, the main risk of carting away medical waste *is that bags may be broken or torn during transport, potentially exposing the worker to the wastes.* Choices **a** and **b** describe the risks of using chutes, not carts, to dispose of medical waste.

20. a. This response relies on an understanding of pathological wastes, which are wastes generated by infectious materials. The seventh paragraph points out that incineration is especially appropriate for pathological wastes. Previously, the sixth paragraph had said that steam sterilization is appropriate for substances contaminated with infectious organisms.

21. d. The second paragraph says that the main risk of manual carts is potential exposure from torn bags, but automated carts can reduce that potential.

22. b. See the next-to-last sentence of the fourth paragraph. Sterilization does not change the appearance of waste. While compacting does change the volume of the waste, it is not appropriate for eliminating hazardous materials.

23. d. According to the final sentence of the sixth paragraph, the fact that steam *sterilization does not change the appearance of the waste* causes problems getting landfills to accept such waste. Therefore, it is logical to conclude that changing the appearance of the waste after sterilization might make it easier to convince landfills to accept it.

24. b. The last paragraph states that the use of grate-type units has been discontinued due to high air emissions. It is the rotary type that is cost prohibitive. No mention of availability or local laws was made.

25. b. The third paragraph of the passage indicates that even the smallest antigens *carry several different kinds of epitopes on their surface; some may even carry several hundred.*

26. b. All of the answers indicate peaceful coexistence. However, according to the fifth sentence of the second paragraph, in this instance, the state is referred to as *self-tolerance.*

27. c. See the last paragraph. Allergens are responsible for triggering an inappropriate immune response to otherwise harmless substances such as ragweed pollen.

28. d. The last paragraph of the passage mentions that an antigen *announces its foreignness* with intricate shapes called *epitopes* that protrude from the surface.

29. a. According to the diagram, the spleen is located in the torso just above the left hip. Choice **b** is not depicted in the diagram at all, and choices **c** and **d** are located in the head.

30. a. According to the second paragraph, the ability to distinguish between self and nonself is the heart of the immune system. This topic is further elucidated throughout the body of the passage.

31. b. The last paragraph states that in abnormal situations the immune system wrongly identifies self as nonself and attacks, resulting in an autoimmune disease like rheumatoid arthritis. The other choices are not abnormal situations.

32. c. The first paragraph introduces the concept of autoimmune attacks before specifying psoriasis as one kind of autoimmune attack. Psoriasis may result in deformity, but it is not a deformity in itself. Although it affects the skin, it is not a form of cancer, so choice **b** is incorrect.

33. a. The third paragraph of the passage discusses the researchers' studies to determine whether psoriasis is an autoimmune disease, or if it is more likely caused by nonimmune epidermal skin cells.

34. b. The second paragraph states that in psoriasis-prone families, genetic markers, known as HLA antigens, are inherited more often than in the general population. The other answer choices refer to Rh antibodies (relate to red blood cells), H1V1 (a flu virus), and CD103 (a mouse antibody).

35. c. The passage indicates that psoriasis can cause all of the conditions in the answer choices except for paralysis, which is not mentioned in the passage at all.

36. c. According to the sixth paragraph of the passage, four out of 10 patients showed *striking* improvement.

37. c. According to the fourth paragraph, *only T cells that are activated to participate in immune reactions carry the IL-2 receptor.*

38. b. The diagram shows that skin suffering from psoriasis contains plaque in the keratin layer while there is no indication of plaque in the keratin layer of the healthy skin cross section.

39. a. Psoriasis does have a genetic link, but that is only one element in the passage. Scientists are still studying the epidermal vs. immune impact. There is no mention of scientists having anything negative to say about the immune-related cause of psoriasis. Therefore, it can be successfully argued that the only viable option is that scientists, based on this new research detailed throughout the passage, are closer to understanding the causes of psoriasis.

40. d. Psoriasis is all of the answers given: a uniquely human disease (see the last paragraph), an autoimmune disease (see paragraph one), and a sometimes disfiguring skin disease (see paragraph two).

41. b. The final paragraph of the passage is chiefly concerned with how gene therapy has been used to treat cancer. Although melanoma is one kind of cancer mentioned in the paragraph, it is just an example of a cancer gene therapy and is not the chief focus of the paragraph.

42. d. According to the first paragraph of the passage, recombinant DNA technology can cause goats to *secrete a clot-dissolving heart attack drug,* tissue plasminogen activator *(TPA), in their milk.*

43. a. Included in the vaccine procedure is taking bits of tumor from a patient, treating those pieces of tumor with immune-cell-activating cytokines, and reinjecting the patient with the cancerous (albeit genetically altered) growths.

44. b. According to the fourth paragraph of the passage, *TILs reinforced with a gene for the anti-tumor cytokine known as* tumor necrosis factor *(TNF) have been administered to patients with advanced melanoma.*

45. d. According to the third paragraph, ADA is delivered to the T cells by a modified retrovirus.

Section 3: Math

1. **a.** The correct answer is 14,600. The incorrect answers are common errors in computation, particularly not carrying digits to the next place.

2. **b.** The correct answer is 375. Multiply $\frac{5}{8}$ by 600 by writing $\frac{5}{8} \times \frac{600}{1} = \frac{3,000}{8} = 375$.

3. **c.** Write the numerator and denominator in terms of their prime factors: $\frac{52}{117} = \frac{(13)(2)(2)}{(13)(3)(3)}$. Cancel out any common factors that the numerator and denominator share. The reduced form is $\frac{(2)(2)}{(3)(3)} = \frac{4}{9}$.

4. **d.** Substitute each value for x in the number sentence. The correct answer is the value that makes a true statement. The answer is $x = 67$.

5. **a.** The correct answer is 2. Because dividing two negatives yields a positive, choices **c** and **d** can be easily ruled out. Choice **b** is the result of dividing in the wrong order.

6. **d.** The answer to this question lies in knowing that there are four quarts in one gallon. There are 20 quarts in a five-gallon container. Multiply 20 by 1.06 quarts per liter to get 21.2 liters, and then round off to 21.

7. **d.** Choice **a** equals 276; choice **b** equals 2,706; choice **c** equals 20,076.

8. **a.** Raise the fraction $\frac{2}{9}$ to 54ths by multiplying both numerator and denominator by 6.

9. **c.** $6(7)(2) = 84$

10. **b.** Choice **a** equals 40,000, choice **c** equals 400, and choice **d** equals 0.40.

11. **c.** Use order of operations to simplify the expression. The first step is to find $18 \div 6$, which equals 3. Then add or subtract from left to right to get $44 + 3 - 9 = 38$.

12. **a.** The first step in solving the problem is to subtract 86 from 148. The remainder, 62, is then divided by 2 to get 31.

13. **b.** You simply add all the numbers together to get the correct answer, $92.61.

14. **b.** $150x = (100)(1)$, where x is the part of a mile a jogger has to go to burn the calories a walker burns in one mile. If you divide both sides of this equation by 150, you get $x = \frac{100}{150}$. Cancel 50 from the numerator and denominator to get $\frac{2}{3}$. This means that a jogger has to jog only $\frac{2}{3}$ of a mile to burn the same number of calories a walker burns in a mile of brisk walking.

15. **c.** The ratio is $\frac{12 \text{ cc}}{100 \text{ lbs.}} = \frac{x \text{ cc}}{175 \text{ lbs.}}$, where x is the number of cc's per 175 lbs. Multiply both sides by 175 in order to get $175 \times \frac{12}{100} = x$, so $x = 21$.

16. **a.** 20% of $1,800 = (0.2)(1,800) = 360$ calories from fat. Since there are 9 calories in each gram of fat, you should divide 360 by 9 to find that 40 grams of fat are allowed.

17. **b.** 5% of 1 liter $= (0.05)(1) = 0.02x$, where x is the total amount of water in the resulting 2% solution. Solving for x, you get 2.5. Subtracting the 1 liter of water already present in the 5% solution, you will find that 1.5 liters need to be added.

18. **b.** 20% of 15 cc $= (0.20)(15) = 3$. Adding 3 to 15 gives 18 cc.

19. **c.** The volume of a cylinder is $\pi r^2 h$, where r is the radius of the cylinder and h is the height. The radius is half the diameter, so the radius of this cylinder is $(\frac{1}{2})(8 \text{ cm}) = 4$ cm. The height of the volume is $10 - 4 = 6$ (the height of the whole cylinder minus the height of space in which the liquid has been poured out). So the volume is $\pi r^2 h = \pi(4)^2(6) = \pi(16)(6) = 96\pi$ cm^3.

20. **c.** The easiest way to calculate the volume is to realize that the shaded figure is made up of half a circle of diameter 4 or radius 2 on top of a rectangle that is 4 units wide and 6 units tall. The area of a rectangle is length times width. The area of a circle is πr^2. So the shaded area $= (4)(6) + \frac{1}{2}\pi 2^2 = 24 + 2\pi$.

21. b. $\overline{PQ}$ and $\overline{RS}$ are intersecting lines. The fact that angle *POR* is a 90° angle means that $\overline{PQ}$ and $\overline{RS}$ are perpendicular, indicating that all the angles formed by their intersection, including angle *ROQ*, measure 90°.

22. d. A line that intersects two parallel lines forms complementary angles on either side of it. Complementary angles are angles whose measures add up to 180°. So $P + Q = 180°$; $P = 40°$, so $40° + Q = 180°$. Subtracting 40° from each side yields $Q = 140°$.

23. d. Multiply 33.55 by 22.75. The total pay is $763.26.

24. a. 72% of 9,125 = (0.72)(9,125) = 6,570 males. If three out of five males were under 25, then two out of five, or $\frac{2}{5}$, were 25 or older, so $(\frac{2}{5})(6,570) = 2,628$ male patients 25 or older.

25. b. $62.5\% = \frac{62.5}{100}$. You should multiply both the numerator and denominator by 10 to move the decimal point, resulting in $\frac{625}{1,000}$, and then factor both the numerator and denominator to find out how far you can reduce the fraction. If you cancel 5 from both the numerator and denominator three times (or cancel 125), you will get $\frac{5}{8}$.

26. b. Simply estimating the value of $\frac{7}{40}$ will probably let you know that 0.0175 is much too small and 1.75 is much too large. If that did not work for you, however, you could divide 7.0 by 40 in order to get 0.175.

27. d. 30 ppm of the pollutant would have to be removed to bring the 50 ppm down to 20 ppm; 30 ppm represents 60% of 50 ppm.

28. a. The drug is 50% effective for half (or 50%) of migraine sufferers, so it eliminates (0.50)(0.50) = 0.25 = 25% of all migraines.

29. d. Division is used to arrive at a decimal, which can then be rounded to the nearest hundredth and converted to a percentage: $11,350 \div 21,500 = 0.5279$; 0.5279 rounded to the nearest hundredth is 0.53, or 53%.

30. c. Since there are two decimal places in each number you are multiplying, you need a total of four decimal places in the answer, 0.2646.

31. b. Write all the numbers as decimals to compare them. $2^{-2} = \frac{1}{2^2} = \frac{1}{4} = 0.25$. $\frac{2}{5} = 0.4$. $\frac{3}{9} = 0.33$. The smallest number is 2^{-2}.

32. a. First, find the least common denominator, 16; $\frac{7}{8} = \frac{14}{16}$, so you can rewrite the problem as $(3 + \frac{9}{16}) - (1 + \frac{14}{16})$. To get a large enough numerator from which to subtract 14, you borrow 1 from the 3 to rewrite the problem as $2\frac{25}{16} - 1\frac{14}{16} = 1\frac{11}{16}$.

33. b. This is a simple multiplication problem, which is solved by multiplying 35×8.2 in order to get 287.

34. c. The problem is solved by dividing 204 by 1,700. The answer, 0.12, is then converted to a percentage, 12%.

35. d. To solve this problem, you must convert $3\frac{1}{2}$ to $\frac{7}{2}$ and then divide $\frac{7}{2}$ by $\frac{1}{4}$, which is the same as multiplying $\frac{7}{2}$ by 4.

36. b. The simplest way to solve this problem is to divide 1 by 1,500, which is 0.0006667, and then count off two decimal places to arrive at the percentage 0.06667%. Since the question asks *about what percentage*, the nearest value is 0.067%.

37. a. You can use trial and error to arrive at a solution to this problem. Using choice **a**, after the first hour, the number would be 20, after the second hour 40, after the third hour 80, after the fourth hour 160, and after the fifth hour 320. The other answer choices do not have the same outcome.

38. a. Since the solution to the problem $x + 25 = 13$ is −12, choices **b**, **c**, and **d** are all too large to be correct.

39. b. A cube has four sides, a top, and a bottom, which means that it has six faces.

40. d. To solve this problem, you should use the formula $A = lw$, or $117 = 9l$. Next, you must divide 117 by 9 to find the answer, 13.

41. b. The patient pays $100\% - 85\% = 15\%$ of the cost. Multiply $830 by 0.15 to get $124.50 as the patient's total cost.

42. c. Add the whole numbers: $2 + 4 = 6$. Use the least common denominator of 8 to add the fractions: $\frac{2}{8} + \frac{5}{8} + \frac{4}{8} = \frac{11}{8} = 1\frac{3}{8}$. Add 1 to the whole number sum: $1 + 6 = 7$, and then add the fraction to get $7\frac{3}{8}$.

43. d. 750 is $n\%$ of 600, expressed as an equation, is $750 = (\frac{n}{100})(600)$. Cancel 100 in the right side of the equation: $750 = 6n$. Divide both sides by 6 to arrive at the answer, $n = 125$.

44. a. Replace r with 65 and t with 12. Then multiply 65 and 12 to find the value of d. The value of d is 780.

45. c. 0.32×10^3 is equal to $0.32 \times (10 \times 10 \times 10)$, or 320.

46. c. The measures of the angles of the triangle add up to 180º. Angle R has a measure of 90° because it is a right angle. Angle S has a measure of 37°. To find the measure of angle Q, first add 90 and 37 to get 127. Then, subtract 127 from 180 to get 53°.

47. c. This is a simple subtraction problem, as long as the decimals are lined up correctly: $3.60 - 1.89 = 1.71$.

48. c. This is a two-step multiplication problem. To find out how many heartbeats there would be in one hour, you must multiply 72 by 60 minutes, and then multiply this result, 4,320, by 6.5 hours in order to get 28,080.

49. a. The unreduced ratio is 8,000:5,000,000 or 8:5,000; $5,000 \div 8 = 625$, for a ratio of 1:625.

50. b. The correct answer is $\frac{1}{24}$. Before subtracting, you must convert both fractions to 24ths.

Section 4: General Science

1. c. Pressure, the force applied over an area, is not a fundamental force. The other three choices are fundamental forces of the universe, with the fourth being the strong nuclear force.

2. c. Van Leeuwenhoek was the famous early microscopist. Benedict Spinoza, though also Dutch, was a philosopher of science who claimed that God was the principle of nature being discovered by science.

3. a. Kepler was the first to state that the planets follow an elliptical path around the Sun.

4. a. The concept that Earth was not the center of the universe was revolutionary for the time and went against religious teachings, which supported the geocentric, or Earth-centered, universe paradigm. This was part of the beginning of the scientific revolution that led to work by Galileo, Kepler, and other astronomers who later proved the heliocentric (Sun-centered) model of the solar system to be correct.

5. c. Mendel used pea plants to conduct his research in trait inheritance. He grew and studied nearly 30,000 pea plants.

6. c. The largest mass extinction of all time occurred at the end of the Permian period, when over 90% of all species went extinct.

7. d. Galileo made himself a small—but for that time powerful—telescope, turned it skyward, and made many discoveries, including the moons of Jupiter, craters of our Moon, and sunspots.

8. a. The control in an experiment is the baseline not subjected to the variable under study. Choices **c** and **d** are not scientific terms.

9. c. One gram is equal to 1,000 milligrams. The prefix *milli-* means thousandth.

10. b. Theories are the biggest concepts, such as Einstein's theory of relativity or Darwin's theory of evolution. Theories can contain more detailed hypotheses and good theories make predictions.

11. b. Famous philosopher of science Karl Popper emphasized the crucial importance that experiments play in falsifying hypotheses and claimed this is the way the best science truly works.

12. b. There are six flavors of quark: up, down, bottom, top, charm, and strange.

13. c. Mars Pathfinder successfully landed on Mars in 1997.

14. d. Reductionism, which most scientists strive for, focuses on how parts interact to form wholes.

15. c. By convention, in an XY graph the *x*-axis (horizontal) is the independent variable and the *y*-axis (vertical) is the dependent variable. When you compare time and distance, time is the independent variable and distance traveled is the dependent variable, because it is the result being measured.

16. d. The prefix *micro-* refers to millionths.

17. d. The prefix *giga-* refers to billions.

18. a. The standard metric unit of energy is joule.

19. b. There are 1,000 or 10^3 meters in a kilometer.

20. d. Oxygen is the second most abundant gas in the atmosphere, making up 21% by volume. This relatively high concentration is due to photosynthesizing organisms, which release oxygen as a byproduct. Life does affect the concentrations of carbon dioxide and methane in the atmosphere, but both of these gases are present in very small amounts, each making up less than 0.05% of the atmosphere.

21. c. The prefix *nano-* refers to a billionth.

22. d. The prefix "milli" means one thousandth (0.001); therefore, it takes 1,000 mL to equal 1 L.

23. a. Small differences in the spatial patterns of temperature of the cosmic background radiation, which originated after the Big Bang but before the formation of galaxies, show the lumpiness that eventually resulted in differences of gravity that could contract matter into galaxies.

24. b. Based upon observable evidence, including redshifted galaxies and cosmic background radiation, most cosmologists (astronomers who study the origin of the universe) currently adhere to the expanding model of the universe.

25. a. N-S-E-P; the order of events is discussed in Chapter 9.

26. d. Patterns from distant galaxies are shifted "red," which means toward longer wavelengths. In this case, going from a pattern in the red toward a pattern in longer wavelengths means the infrared.

27. d. Oxygen is formed last because it is the most massive and complex. Fusion reactions build from the simplest to the most complex, and the stages of fusion use hydrogen and then the other elements built in sequence as starting points for more complex elements.

28. a. Supernova explosions, which are catastrophic events at the end of the lives of giant stars, scatter elements previously made by fusion reactions in the star over their lifetimes, as well as elements born in the intense temperatures and pressures of the supernova explosion itself.

29. c. Agriculture allowed the human population to grow from 10 million people 10,000 years ago to over 100 million people 5,000 years ago. The Industrial Revolution did help the population to reach the 1 billion mark, but this was much later, in the 1800s.

30. c. Helium is both primordial and made during fusion reactions when two hydrogen nuclei are fused together inside stars. This fusion reaction is the main source of energy for stars.

31. d. Carbon increases in density because as time passes, more and more carbon is made in the fusion reactions inside stars. Choices **a** and **b** actually decrease in density as the universe expands, and choice **c** also decreases in density as hydrogen is consumed in fusion reactions.

32. a. Venus is the closest planet to Earth. It is 38 million kilometers from Earth at its closest approach. Mars, the second-nearest planet to Earth, is 54 million kilometers at its closest approach.

33. b. The time when the Big Bang occurred was 13.7 billion years ago, and the formation of Earth occurred about 4.5 billion years ago. Therefore, taking 1 EFU as 4.5 billion years (by definition from the question), there were $\frac{13.7}{4.5}$ or about 3 EFUs back to the Big Bang.

34. c. Meteorites formed along with Earth at the beginning of the solar system. But on Earth, no rocks go back that far. The dates from meteorites give us the best estimate of the origin of our solar system.

35. d. Mercury is the smallest planet in the solar system and its small mass does not provide enough gravitational pull to retain an atmosphere. Neptune is one of the "gas giants" of the outer solar system, Mars has a thin atmosphere consisting primarily of carbon dioxide, and Venus has a thick carbon dioxide atmosphere with a runaway greenhouse effect.

36. b. Of the possibilities, the only one in space right now is the International Space Station. Choices **a** and **d** are inactive, and choice **c** is unmanned.

37. b. Eris is the most massive known dwarf planet in the solar system.

38. b. In 2004, rovers on the surface of Mars discovered types of minerals that, as far as we know, could have been formed only with the activity of water. Also, previously, channels on Mars had been seen that looked much like the branching patterns of Earth's slow rivers.

39. a. Since its discovery by Clyde Tombaugh in 1930, astronomers noted that Pluto's eccentric orbit and small size didn't quite fit the properties of the other eight planets. During the International Astronomical Union meeting in 2006, astronomers refined the meaning of a "planet," thus downgrading Pluto's status from a planet to a "dwarf planet."

40. d. The spins of galaxies cannot be explained by the amount of known, ordinary matter. Something out there (the "dark matter") is creating more gravity than we can account for with the known, ordinary matter.

41. b. 73% of the universe is dark energy.

42. c. Carbon is made by fusion reactions in stars. Therefore, before stars and supernovas had dispersed that carbon, there would have been no carbon in the earliest planets (in fact, planets as solid bodies could not have formed either). Life is so dependent on carbon that without carbon it seems likely there could not have been life.

43. c. The continental slope is still part of the continent, but it does head downward to the ocean floor itself.

44. a. The word *atom* came from the Greek word that meant indivisible. Though atoms are now known to have parts (they are divisible), they still are the fundamental units of any element.

45. d. Carbon-14 is the radioactive form of carbon (the most common form is carbon-12). Carbon-14 is formed in the atmosphere when cosmic rays hit nitrogen and convert small amounts of it (by changing a proton to a neutron—a nuclear change). Using its decay rate, we can measure the amount of carbon-14 in ancient organic materials to determine their ages. For example, we can date the wood architecture of ancient peoples as well as their campfires and even bones.

46. c. Protons are positively charged, electrons are negatively charged, and neutrons have no charge. Quarks make up protons and neutrons.

47. d. Neutrons and protons are the parts of the nucleus of an atom.

48. b. The unit of resistance is the ohm.

49. a. Electromagnetism describes the interaction between charged particles. Answer choices **b**, **c**, and **d** correspond to the strong, weak, and gravitational forces, respectively.

50. a. The following are the SI units: 10^{-1} = *deci*; 10^{-2} = *centi*; 10^{-3} = *milli*; 10^{-6} = *micro*; 10^{-9} = *nano*; 10^{-12} = *pico*; 10^{-15} = *femto*; 10^{-18} = *atto*.

Section 5: Biology

1. d. Guanine is a purine. Thymine, cytosine, and uracil are the major pyrimidines.

2. d. The lining of the uterus, shed during menstruation, is referred to as the endometrium. Fimbria are found at the ends of the fallopian tubes in mammals. The cervix is the narrow neck of the uterus. The myometrium is the layer of smooth muscles of the uterine wall.

3. c. The prefix *dys-* means abnormal; *plasis* is Greek for formation.

4. a. Genetic engineering is the physical manipulation of genes in the laboratory, which can include inserting, deleting, or changing genes.

5. d. A capsid is the protein coat of a viral genome. Some viruses also have a lipid and protein envelope that covers the capsid, but the capsid is the protein layer that directly encloses the viral genome.

6. b. Organisms have two genes for each trait. If both genes are the same, the organism is homozygous for that trait. If both genes are different, the organism is heterozygous for that trait.

7. b. Chloroplasts are found only in plants. Both plants and animals have mitochondria and nuclei, and both bacteria and plants possess cell walls.

9. b. A compartment filled with air or watery fluid in the cytoplasm is referred to as a vacuole. Centrioles and centrosomes are associated with the process of cell division.

8. c. Mendel is known as the founder of modern genetics because of his work showing how the inheritance of certain traits in pea plants follows a pattern. This is now called Mendelian inheritance.

10. a. Hormones can be divided into three classes: steroid hormones, amino acid derivatives, and peptides. Insulin is a peptide, testosterone is a steroid hormone, and adrenaline and thyroxine are amino acid derivatives.

11. a. Mitochondria are known as the power plants of the cell and are responsible for most ATP generation.

12. a. Prophase is the first phase of mitosis, or cell division. Telophase is the fourth stage.

13. a. A gamete is a unique cell because it is haploid—that is, it contains only one set of chromosomes instead of the two sets that are found in most somatic cells, which are diploid.

14. c. The lysosome is the garbage truck of the cell, handling waste and breaking it down.

15. a. During prophase I, chromosomes pair up close to their homologues. The chromosomes then break at identical sites and swap segments. This process is known as crossing over.

16. d. The figure is the cell body of a nerve cell. Note the long extensions (dendrites) unique to neurons. Blood, fat, and muscle cells have very different shapes.

17. c. Hepatitis is a disease marked by a inflammation of the liver, as indicated by the Greek roots *hepato* meaning liver and *itis* meaning inflammation.

18. d. Bacteria reproduce by binary fission. All the other answer choices relate to eukaryotic cell division.

19. a. The primary function of a blood platelet is to aid in the blood clotting process. Platelets scrape against the rough edges of broken tissue and release a substance to promote clotting. Red blood cells carry oxygen. Antibodies are produced by B lymphocytes. Phagocytic cells include neutrophils and macrophages (monocytes).

20. d. An expressed trait is determined by two alleles. A phenotype is the physical or visual expression of the genotype.

21. c. Bacteria reproduce asexually but can exchange DNA with other bacteria and undergo genetic recombination through conjugation, transduction, or transformation.

22. a. When a mutation occurs, a gene is changed.

23. c. Choice **c** has the proper complementary bases—including the use of U instead of T as the complement to A in RNA; the other choices are either nonsense or they use T and not U.

24. d. Incomplete dominance is a condition in which the heterozygous genotype for certain alleles gives rise to a phenotype intermediate between dominant and recessive traits because both traits are expressed and blended.

25. d. Enzymes are catalysts that allow chemical reactions to proceed more rapidly.

26. c. Kelp is a brown algae; the others are fungi.

27. b. Blood needs to maintain osmotic pressure to keep water in the bloodstream. Albumin makes up around 60% of blood proteins and is mainly responsible for maintaining the osmotic pressure of the plasma.

28. b. Bacteria can be placed in three groups (cocci, bacilli, spirilla) based on their shape.

29. c. Malaria is caused by *Plasmodium*, which is a protist. The others are viruses.

30. b. All bacteria have double-stranded DNA making up their genomes, as do some viruses. Viruses can also have single-stranded DNA or RNA genomes, or double-stranded RNA genomes.

31. a. Transcription describes the copying of DNA to messenger RNA, which travels out of the nucleus before being translated into proteins.

32. a. Plants are first classified broadly as either vascular or nonvascular. Vascular plants can then be divided into seeded or seedless plants. Seeded plants are further divided into angiosperms or gymnosperms. Finally, angiosperms are either monocots or dicots.

33. b. A zygote is the product of a sperm nucleus fused with an ovum nucleus. A zoospore is found in certain fungi. Ova is the plural of ovum, a female egg, while an oocyte is a cell in the ovary that produces an ovum after undergoing meiosis.

34. a. Glycolysis is a combination of *glucose* and *lysis* (meaning breaking down).

35. a. When there is a shortage of oxygen in muscle tissue, pyruvic acid produces lactic acid to be converted to glucose by the liver. Lactose is milk sugar. Adrenaline is a hormone produced in the adrenal medulla that stimulates the sympathetic nervous system, while serotonin, also a hormone, is produced in many parts of the body.

36. c. The large intestine's main functions are water absorption and feces production. The large intestine consists of the rectum, colon, and caecum. Almost all the digestion and absorption of nutrients occur in the small intestine. The liver has numerous functions including the metabolism of carbohydrates, lipids, and proteins, as well as the removal of drugs and hormones and the production of bile. The stomach is the holding reservoir in which saliva, food, and gastric juices mix prior to passing into the small intestine.

37. a. Calcium ions are released between the time when a stimulus is received and a response occurs in muscle tissue.

38. a. Beriberi, most common in countries where white rice is the main food source, is caused by a lack of vitamin B_1. Deficiencies in vitamin C can cause scurvy and deficiencies in vitamin D can cause rickets. Hemolytic anemia is a possible consequence of vitamin E deficiency.

39. c. Chlorophyll is the pigment that absorbs light energy and is critical for photosynthesis.

40. d. Anaphylaxis is an immune system response such as that which occurs in a person who gets stung by a bee and is allergic to the venom. Hypertension is another term for high blood pressure.

41. a. The correct answer is analgesic. Anesthetics block perception of *all* sensory stimuli either generally (all over) or locally (in a specific area). Acetycholine is a neuro-transmitter.

42. c. Thymine is a DNA nucleotide that pairs with adenine.

43. a. Flagella are structures that project from a bacterium. The movement of the flagella allows the bacterium to move.

44. a. The first law of thermodynamics describes the conservation of energy.

45. b. Complementary base pairing describes how the bases in DNA pair in set ways. Cytosine pairs only with guanine, and adenine pairs only with thymine.

46. d. Ethanol or ethyl alcohol depresses the CNS, thereby affecting the neural activity of the consumer. Isopropyl alcohol is for external use only and is found in cosmetics. Methanol is wood alcohol used as a solvent. Methionine is an amino acid used in dietary supplements.

47. a. The primary structure describes a protein's amino acid sequence. Answer choices **b** and **c** describe a protein's secondary and tertiary structures, respectively.

48. a. Warts are usually insignificant growths caused by a virus. Sarcomas are malignant tumors arising from connective tissue, while adenomas are glandlike benign tumors. A cold sore is a lesion caused by the herpes simplex virus.

49. c. Rhodopsin or visual purple is the light-sensitive pigment in vertebrate eyes. Cytochrome is a respiratory enzyme, hemoglobin is the oxygen-bearing protein in red blood cells that gives them their red color, and melanin is the dark pigment found in skin, hair, and the retina.

50. b. People suffering from high blood pressure, or hypertension, have an increased risk of stroke and heart attack. Cardiomyopathy is a form of muscle damage that leads to heart failure.

Section 6: Chemistry

1. b. It is very important for blood to be close to neutral, as variance outside a small pH range can cause death. Ammonia is a well-known base, while lemon juice and vinegar contain citric and acetic acids, respectively, giving them low pH.

2. a. If more chloride ions are added to the solution, this will drive the equilibrium reaction to the left. Less AgCl will dissolve, so fewer silver and chloride ions form.

3. c. NH_2 is an amino group, which gives an amino acid the first part of its name. It is found in 19 of the 20 amino acids. The other prevalent group is carboxylic acid, or COOH, which is not one of the answer choices.

4. a. When two amino acids come together, the carboxylic acid group of one reacts with the amine group of the other. An OH from the carboxylic acid combines with an H from the amine group to form H_2O. The remaining C=O of the carboxylic acid then bonds with the remaining N-H of the amine to form a peptide bond.

5. b. The secondary structure describes the geometry of segments of the protein, such as α-helices and β-sheets. The amino acid sequence describes the primary structure, while the three-dimensional fold of the protein describes the tertiary structure.

6. b. The mass number (35) is equal to the number of protons plus neutrons; $35 - 17 = 18$ neutrons.

7. a. A catalyst is a substance that increases the rate of a reaction without being consumed in the reaction. It decreases the amount of energy necessary for the reaction to occur.

8. b. The number of neutrons in an atom can be found by subtracting the atomic number from the mass number.

9. c. This is the only choice where all atoms have a full octet and no formal charges. The other three choices have either or both, and unfilled octets and formal charges are undesirable in a stable molecule.

10. d. A butyl is an alkane with four carbon atoms. The *t* in *t*-butyl stands for a tertiary carbon. The central carbon of choice **d** is tertiary because it has three other carbon atoms bonded to it. Choice **a** is also a butyl molecule, but it is *n*-butyl. Choices **b** and **c** are not butyls.

11. c. Neutral oxygen possesses eight electrons (the same as the number of protons). The −2 charge on the ion means that there are two additional electrons for 10 total.

12. c. The halogens, group VIIA (group 17) on the periodic table, form negative ions by gaining one more electron in their outer shells to achieve a stable noble gas configuration. The alkali and alkaline earth metals lose electrons to form positive ions.

13. b. Combustion is a reaction in which an alkane burns in excess oxygen to give carbon dioxide and water. Hydrogen gas, present in all three incorrect equations, is not a participant in combustion reactions.

14. d. The configuration of a chlorine atom in the ground state is $[Ne]3s^23p^5$. A Cl^- ion has an additional electron, giving it the same electron configuration as an argon atom in the ground state, which can also be written as $[Ne]3s^23p^6$.

15. c. The carbon atom in methane has four sigma bonds around it, meaning that it uses its *s* atomic orbital and all three *p* atomic orbitals to form four sp^3 molecular orbitals. The number of atomic orbitals combining always equals the number of molecular orbitals formed.

16. b. In electron configurations, the *s* orbitals have a maximum of two electrons and the *p* orbitals have a maximum of six electrons. The electron configuration $1s^2 2s^4$ is not possible because the second *s* orbital has four electrons.

17. b. This is the definition of the boiling point. At temperatures higher than the boiling point, the vapor pressure of the liquid is greater than external pressure and molecules begin to escape in the gaseous phase.

18. c. Fe_2O_3 contains three oxygen atoms, each with a –2 charge. To balance this –6 overall charge, each iron atom must have an oxidation state of +3.

19. a. The empirical formula of a compound is the formula written with the simplest whole number ratios possible. $C_2H_6O_2$ has one molecule of both C and O for every three molecules of H, so the empirical formula is CH_3O.

20. a. Neutral magnesium possesses two valence electrons. To reach its nearest full valence shell, it loses those electrons, giving it an oxidation state of +2.

21. d. The complete chemical symbol includes two numbers. The lower number is the atomic number, or the number of protons in the nucleus. The upper number is the mass number, or the sum of the protons and neutrons in the nucleus. Therefore, the answer is $^{33}_{16}S^{2-}$, because there are 18 electrons present.

22. b. Nonmetal oxides (SO_3) and bases (KOH) react to form salts and water. The solution in choice **a** forms an acid and that in choice **c** forms a salt, but such a reaction would not give off oxygen.

23. d. Lewis acids are electron-pair acceptors, whereas Bronsted acids are proton donors. HCl and H_2SO_4 are proton donors. CH_4 is not an acid of any type. The aluminum atom in $AlCl_3$ has the ability to accept two electrons (to give it eight electrons in its valence shell), making it a Lewis acid.

24. d. This problem is simply an equation-balancing problem. The number of molecules of each element must be the same on each side of the equation. Choice **d** has 8 carbons, 20 hydrogens, and 26 oxygens on each side of the equation.

25. a. The molar mass of the compound NaCl is approximately 58.4 g/mol; 29.2 grams is one-half the molar mass of NaCl, so the solution is 0.5 M because there is one liter of the solution. Molarity is moles/liter.

26. a. Ethers have the formula $R_1–O–R_2$. Answer choices **b**, **c**, and **d** are a carboxylic acid, amine, and alkene, respectively.

27. c. The sum of the oxidation numbers must be equal to the net charge on the compound, so the sum must be equal to zero. The charge on the cation is the same as its oxidation number, so the oxidation number of Na is +1 and the oxidation number for S_2O_3 is –2. Oxygen almost always has an oxidation number of –2, so the oxidation number of sulfur must be +2.

28. b. The formula $P_1V_1 = P_2V_2$ must be used. Solving $2(2\text{ L}) = P_2(0.5\text{ L})$ for P_2 gives 8 atm.

29. d. The sum of the partial pressures is the total pressure, or in this case the air pressure. Since the sample is 21% oxygen, and there is a total pressure of 800 torr, the partial pressure is 800×0.21, or 170 torr.

30. a. One factor that affects reaction rate is the concentration of the reactants. The second reaction uses an acid solution with a lower concentration of acid. This reaction would proceed at a slower rate than the first reaction.

31. d. P possesses 15 electrons total and this is its electronic structure according to Hund's rule.

32. b. The molecules move faster when heated, causing more collisions, which in turn increases the pressure.

33. a. The formula $q = $ (specific heat) $\times$ (mass of water) $\times \Delta T$ is used. Because the units in the specific heat involve grams, the mass is left as grams instead of changed to kilograms; $(100 \text{ g})(4.2 \text{ J/g·K})(75 \text{ K}) = 3.2 \times 10^4$ J.

34. d. The Kelvin temperature scale starts at absolute zero, which is equivalent to $-273.15°$ C. Temperature in degrees Celsius is converted to K by adding 273.15 to the temperature.

35. c. Ion-dipole forces act between an ion and a polar molecule. Dipole-dipole forces act between two polar molecules. Because K^+ is an ion, this can be ruled out. Hydrogen bonds are a special type of dipole-dipole interaction. London forces are generally weak attractions between temporary dipoles.

36. b. A decomposition reaction occurs when a reactant breaks down into smaller molecules. If one reactant results in two products, a decomposition reaction must have occurred.

37. b. Compounds are solids in the upper left portion of the diagram, above and to the left of the line that connects A, B, and D.

38. c. To sublime is to go directly from the solid to the gas state. The gas state is the bottom portion of the phase diagram, below and to the right of the lines that connect A, B, and C.

39. a. NH_3 and O_2 form NO. Choice **a** is the only equation that is balanced.

40. b. 36 grams of O_2 are needed; the molar mass of O_2 is 32 g/mol.
1.5 mole Al $\times \frac{3 \text{ moles } O_2}{4 \text{ moles Al}} \times \frac{32 \text{ g } O_2}{\text{mole } O_2} = 36$ g O_2

41. d. If an equation is
$aA + bB \rightleftharpoons cC + dD$, $K_c = \frac{[C]^c[D]^d}{[A]^a[B]^b}$

42. b. pOH = $-$log $[OH^-]$ = 8. pH = 14 $-$ pOH = $14 - 8 = 6$.

43. c. Electronegativity increases up and to the right on the periodic table.

44. c. 0.04 moles of acid are needed to titrate the NaOH: 0.4 M $\times$ 0.100 l = 0.04 moles.

45. a. LiF is the only ionic crystal. SiO_2 (glass) is a covalent crystal, while the other two are molecular.

46. b. A neutral chlorine atom has 17 electrons. For it to have the same stable configuration as argon, it would have to gain one electron and form an ion with a charge of -1.

47. d. Electronegativity increases on the periodic table traveling up and to the right, making F the most electronegative element.

48. b. The balanced reaction for the formation of $PbCl_2$ is $Pb^{2+}_{(aq)} + 2Cl^-_{(aq)} \rightarrow PbCl_{2(s)}$. There are (0.1 M)(0.1 L) = 0.01 mol $Pb(NO_3)_2$ = 0.01 mol Pb^{2+} and (0.1 M)(0.1 L) = 0.01 mol $BaCl_2$ = 0.02 mol Cl^-. So the theoretical yield should be 0.01 mol $PbCl_2$ = (0.01 mol)(278 g/mol) = 2.78 g. So, percent yield = $\frac{\text{actual yield}}{\text{theoretical yield}} \times 100\%$ = $\frac{1.67 \text{ g}}{2.78 \text{ g}} \times 100\% = 60\%$.

49. a. The empirical formula describes the simplest relative ratios of the atoms in a molecule.

50. b. The molecular weight of a compound is the sum of the atomic weights of the elements making up the compound. The molecular weight of $CaCl_2$ is found by adding 40.078, 35.4527, and 35.4527.

Scoring

Your score on each section is reported both as a raw score (the number of questions you got right in that section) and as a percentile (a number that indicates what percent of other test takers scored lower than you did on this section). No total score is reported, only scores for individual sections. Furthermore, there is no such thing as a "passing" raw or percentile score. Individual schools and agencies set their own standards.

For purposes of comparison, you'll work with raw scores in this book. So the first thing you should do is count up the number of questions you got right in each section, and record them in the following blanks.

Section 1: _____ of 50 questions right
Section 2: _____ of 45 questions right
Section 3: _____ of 50 questions right
Section 4: _____ of 50 questions right
Section 5: _____ of 50 questions right
Section 6: _____ of 50 questions right

Your purpose in taking this first practice exam—in addition to getting practice in answering the kinds of questions found on health occupations entrance exams—is to identify your strengths and weaknesses. In order to do so, convert your raw scores above into percentages. (Note that this *percentage* is not the same as the *percentile* that will appear on your score report. The percentage is simply the number you would have gotten right if there had been 100 questions in the section; it will enable you to compare your raw scores among the various sections. The percentile compares your score with that of other candidates.)

To get percentages for the sections with 50 questions, simply multiply your raw score by two. (Since each section has 50 questions, your percentage is twice your raw score.)

For section 2, divide your raw score by 45, and then move the decimal point two places to the right to arrive at a percentage.

Now that you know what percentage of the questions on each section you got right, you're ready to outline your study plan. The sections on which you got the lowest percentages are the ones you should plan on studying hardest. Sections on which you got higher percentages may not need as much of your time. However, unless you scored over 95% on a given section, you can't afford to skip studying that section altogether. After all, you want the highest score you can manage in the time left before the exam.

Use your percentage scores in conjunction with the Health Occupations Entrance Exam Planner in Chapter 1 of this book to help you devise a study plan. Then turn to the chapters that follow this one, which cover each of the areas tested on the health occupations entrance exam. These chapters contain valuable information on each section of the exam, along with study and test-taking tips and lots of practice questions, to help you score your best.

4 ▶ VERBAL ABILITY

CHAPTER SUMMARY
To be successful in the health profession of your choice, you must be able to communicate ideas clearly and accurately. Because written expression is an important part of communicating, your health occupations entrance exam will include a spelling section. You won't be required to spell words, but you will be asked to *identify* which of four words is spelled correctly.

This chapter is designed to help you refresh your spelling skills by pointing out rules that can help you spell your best. You'll review strategies for spelling words with tricky letter combinations, unusual plurals, or prefixes, and suffixes.

What Spelling Questions Are Like

If you are only taking the TEAS, you won't have to concern yourself with this chapter very much, but spelling constitutes an entire section of the HOAE. These questions are slightly unusual in that they only have three answer choices rather than the usual four. In the spelling section of the HOAE, you're tested on your ability to recognize properly and improperly spelled words. You will be given a set of differently spelled versions of the same word and asked to find the one that is spelled correctly. For example:

1. Choose the correctly spelled word.
   a. peice
   b. piece
   c. peece

The correct answer is choice **b**, *piece*. Knowing the rule for when to use *ie* or *ei* could have helped you if you weren't sure of the answer. Read on to learn the rule.

How to Prepare for Spelling Questions

Reading as much as you can, looking at words carefully, visualizing words, listening for the sounds of words, knowing the most common prefixes, suffixes, and roots—all of these are simple and effective ways to naturally improve your spelling skills. But if you want to ensure that you ace the spelling portion of your entrance exam, nothing beats learning these important spelling rules.

Spelling Rules

Most of the spelling items on your health occupations entrance exam test your knowledge of spelling rules, so getting a good grasp on them is essential. The following are some common rules you'll likely be tested on.

ie *and* ei
There's an old phonics rhyme, "*I before e except after c,* or when sounding like *a* as in *neighbor* or *weigh*." If you've never heard it before, learn it now because it works. Another rule about *ie* vs. *ei* is to remember that *ie* makes a long *e* sound and *ei* makes a long *a* sound. Words with the long *e* sound include: *wield*, *fierce*, and *cashier*. Words with the long *a* sound include: *eight*, *vein*, and *deign*.

2. Choose the correctly spelled word.
   a. yeild
   b. mischeivous
   c. achieve

If you remember the rhyme and rule above, it's easy to see the correct answer is choice **c**, *achieve*.

But beware! There are some words that are exceptions to this rule; be sure to memorize them:

friend	*piety*	*fiery*
quiet	*notoriety*	*society*
science	*ancient*	*deficient*
conscience	*either*	*seize*
weird	*sheik*	*seizure*
leisure	*height*	*sleight*
stein	*seismology*	*heifer*
their	*foreign*	*forfeit*
neither	*protein*	*Fahrenheit*
codeine		

ia *and* ai
The vowel combination *ai* has the sound "uh," as in the word *villain*. For *ia*, each vowel is pronounced separately, as in the word *median*.

3. Choose the correctly spelled word.
   a. guardian
   b. guardain
   c. guardean

Choice **a** is spelled correctly. In *guardian*, the *i* and *a* are pronounced separately—*GUARD-ē-uhn*, so *ia* is the right combination.

Other Two-Vowel Combinations
Another phonics rhyme goes: "When two vowels go walking, the first one does the talking." This holds true most of the time. Let's break down the rhyme to fully understand it. "When two vowels go walking" refers to a two-vowel combination in a word. For ex-

ample, abst*ai*n, ch*ea*p, f*oe,* and j*ui*ce. "The first one does the talking" means that only the first vowel in the two-vowel combination is pronounced, and the second vowel is silent. In the case of our examples, you hear the *a* in *abstain,* but not the *i.* In *cheap,* you hear the *e* but not the *a.* Similarly, in *foe,* you hear the *o* but not the *e,* and in *juice,* you hear the *u* but not the *i.*

Here are a few more examples of words that follow the two-vowel rule:

plead	float
woe	repeat
boat	gear
treat	suit
steal	read
chaise	lead
moat	heat

4. Choose the correctly spelled word.
   a. nuisance
   b. niusance
   c. nuicanse

The correct answer is choice **a,** *nuisance.* Say this word out loud. It sounds like *NEW-sance,* right? That's because you hear the *u* sound, but not the *i.* The first vowel is doing the talking here.

When to Drop a Final e

You should drop a final *e* before adding any ending beginning with a vowel, like *-ed, -ing,* and *-able.* Keep the final *e* when adding an ending that begins with a consonant, like *-ly* or *-ful.*

There are a few exceptions to this rule. You keep a final *e* when adding an ending that begins with a vowel if:

■ The *e* follows a soft *c* or *g.* A soft *c* sounds like an *s*; a soft *g* sounds like a *j.*

■ You need to protect pronunciation like showing that a preceding vowel needs to be long, as in *hoe + ing = hoeing,* not *hoing.*

You drop a final *e* when adding an ending that begins with a consonant if:

■ The *e* follows a *u* or *w.*

5. Choose the correctly spelled word.
   a. trully
   b. truely
   c. truly

The correct word is choice **c,** *truly.* The correct spelling is *truly.* The rule says to keep a final *e,* when adding a consonant ending like *-ly* unless it follows a *u* or *w.* In *true,* the *e* does indeed follow the letter *u,* so you drop the final *e: truly.*

When to Keep a Final y or Change it to i

When a final *y* follows a consonant, change the *y* to *i* before adding an ending, except *-ing.* When the final *y* follows a vowel, the *y* does not change. This rule applies to **all** endings, even plurals.

Change the *y* to an *i*:

early—earlier	fly—flier, flies
party—partied,	weary—wearied, wearies
partier, parties	pretty—prettier,
sorry—sorrier	prettiness
worry—worried,	try—tried, tries
worrier, worries	

Remember to keep the *y* when adding *-ing*:

fly—flying	party—partying
weary—wearying	worry—worrying
try—trying	

Don't change the final *y* to an *i* when it's preceded by a vowel. For example:

enjoy—enjoyed,   employ—employed,
   enjoying, enjoys   employing, employs
pray—prayed,   delay—delayed,
   praying, prays   delaying, delays

6. Choose the correctly spelled word.
   a. queasyness
   b. queasiness
   c. queaseyness

The rule states that when a final *y* follows a consonant, you must change the *y* to *i* before adding an ending (except -*ing*). The final *y* in *queasy* is preceded by a consonant (*s*), so when adding -*ness*, the *y* changes to *i*: *queasiness*. Therefore, choice **b** is correct.

Adding Endings to Words That End with a c

Add a *k* after a final *c* before any ending that begins with *e*, *i*, or *y*. All other endings do not require a *k*.
   For example:

traffic + -*er* = trafficker
traffic + -*able* = trafficable

Other examples of when to add a *k* are:

panic—panicking, panicked, panicky
mimic—mimicking, mimicked, mimicker
picnic—picnicking, picnicked, picnicker

7. Choose the correctly spelled word.
   a. historickal
   b. historikal
   c. historical

Only choice **c**, *historical*, is spelled correctly. Remember, a *k* is required after a final *c* when the ending begins with *e*, *i*, or *y*.

In English, one of the difficulties of spelling is in making plurals. Unfortunately, you can't always simply add the letter -*s* to show more than one!

When to Use -s or -es to Form Plurals

There are two simple rules that govern most plurals.

1. To make most nouns plural, add -*s*.
2. If a noun ends in a sibilant sound (*s*, *ss*, *z*, *ch*, *x*, *sh*), add -*es*.

Here are some examples of plurals:

cars	faxes	dresses
computers	indexes	churches
books	lunches	guesses
skills	dishes	buzzes

Exceptions

In the last lesson, you learned that when a word ends in a *y* preceded by a consonant, you change the *y* to *i* before adding -*es*.

SINGULAR	PLURAL
fly	flies
rally	rallies

Plurals for Words That End in o

There is just one quick rule that governs a few words ending in *o*.
   If a final *o* follows another vowel, it takes -*s*.
   Here are some examples:

patios	radios
studios	videos

When the final *o* follows a consonant rather than a vowel, there is no rule to guide you in choosing -*s* or -*es*. You just have to learn the individual words.

The following words form a plural with -*s* alone:

albinos   *pianos*
altos   *silos*
banjos   *sopranos*
logos   *broncos*

The following words take -*es*:

heroes   *tomatoes*
potatoes   *vetoes*

When in doubt about whether to add -*s* or -*es*, look the word up in the dictionary until you memorize it.

Plurals That Don't Use -s or -es

There are many words that don't simply use -*s* or -*es* to form plurals. These are usually words that still observe the rules of the languages from which they were adopted. Most of these plurals are part of your reading, speaking, and listening vocabularies. You can see that there are patterns that will help you. For instance, in Latin words, -*um* becomes -*a*, -*us* becomes -*i*, and in Greek words, -*sis* becomes -*ses*. A good way to remember these plurals is by saying the words aloud, because for the most part, they do not change form and you may remember them more easily if you listen to the sound of the spelling.

SINGULAR	PLURAL
child	children
deer	deer
goose	geese
man	men
mouse	mice
ox	oxen
woman	women
alumnus	alumni
curriculum	curricula
datum	data
fungus	fungi
medium	media
stratum	strata
analysis	analyses
axis	axes
basis	bases
oasis	oases
parenthesis	parentheses
thesis	theses

8. Choose the correctly spelled word.
   a. spyes
   b. spys
   c. spies

Only choice **c**, *spies*, is spelled correctly. It is the plural of *spy*, and words that end in —*y* always end in —*ies* in the plural form.

Homonyms

Homonyms are words that sound the same but have different spellings and meanings. Many of these words have just one change in the vowel or vowel combination. There's no rule about these words so you'll simply have to memorize them. Sometimes it helps to learn each word in terms of the job it does in a sentence. Often, the two words in a homophone pair are different parts of speech. Here are a few examples:

affect/effect	led/lead
altar/alter	minor/miner
bare/bear	passed/past
bloc/block	peal/peel
cite/site	piece/peace
cord/chord	sheer/shear
coarse/course	stationery/stationary
descent/dissent	weak/week
dual/duel	which/witch
heal/heel	write/right

Since the meanings of these homonyms are different, context is probably the best way to differentiate between them.

Examples in Context

He led a **dual** (*adjective*) life as a spy.
He fought a **duel** (*noun*) with his great enemy.

He had to **alter** (*verb*) his clothes after he lost weight.
The bride smiled as she walked toward the **altar** (*noun*).

Prefixes

Generally, when you add a prefix to a root word, neither the root nor the prefix changes spelling:

un- + prepared = unprepared
mal- + nutrition = malnutrition
sub- + traction = subtraction
mis- + informed = misinformed

This rule applies even when the root word begins with the same letter as the prefix. Generally, you use both consonants, but let your eye be your guide. If it looks funny, it's probably not spelled correctly. The following are some examples of correctly spelled words:

dissatisfied	irreverent
disservice	misspelled
illegible	misstep
irrational	unnatural

9. Choose the correctly spelled word.
  a. ilogical
  b. illogicall
  c. illogical

Only choice **c**, *illogical*, is spelled correctly. Remember, when you add a prefix to a root word (*il-* + logical), neither the root nor the prefix changes spelling, even when the root begins with the same letter as the prefix.

Practice Questions

Here are some practice spelling questions. Answers follow.

Choose the correctly spelled word.

10. **a.** magically
    b. magickelly
    c. majicelly
    d. magicaly

11. **a.** beleif
    b. bilief
    c. belief
    d. beleaf

12. **a.** nieghbor
    b. neihbor
    c. niehbor
    d. neighbor

13. **a.** eficient
    b. eficeint
    c. efficient
    d. efficeint

14. **a.** collaborate
    b. colaborate
    c. collaborat
    d. colabarate

15. **a.** babys
    b. babis
    c. babies

16. **a.** leafes
    b. leaves
    c. leeves

17. **a.** announcement
    b. anouncement
    c. announcemant

18. **a.** litrature
    b. literatore
    c. literature

19. **a.** goos
    b. geeses
    c. geese

Answers to Practice Questions

10. **a.** magically
11. **c.** belief
12. **d.** neighbor
13. **c.** efficient
14. **a.** collaborate
15. **c.** babies
16. **b.** leaves
17. **a.** announcement
18. **c.** literature
19. **c.** geese

Tips for Answering Verbal Ability Questions

- **Practice** using the sample questions in this chapter.
- **Read widely** to improve your general vocabulary and spelling.
- **Say the words** silently to yourself.
- **Dissect the words** to find their roots, prefixes, and suffixes.
- **Learn the rules** of spelling and memorize words that are exceptions.

5 ▶ READING COMPREHENSION

CHAPTER SUMMARY

Because reading is such a vital skill, many health occupations entrance exams include a reading comprehension section that tests your ability to understand what you read. The tips and exercises in this chapter will help you improve your comprehension of written passages so that you can increase your score in this area.

As a health services professional, you will do a lot of reading—memos, policies, and manuals, as well as medical and technical reports, charts, and procedures. Understanding written material is a key part of the job. So reading comprehension is an essential skill for students of health education programs—most likely, you will need to read and understand scientific and medical textbooks as you train for your career. Because reading is so important, health occupations entrance exams include a reading comprehension section that tests your ability to understand what you read.

The reading comprehension section of the test looks much like other reading comprehension tests you've completed on other standardized tests. You're asked to read a passage and then answer questions based on what you have just read. You don't need to have any prior knowledge to answer the questions—you need only the information presented in the passage. You *will* be asked to interpret passages, identify the author's purpose, look at how ideas are organized and presented, and draw conclusions based on information in the passage.

You may notice a wide variation in the complexity of the reading comprehension questions in this book. That's because these questions appear very differently on the two main health occupations entrance exams. HOAE reading comprehension questions tend to be worded very simply with one-word answer choices, while TEAS ones are longer and more complex.

Types of Reading Comprehension Questions

As a test taker, you have two advantages when answering multiple-choice questions about reading passages:

1. You don't have to know anything about the topic of the passage.
2. You're being tested only on the information the passage provides.

The disadvantage is that you have to know where and how to find that information quickly in an unfamiliar text. This makes it easy to fall for one of the wrong answer choices, especially since they are designed to mislead you.

The best way to do well on this passage/question format is to be very familiar with the kinds of questions that are typically asked on the test. Questions most frequently ask you to:

- Identify a specific **fact or detail** in the passage.
- Note the **main idea** of the passage.
- Make an **inference** based on the passage.
- Define a **vocabulary** word from the passage.
- Interpret information in a **graphic**.

Facts and details are the specific pieces of information that support the passage's **main idea**. The main idea is what the passage is mostly about. Generally speaking, facts and details are indisputable—things that don't need to be proven, like statistics (18 million people) or descriptions (a green overcoat). Let's say, for example, you read a sentence that says, "After the department's reorganization, workers were 50% more productive." A sentence like this, which gives you the **fact** that 50% of workers were more productive, might support a **main idea** that says, "Every department should be reorganized." Notice that this main idea is not something indisputable; it is an opinion. The writer thinks all departments should be reor-

ganized, and because this is his opinion (and not everyone shares it), he needs to support his opinion with facts and details.

An **inference**, on the other hand, is a conclusion or judgment that can be drawn based on facts or evidence. For example, you can infer—based on the fact that workers became 50% more productive—that the department wasn't efficiently organized before the change. The fact also implies that the reorganization was the reason workers became more productive. Of course, there may have been other reasons, but we can infer only one from the sentence.

As you might expect, **vocabulary** questions ask you to determine the meanings of particular words. Often, if you have read carefully, you can determine the meaning of such words from their context: how the word is used in the sentence or paragraph.

Some questions will require you to interpret information in a **graphic**, such as a chart, table, graph, or even a tool or instrument, such as a thermometer. Although these graphics often include numerical information, graphic questions do not really require you to perform complex mathematical equations. They will merely test your comprehension and interpretive skills as any traditional reading passage would. Graphics do not appear on every health occupations entrance exam, but it is still valuable to become familiar with them since many of the texts you will read as a student will feature graphics.

Because most of the texts you will read as a health occupations student and professional are scientific in nature, you are most likely to find fact or detail and vocabulary questions on your entrance exam. However, not all scientific texts are filled with only objective facts, and because analysis and interpretation are important parts of the scientific process, you will find main idea and inference questions on the tests as well.

The following is a sample test passage, accompanied by five sample questions. Read the passage carefully, and then answer the questions by circling your choices. Note under your answer which type of question was asked (fact or detail, main idea, inference, graphic, or vocabulary). Correct answers are given immediately after the questions.

Practice Passage 1:
Using the Five Question Types

The immune system, which protects the body from infections, diseases, and other injuries, is composed of the lymphatic system and the skin. The lymphatic system includes the lymph nodes, which measure about one to 25 centimeters across, and small vessels called lymphatics. The nodes are located in the groin, armpits, throat, and trunk, and are connected by the lymphatics. The nodes work with the rest of the body's immune system to fight off infectious agents like bacteria and fungus. When infected, lymph nodes are often swollen and sensitive. The skin, the largest organ of the human body, is also part of the immune system. Hundreds of small nerves in the skin send messages to the brain, communicating pressure, pain, and other sensations. The skin surrounds the body's organs to prevent injuries and forms a protective barrier that repels dirt and water and stops the entry of most harmful chemicals. Sweat glands in the skin help regulate the body's temperature, and other glands release oils that can kill or impede the growth of certain bacteria. Hair follicles in the skin also provide protection, especially for the skull and groin.

1. Lymph nodes are connected by
   a. blood vessels.
   b. smaller nodes.
   c. nerves.
   d. small vessels.
   Question type: _____

2. According to the passage, pain in the lymph nodes most likely indicates that the
   a. skin is dirty or saturated with water.
   b. nodes are battling an infection.
   c. brain is not responding properly to infection.
   d. lymphatics are not properly connected to the nodes.
   Question type: _____

3. Which of the following best expresses the main idea of the passage?
   a. The immune system is very sensitive and registers minute sensations.
   b. The skin and its glands are responsible for preventing most infections.
   c. The lymphatic system and the skin work together to protect the body from infection.
   d. Communication between the lymphatic system and the brain is essential in preventing and fighting infection.
   Question type: _____

4. As used in this passage, the word *compose* most nearly means
   a. create
   b. arrange
   c. control
   d. constitute
   Question type: _____

**Thermometer Reading of Patient
with Lowered Immune System**

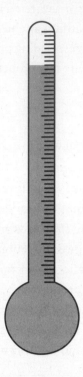

5. On the thermometer above, what is the current
temperature in degrees Fahrenheit?
a. 104 degrees
b. 102 degrees
c. −104 degrees
d. −102 degrees

Answers and Explanations for Practice Passage 1

Don't just look at the correct answers and move on.
The explanations are the most important part, so
read them carefully. Use these explanations to help
you understand how to tackle each kind of question
the next time you come across it.

1. d. Question type: fact or detail. The third
sentence of the passage says that the nodes
are connected by the lymphatics, which are
defined in the second sentence as *small
vessels.* You may know that nerves and blood
vessels make a web of connections in our
bodies, but the passage specifically states
that lymphatics—*small* vessels, not *blood*
vessels—connect the nodes.

2. b. Question type: inference. The passage says
that when lymph nodes are infected, they
are *often swollen and sensitive.* Thus, if nodes
are painful, they are probably swollen and
sensitive, and they are swollen and sensitive
because they are fighting an infection. This
is also the best answer because none of the
other answers are clearly connected to pain
in the lymph nodes. Dirty or saturated skin
(choice **a**) may indeed result in infection,
but that is not what the question is asking.
Choices **c** and **d** describe malfunctions of
the immune system, a subject that is not
discussed in the passage.

3. c. Question type: main idea. The idea that the
lymphatic system and the skin work together
to protect the body from infection is the
only answer that can serve as a "net" for the
whole passage. The other three answers are
limited to specific aspects of the immune
system and therefore are too restrictive to be
the main idea. For example, choice **b** refers
only to the skin, so it does not encompass
all of the ideas in the passage.

4. d. Question type: vocabulary. Although all of the answers can mean *compose* in certain circumstances, choice **d** is the only meaning that really works in the context of the passage, which says that the lymph nodes and the lymphatics *compose* the lymphatic system. The passage makes it clear that the lymph nodes and the lymphatics are the two parts of the lymphatic system. Thus, they *constitute* the lymphatic system. They don't create it, arrange it, or control it; they are it.

5. a. Question type: graphic. Like many graphic questions you will encounter on the health occupations exam, this one is basically independent of the passage and requires nothing more than interpreting its information correctly. The key to interpreting this thermometer correctly is recognizing that every degree is not represented on the thermometer; there are only lines for every other degree. Therefore, choice **a** is the correct answer. Selecting choice **b** indicates a failure to comprehend this pattern. Choices **c** and **d** cannot be correct since the numbers on the thermometer rise; they do not descend.

Detail, Main Idea, and Graphic Questions

Detail or fact questions and main idea questions both ask you for information that is right there in the passage. All you have to do is find it. The same is generally true of graphic questions, which most often require you to find and identify information displayed explicitly on images.

Detail or Fact Questions

Detail or fact questions are usually the simplest kinds of questions: You're asked to identify a specific item of information from the text. You just have to be able to separate important information from less important information. However, the choices may often be very similar, so you must be careful not to get confused.

Be sure you read the passage and questions carefully. In fact, it is usually a good idea to read the questions first, *before* you even read the passage, so you will know what details to look out for.

Main Idea Questions

The main idea of a passage, like that of a paragraph or a book, is what it is *mostly* about. The main idea is like an umbrella that covers all of the ideas and details in the passage, so it is usually something general, not specific. For example, in Practice Passage 1, question 3 asked about the main idea, and the correct answer was the only one that included both the skin and the lymphatic system, both of which were discussed in the passage.

Sometimes, the main idea is stated clearly, often in the first or last sentence of the passage. The main idea is expressed in the first sentence of Practice Passage 1, for example. The sentence that expresses the main idea is often referred to as the **topic sentence**.

At other times, the main idea is not stated in a topic sentence but is *implied* in the overall passage, and you will need to determine the main idea by inference. Because there may be much information in the passage, the trick is to understand what all that information adds up to—the gist of what the author wants you to know. Often, some of the wrong answers on main idea questions are specific facts or details from the passage. A good way to test yourself is to ask, "Can this answer serve as a *net* to hold the whole passage together?" If not, chances are you have chosen a fact or detail, not a main idea.

Practice answering main idea and detail questions by working on the questions that follow this passage. Circle the answers to the questions, and then check your answers against the key that appears immediately after the questions.

Graphic Questions

Graphic questions are only unique in presentation. In essence, they're a lot like detail questions. Basically, you will be presented with an image of a table, chart, graph, or even a machine or instrument with some form of readout, and simply have to locate the information the question requires you to find. Very often, these graphics will have little direct relationship with the reading passage, and they are exclusive to the TEAS. So if you plan to take the HOAE, you will not have to worry about graphic questions at all.

Like any reading comprehension question, reading carefully is the key. For example, if you did not recognize that the thermometer in Practice Passage 1, question 5 only had lines representing even numbers, you may have selected the wrong answer choice. Since graphics often contain numerical information, they may require you to perform equations, but remember that this is not the math section of the health occupations exam. These equations will be extremely basic.

Practice Passage 2: Detail, Main Idea, and Graphic Questions

Because the body responds differently to different allergens, allergic reactions have been divided into four categories. Type I allergies, the most common, are characterized by the production of immunoglobulin E (IgE), a type of antibody the immune system releases when it thinks a substance is a threat to the body. IgE releases chemicals called mediators, like histamine, which cause blood vessels to dilate and release fluid into the surrounding tissues, usually resulting in a runny nose and sneezing. Type I allergies include allergic asthma and hay fever as well as reactions to insect stings and dust. Type II allergies, far more rare, are usually reactions to medications and can cause liver and kidney damage or anemia. The body sends immunoglobulin M (IgM) and immunoglobulin G (IgG) to the site to fight the infection.

Type III allergies are usually caused by reactions to drugs like penicillin. The body releases IgM and IgG, but these allergens cause IgM and IgG to bind away from cell surfaces. This creates clumps of allergens and antibodies that get caught in the tissues and cause swelling, which can affect the kidneys, joints, and skin. Type IV allergies cause the release of mediators that create swelling as well as itchy rashes. These are usually skin reactions to irritants like poison ivy, soaps, cosmetics, and other contact allergens.

1. Which type(s) of allergic reactions result(s) in swelling?
   a. Types I and III
   b. Types III and IV
   c. Type III only
   d. Types II and IV

2. IgE, IgG, and IgM can be classified as
   a. allergens.
   b. mediators.
   c. antibodies.
   d. medications.

3. Which of the following best expresses the main idea of the passage?
   a. Allergies cause different responses in the body.
   b. People should avoid things that may cause allergic reactions.
   c. Type I allergies affect the most people.
   d. Mediators play an important role in allergic reactions.

ALLERGEN CALENDAR	
ALLERGEN	ACTIVE PERIODS
Fungal Spores	All Year
Grasses	September–February
Trees	All Year
Weeds	October–March

4. If a patient takes Telfast 60mg to relieve weed allergies, when would she most likely have to take it?

    a. April

    b. July

    c. September

    d. January

Answers and Explanations for Practice Passage 2

1. b. The passage says that both Type III and Type IV allergic reactions cause swelling. In Type III allergies, IgM and IgG *bind away from cell surfaces. This creates clumps of allergens and antibodies that . . . cause swelling.* Type IV allergies also *cause the release of mediators that create swelling as well as itchy rashes.*

2. c. The passage says that immunoglobulin E (IgE) is *a type of antibody the immune system releases.* The Ig in IgE, IgG, and IgM stands for immunoglobulin; all three are different types of immunoglobulin and therefore different types of antibodies. The immunoglobulins then release the mediators, like histamine, so choice **b** is incorrect. Further, immunoglobulins are produced in response to allergens, so choice **a** cannot be correct. And the passage clearly indicates that immunoglobulins are produced by the body, so choice **d** is also incorrect.

3. a. This choice best expresses the main idea of the passage because it restates the topic sentence, which tells us the body *responds differently* to different allergens. Choice **b** is not a good answer because the passage does not discuss ways to avoid allergic reactions, and although choices **c** and **d** are mentioned in the passage, they are too specific to encompass the whole passage. Remember, the main idea should be general enough to include all of the ideas in the passage.

4. d. According to the calendar, weed allergies are most active from October through March, and choice **d** is the only answer representing a month that falls within this time period. A failure to read the entire calendar may have led to the assumption that fungal spores or grasses are kinds of weeds, resulting in the incorrect selection of one of the other answer choices.

Inference and Vocabulary Questions

Questions that ask you about the meaning of vocabulary words in the passage and those that ask what the passage *suggests* or *implies* (inference questions) are different from detail or main idea questions. In vocabulary and inference questions, you usually have to pull ideas from the passage, sometimes from more than one place in the passage.

Inference Questions

Inference questions can be the most difficult to answer because they require you to draw meaning from the text when that meaning is implied rather than directly stated. Inferences are conclusions that we draw based on the clues the writer has given us. When you draw inferences, you have to be something of a detective, looking for clues such as word choice, tone, and specific details that suggest a certain conclusion, attitude, or point of view. You have to read between the lines in order to make a judgment about what an author was implying in the passage.

    A good way to test whether you have drawn an acceptable inference is to ask, "What evidence do I have for this inference?" If you can't find any, you probably have the wrong answer. You need to be sure that your inference is logical and that it is based on something that is suggested or implied in the passage itself—not by what you or others might think. Like a good detective, you need to base your conclusions on evidence—facts, details, and other information—not on random hunches or guesses.

Vocabulary Questions

There are generally two types of vocabulary questions. The first tests to see how carefully you have read a passage that may contain a number of new or technical terms and definitions. If you see that a passage has a number of unfamiliar terms, mark each term as it is defined. This will make it easier for you to go back and find the right answer.

The second type of vocabulary question is designed to measure how well you can figure out the meaning of a word from its context. *Context* refers to how the word is used in the sentence—how it works with the words and ideas that surround it. If the context is clear enough, you should be able to substitute a nonsense word for the one being sought, and you would still make the right choice because you could determine meaning strictly from the sense of the sentence. For example, you should be able to determine the meaning of the following italicized nonsense word based on its context:

> The speaker noted that it gave him great *terivinix* to announce the winner of the Outstanding Leadership Award.

In this sentence, *terivinix* most likely means
- **a.** pain.
- **b.** sympathy.
- **c.** pleasure.
- **d.** anxiety.

Clearly, the context of an award makes choice **c,** *pleasure,* the best answer. Awards don't usually bring pain, sympathy, or anxiety.

When confronted with an unfamiliar word, try substituting a nonsense word and see if the context gives you the clue. If you are familiar with prefixes, suffixes, and word roots, you can also use this knowledge to help you determine the meaning of an unfamiliar word.

More often, however, you will be asked about how familiar words or phrases are used in context. These questions can be very tricky because words often have more than one acceptable meaning. Your job is to figure out which meaning makes the most sense in the context of the sentence. For example, the word *manipulate* can mean either (**a**) *to handle* or *manage skillfully* or (**b**) *to arrange* or *influence cleverly or craftily.* The meaning of this word depends entirely upon the context in which it is used, as you can see from the following sentences.

> **a.** The patient *manipulated* the wheelchair around the obstacles.
> **b.** The media's *manipulation* of the facts has a powerful effect on politics.

Sentence **a** uses the first definition of the word, while sentence **b** uses the second.

When you are confronted with this type of question, your best bet is to take each possible answer and substitute it for the word in question in the sentence. Whichever answer makes the most sense in the context of the sentence should be the correct answer.

The questions that follow this passage are strictly vocabulary and inference questions. Circle the answers to the questions, and then check your answers against the key that appears immediately after the questions.

Practice Passage 3: Inference and Vocabulary Questions

The rise of science in the seventeenth century ushered in the modern world. Four men are primarily responsible for the discoveries that form the foundation of scientific and philosophical thought today: Copernicus, Kepler, Galileo, and Newton. Copernicus overthrew the geocentric notion of the universe which held that Earth—and therefore humanity—was at the center of the universe and showed that the planets revolve around the Sun. Kepler, the first major astronomer to adopt Copernicus's heliocentric theory, discovered three laws of planetary motion that helped validate Copernicus's theory. Galileo revealed the role of acceleration in dynamics and established the law of falling bodies. Finally, Newton's studies of motion—made possible only by the work of these three scientists—led to his laws of motion and the universal law of gravitation: "Every body attracts every other body with a force directly proportional to the product of their masses and inversely proportional to the square of the distance between them." It is these theories upon which much of modern science is based.

1. As it is used in the passage, the word *adopt* most nearly means to
   a. use
   b. accept
   c. change
   d. take

2. From the passage, which of the following can be inferred about Copernicus's heliocentric theory?
   a. It supported the religious doctrine of the time.
   b. It was accepted only because of Kepler.
   c. It went against established ideas.
   d. It revealed the laws of planetary motion.

3. Information contained in the passage supports which of the following statements about the four scientists?
   a. Their scientific discoveries contributed to the philosophical and social turmoil of the seventeenth century.
   b. Of the four, Newton's theories have been most instrumental in modern science.
   c. Their primary goal was to refute the theory that Earth was the center of the universe.
   d. They recognized that their achievements were based on the achievements of those before them.

4. As it is used in the passage, the word *established* most nearly means
   a. ordained
   b. set up legally
   c. settled
   d. secured

Answers and Explanations for Practice Passage 3

1. **b.** Look at how *adopt* is used in the sentence: *Kepler, the first major astronomer to* adopt *Copernicus's heliocentric theory, discovered three laws of planetary motion that helped validate Copernicus's theory.* Because Kepler helped validate this theory, choice **a** can't be correct, and neither can choice **d**; the passage clearly indicates that it's Copernicus's theory, not Kepler's. Furthermore, there's no indication from the context that Kepler changed the theory to make it suitable for another situation, so choice **c** cannot be correct either.

2. **c.** We can infer that Copernicus's theory went against established ideas because the passage says that Copernicus *overthrew* the notion that humanity was at the center of the universe, suggesting that the geocentric theory was the accepted theory of the time and that Copernicus's idea was revolutionary. There is no suggestion in the passage that Copernicus's theory supported the religious doctrine of the time, so choice **a** cannot be correct. Furthermore, the passage says that Kepler's discovery *helped* validate Copernicus's theory, but this does not imply that it was accepted only because of Kepler (choice **b**). Finally, the laws of planetary motion were discovered by Kepler, not Copernicus, so choice **d** cannot be correct.

3. a. The passage discusses scientific discoveries that challenged and changed the way human beings saw themselves in the universe and how the motion of bodies on Earth and in the universe was understood. We can thus infer that these discoveries greatly altered ideas in both philosophy and, of course, in science. Again, the word *overthrew* suggests upheaval, so choice **a** is the best answer. Choice **b** cannot be correct because the passage does not favor one scientist over the others; in fact, the passage tells us that Newton could not have done his work without those who came before him. Furthermore, although these scientists did refute the theory that Earth was the center of the universe, there's no indication in this passage that that was what they were out to prove, as in choice **c**. Finally, while the *writer* of the passage recognizes that the achievements of these scientists were based only on the achievements of the others before them, there is no indication here of what they themselves thought, so choice **d** cannot be correct.

4. d. If you insert the possible answers into the sentence, it should be clear that choice **d** makes the most sense in the context of the sentence. Galileo *"established* the law of falling bodies"—a law of gravity and motion in the universe—so he could not have instituted these laws by law or agreement (choice **a**), set them up or brought them into existence (choice **b**), or settled them in a place or position (choice **c**). Instead, he introduced them and secured acceptance of them by revealing the role of acceleration in dynamics (choice **d**).

If English Is Not Your First Language

Non-native speakers of English may have difficulties with some questions on reading comprehension tests. People who live in and are educated in the United States are familiar with idioms and other word usage from reading American newspapers, magazines, and textbooks. Such idioms and colloquial expressions may not be immediately clear to non-native speakers.

A second problem for non-native English speakers is difficulty in recognizing vocabulary and idioms (expressions like "chewing the fat") that assist comprehension. In order to read with good understanding, it's important to have an immediate grasp of as many words as possible in the text. Test takers need to be able to recognize vocabulary and idioms immediately so that the ideas those words express are clear.

The Long View

Read newspapers, magazines, and other periodicals that deal with current events and matters of local, state, and national importance. Pay special attention to articles related to the career you want to pursue.

Be alert to new or unfamiliar vocabulary or terms that occur frequently in the popular press. Use a highlighter pen to mark new or unfamiliar words as you read. Keep a list of those words and their definitions. Review them every day. At first, you may have to look up a lot of words, but before long you'll be looking up fewer and fewer as your vocabulary expands.

During the Test

When you are taking the test, make a picture in your mind of the situation being described in the passage. Ask yourself, "What did the writer mostly want me to think about this subject?"

Locate and underline the topic sentence that carries the main idea of the passage. Remember that the topic sentence—if there is one—may not always be the first sentence. If there doesn't seem to be one, try to determine what idea summarizes the whole passage.

Review: Putting It All Together

A good way to solidify what you have learned about reading comprehension questions is for *you* to write the questions. Here is a passage, followed by space for you to write your own questions. Write one question for each of the five types: fact or detail, main idea, inference, vocabulary, and graphic.

In the years since it was first proposed, the free radical theory of aging has gained wide acceptance. But hypotheses that attempt to explain exactly how free radicals are involved in the aging process are troubled by the lack of a clear definition of aging. Is aging a programmed stage of cellular differentiation, or is it the result of physiological processes impaired by free radical or other damage to cells? Despite the want of a clear definition, few question that free radical damage to cell nucleic acids and lipids are an important factor in aging. A recent study shows that oxygen-free radicals cause approximately 10,000 DNA base modifications per cell per day. Perhaps the accumulation of unrepaired damage of this type accounts for the deterioration of physiological function. A new theory, however, indicates that free radicals also damage cell proteins and that the accumulation of oxidized protein is an important factor in aging.

1. Detail question:_____

_____

a.

b.

c.

d.

2. Main idea question:_____

_____

a.

b.

c.

d.

3. Inference question:_____

_____

a.

b.

c.

d.

4. Vocabulary question:_____

_____

a.

b.

c.

d.

5. Graphic question:_____

_____

a.

b.

c.

d.

POTENTIAL RESULTS OF FREE RADICAL DAMAGE
Asthma
Arthritis
Atherosclerosis
Cataractogenesis
Dermatitis
Cancer
Periodontis
Retinal damage
Stroke
Heart Attack

Possible Questions

Here is one question of each type based on the previous passage. Your questions may be very different, but these will give you an idea of the kinds of questions that could be asked.

1. **Detail:** DNA modification can occur
   a. 10,000 times in the life of a cell.
   b. 1,000 times every second.
   c. thousands of times a day.
   d. once a day.

2. **Main idea:** Which sentence best sums up this passage?
   a. There are many theories, but no one knows how free radicals really affect aging.
   b. Free radicals are deadly.
   c. Scientists need a clearer definition of aging.
   d. Free radicals will lead scientists to the fountain of youth.

3. **Inference:** The passage suggests which of the following about the aging process?
   a. A clear definition of aging must be found in order to determine the cause of aging.
   b. DNA controls the aging process.
   c. Free radical damage to proteins increases with aging.
   d. Aging is somehow related to free radical damage to cells.

4. **Vocabulary:** The phrase *want of* as used in the fourth sentence most nearly means
   a. desire for.
   b. lack of.
   c. requirement of.
   d. falling short of.

5. Which of the following is true based on the table?
   a. Free radicals are the most common cause of heart attacks.
   b. Free radicals can be suppressed with chemotherapy.
   c. Free radicals have the potential to cause organ damage.
   d. Free radical damage is consistently fatal.

Answers

1. c.
2. a.
3. d.
4. b.

Additional Resources

Here are some other ways you can build the vocabulary and knowledge that will help you do well on reading comprehension questions.

- Practice asking the four sample question types about passages you read for information or pleasure.
- If you have Internet access, search out articles and forums related to the career you would like to pursue. Exchange views with others online. All of these exchanges will help expand your knowledge of job-related material that may appear in a passage on the test.
- Begin now to build a broad knowledge of your potential profession. Get in the habit of reading articles in newspapers and magazines on job-related issues. Keep a clipping file of those articles. This will help keep you informed of trends in the profession and familiarize you with pertinent vocabulary.
- Consider reading or subscribing to professional journals. They are usually available for a reasonable annual fee. They may also be available in your library.

6 ▶ MATH REVIEW

CHAPTER SUMMARY

This chapter gives you important tips for dealing with math questions on your health occupations entrance exam and reviews some of the most commonly tested concepts. If you have forgotten some of your high school math or have math anxiety, this chapter is for you.

The math section covers concepts that you probably studied in high school, with an emphasis on arithmetic, algebra, and geometry, often using word problems. Health professionals need to be comfortable with numbers and be able to perform accurate mathematical computations quickly. Your ability to learn the scientific concepts that form the foundation of your work, as well as your on-the-job performance, will depend on your ability to reason logically using numbers.

For an entrance exam to the educational program of your choice, not only do you need to know how to work with whole numbers, but it is even more important that you are comfortable with and proficient at performing operations with fractions and decimals. You will have to be able to figure percentages, solve algebraic equations, and work with geometric figures. The tests assume that you know some basic terminology—words such as sum and perimeter—and some basic formulas, such as the area of a square or circle. Some admissions tests have a separate analytical reasoning section that measures your ability to recognize relationships between shapes or objects through visualization. This chapter will also prepare you for these types of questions.

Here are some terms that you must know in order to be successful on your exam. Review them and make sure you are familiar with all of these concepts before continuing on to the different math strategies that are discussed next.

Before you review those concepts, however, take a look at some strategies you can use to help you answer multiple-choice math questions.

GLOSSARY OF TERMS

Area	the space within a two-dimensional shape, which is measured in units squared (ft.^{2}, in.^{2}).
Denominator	the bottom number in a fraction. *Example*: 2 is the denominator in $\frac{1}{2}$.
Difference	The difference of two numbers is the result of subtracting one number from the other.
Divisible by	a number is divisible by a second number if that second number divides evenly into the original number. *Example*: 10 is divisible by 5 (10 ÷ 5 = 2, with no remainder). However, 10 is not divisible by 3. (See *multiple of*)
Even Integer	integer that is divisible by 2, like . . . –4, –2, 0, 2, 4, . . . (See *integer*)
Integer	a number that is not a fraction. It can be positive, negative, or zero. Integers include the whole numbers and their opposites. (See *whole number*)
Multiple of	a number is a multiple of a second number if that second number can be multiplied by an integer to get the original number. *Example*: 10 is a multiple of 5 (10 = 5 × 2); however, 10 is not a multiple of 3. (See *divisible by*)
Negative Number	a number that is less than zero, like . . . –1, –18.6, $-\frac{3}{4}$, . . .
Numerator	the top part of a fraction. *Example*: 1 is the numerator of $\frac{1}{2}$.
Odd Integer	an integer that is not divisible by 2, like . . . –5, –3, –1, 1, 3, . . .
Perimeter	the distance around the outside of a one-dimensional shape.
Positive Number	a number that is greater than zero, like . . . 2, 42, $\frac{1}{2}$, 4.63, . . .
Prime Number	an integer larger than 1 that is divisible only by 1 and itself, like . . . 2, 3, 5, 7, 11, . . . (1 is not a prime number)
Product	The product of two numbers is the result of multiplying two numbers together.
Quotient	the answer you get when you divide. *Example*: 10 divided by 5 is 2; the quotient is 2.
Real Number	any number you can think of, like . . . 17, –5, $\frac{1}{2}$, –23.6, 3.4329, 0, . . . Real numbers include the integers, fractions, and decimals. (See *integer*)
Remainder	the number left over after division. *Example*: 11 divided by 2 is 5, with a remainder of 1.
Sum	The sum of two numbers is the result of adding the numbers together.
Volume	the three-dimensional space that is held within a three-dimensional object, which is measured in units cubed (ft.^{3}, in.^{3}).
Whole Number	All positive counting numbers, like . . . 1, 2, 3, . . . (not including fractions or decimals).

Math Strategies

- **Don't work in your head! Use your test book or scratch paper to take notes, draw pictures, and calculate.** Although you might think that you can solve math questions more quickly in your head, that's a good way to make mistakes. Write out each step.

- **Read a math question in *chunks* rather than straight through from beginning to end.** As you read each chunk, stop to think about what it means and make notes or draw a picture to represent that chunk.

- **When you get to the actual question, circle it.** This will keep you more focused as you solve the problem.

- **Glance at the answer choices for clues.** If they're fractions, you probably should do your work in fractions; if they're decimals, you should probably work in decimals.
- **Make a plan of attack to help you solve the problem.**
- **If a question stumps you, try one of the backdoor approaches explained in the next section.** These are particularly useful for solving word problems.
- **When you get your answer, reread the circled question to make sure you've answered it.** This helps avoid the careless mistake of answering the wrong question.
- **Check your work after you get an answer.** Test takers get a false sense of security when they get an answer that matches one of the multiple-choice answers. Here are some good ways to check your work *if you have time*:
  - Ask yourself if your answer is reasonable, if it makes sense.
  - Plug your answer back into the problem to make sure the problem holds together.
  - Do the question a second time, but use a different method.
- **Approximate when appropriate.** For example:
  - $5.98 + $8.97 is a little less than $15. (Add: $6 + $9)
  - 0.9876 × 5.0342 is close to 5. (Multiply: 1 × 5)
- **Skip hard questions and come back to them later.** Mark them in your test book so you can find them quickly.

Backdoor Approaches for Answering Questions That Puzzle You

Remember those word problems you dreaded in high school? Many of them are actually easier to solve by backdoor approaches. The two techniques that follow are terrific ways to solve multiple-choice word problems that you don't know how to solve with a straightforward approach. The first technique, *nice numbers*, is useful when there are unknowns (like *x*) in the text of the word problem, making the problem too abstract for you. The second technique, *working backward*, presents a quick way to substitute numeric answer choices back into the problem to see which one works.

Nice Numbers

1. When a question contains unknowns, like *x*, plug nice numbers in for the unknowns. A nice number is easy to calculate with and makes sense in the problem.
2. Read the question with the nice numbers in place. Then solve it.
3. If the answer choices are all numbers, the choice that matches your answer is the right one.
4. If the answer choices contain unknowns, substitute the same nice numbers into **all** the answer choices. The choice that matches your answer is the right one. If more than one answer matches, do the problem again with different nice numbers. You'll only have to check the answer choices that have already matched.

Example:

Judi went shopping with *p* dollars in her pocket. If the price of shirts was *s* shirts for *d* dollars, what is the maximum number of shirts Judi could buy with the money in her pocket?

a. *psd*

b. $\frac{ps}{d}$

c. $\frac{pd}{s}$

d. $\frac{ds}{p}$

To solve this problem, let's try these nice numbers: $p = \$100$, $s = 2$; $d = \$25$. Now reread it with the numbers in place:

Judi went shopping with **$100** in her pocket. If the price of shirts was **2** shirts for **$25**, what is the maximum number of shirts Judi could buy with the money in her pocket?

Since 2 shirts cost $25, that means that 4 shirts cost $50, and 8 shirts cost $100. So our answer is 8. Let's substitute the nice numbers into all four answers:

    a. $100 \times 2 \times 25 = 5,000$

    b. $\frac{100 \times 2}{25} = 8$

    c. $\frac{100 \times 25}{2} = 1,250$

    d. $\frac{25 \times 2}{100} = \frac{1}{2}$

The correct answer is choice **b** because it is the only one that matches our answer of **8**.

Working Backward

You can frequently solve a word problem by substituting the answer choices back into the text of the problem to see which one fits all the facts stated in the problem. The process is faster than you think because you'll probably only have to substitute one or two answers to find the right one.

This approach works only when:

- All of the answer choices are numbers.
- You're asked to find a simple number, not a sum, product, difference, or ratio.

Here's what to do:

1. Look at all the answer choices and begin with a choice that is in the middle of the range of answers. For example, if the answers are 14, 8, 2, and 20, begin by substituting either 8 or 14 into the problem since they are the two middle choices when listed in numerical order: 2, 8, 14, 20.
2. If your choice doesn't work, eliminate it. If your answer needs to be bigger, then select a bigger answer choice to try next. If your answer needs to be smaller, try a smaller choice next. (This is the benefit of having started with one of the middle numbers!)

3. Substitute in one of the remaining choices.
4. If none of the answers works, you may have made a careless error. Begin again or look for your mistake.

Example:

Juan ate $\frac{1}{3}$ of the jelly beans. Maria then ate $\frac{3}{4}$ of the remaining jelly beans, which left 10 jelly beans. How many jelly beans were there to begin with?
a. 60 jelly beans
b. 80 jelly beans
c. 90 jelly beans
d. 120 jelly beans

Starting with one of the middle answers, let's assume there were 90 jelly beans to begin with:

Since Juan ate $\frac{1}{3}$ of them, that means he ate 30 ($\frac{1}{3} \times 90 = 30$), leaving 60 of them ($90 - 30 = 60$). Maria then ate $\frac{3}{4}$ of the 60 jelly beans, or 45 of them ($\frac{3}{4} \times 60 = 45$). That leaves 15 jelly beans ($60 - 45 = 15$).

The problem states that there were **10** jelly beans left, and we wound up with **15** of them. That indicates that we started with too big a number, so that means that 120 could not be correct, either. With only two choices of 80 or 60 left, let's use common sense to decide which one to try next. Since 80 is only a little smaller than 90 and may not be small enough, let's try 60:

Since Juan ate $\frac{1}{3}$ of them, that means he ate 20 ($\frac{1}{3} \times 60 = 20$), leaving 40 of them ($60 - 20 = 40$). Maria then ate $\frac{3}{4}$ of the 40 jelly beans, or 30 of them ($\frac{3}{4} \times 40 = 30$). That leaves 10 jelly beans ($40 - 30 = 10$).

Because this result of 10 jelly beans left agrees with the problem, the correct answer is choice **a**.

Word Problems

Many of the math problems on tests are word problems. A word problem can include any kind of math, including simple arithmetic, fractions, decimals, percentages, even algebra and geometry.

The hardest part of any word problem is translating English into math. When you read a problem, you can frequently translate it *word for word* from English statements into mathematical statements. At other times, however, a key word in the word problem hints at the mathematical operation to be performed. Here are the translation rules:

EQUALS key words: is, are, has

English	Math
Bob **is** 18 years old.	$b = 18$
There **are** 7 hats.	$h = 7$
Judi **has** 5 books.	$j = 5$

ADDITION key words: sum; more, greater, or older than; total; altogether

English	Math
The **sum** of two numbers is 10.	$x + y = 10$
Karen has $5 **more than** Sam.	$k = 5 + s$
The base is 3" **greater than** the height.	$b = 3 + h$
Judi is 2 years **older than** Tony.	$j = 2 + t$
The **total** of three numbers is 25.	$a + b + c = 25$
How much do Joan and Tom have **altogether**?	$j + t = ?$

SUBTRACTION key words: difference; fewer, less, or younger than; remain; left over (WARNING! Often with subtraction key words like *less than* or *younger than*, you will need to switch the order of the information presented. Notice this in the following examples!)

English	Math
The **difference** between two numbers is 17.	$x - y = 17$
Mike has 5 **fewer** cats **than** twice the number Jan has.	$m = 2j - 5$
Jay is 2 years **younger than** Brett.	$j = b - 2$
After Carol ate 3 apples, r apples **remained**.	$r = a - 3$

MULTIPLICATION key words: of, product, times, each

English	Math
20% **of** the samples	$0.20 \times s$
Half **of** the bacteria	$\frac{1}{2} \times b$
The **product** of two numbers is 12.	$a \times b = 12$

DIVISION key word: per, over

English	Math
15 drops **per** teaspoon	$\frac{15 \text{ drops}}{\text{teaspoon}}$
22 miles **per** gallon	$\frac{22 \text{ miles}}{\text{gallon}}$
60 pills **over** 30 days	$\frac{60 \text{ pills}}{30 \text{ days}}$

Distance Formula:
Distance = Rate × Time

The key words are movement words like *distance*, *speed*, *rate*, *how fast*, *how far*, *how long*, *miles per hour*.

In order to solve problems that involve distance, rate, and time, follow these three steps:

1. Write the formula "Distance = rate × time."
2. Fill in the information that is given where appropriate.
3. Solve for the missing piece of information using division or multiplication.

- **How far** did the plane travel in 4 hours if it averaged 300 miles per hour?

  $D = R \times T$

  $D = 300 \times 4$

  $D = 1,200$ miles

- Ben walked 20 miles in 4 hours. What was his average **speed**?

  $D = R \times T$

  $20 = r \times 4$

  5 miles per hour $= r$

Solving a Word Problem Using Translation

Remember the problem at the beginning of this chapter about the jelly beans?

> Juan ate $\frac{1}{3}$ of the jelly beans. Maria then ate $\frac{3}{4}$ of the remaining jelly beans, which left 10 jelly beans. How many jelly beans were there to begin with?
>
> **a.** 60 jelly beans
> **b.** 80 jelly beans
> **c.** 90 jelly beans
> **d.** 120 jelly beans

We solved it by *working backward*. Now let's solve it using our translation rules.

Assume Juan started with J jelly beans. If Juan ate $\frac{1}{3}$ **of** them, that means there were $\frac{2}{3}$ of them left, or $\frac{2}{3} \times J$ jelly beans. Maria then ate $\frac{3}{4}$, leaving $\frac{1}{4}$ **of** the $\frac{2}{3} \times J$ jelly beans, or $\frac{1}{4} \times \frac{2}{3} \times J$ jelly beans. Multiplying out $\frac{1}{4} \times \frac{2}{3} \times J$ gives $\frac{1}{6}J$ as the number of jelly beans left. The problem states that there were 10 jelly beans left, meaning that we set $\frac{1}{6} \times J$ **equal** to 10:

$$\frac{1}{6} \times J = 10$$

Solving this equation for J gives $J = \mathbf{60}$. Thus, the correct answer is choice **a** (the same answer we got when we *worked backward*). As you can see, both methods—working backward and translating from English to math—work. You should use whichever method is more comfortable for you.

Practice Word Problems

You will find word problems using fractions, decimals, and percentages in those sections of this chapter. For now, practice using translation on problems that just require you to work with basic arithmetic. Answers are at the end of the chapter.

_____ **1.** Joan went shopping with $100 and returned home with only $18.42. How much money did she spend?
  a. $81.58
  b. $72.68
  c. $72.58
  d. $71.68
  e. $71.58

2. Each of five physical therapists at the therapy center works six hours per day. Each therapist can work with three patients per hour. In total, how many patients can be seen each day at the center?

   a. 18 patients

   b. 30 patients

   c. 60 patients

   d. 75 patients

   e. 90 patients

3. A speech therapist who charges $115 per hour, billed $373.75 for a session. How many hours did the therapist work?

   a. 3

   b. 3.25

   c. 2.5

   d. 3.5

   e. 4

4. Mr. Wallace is writing a budget request to upgrade his personal computer system. He wants to purchase a wireless router, which will cost $100, two new software programs at $350 each, a color printer for $249, and an additional color cartridge for $25. What is the total amount Mr. Wallace should write on his budget request?

   a. $724

   b. $974

   c. $1,049

   d. $1,064

   e. $1,074

Fraction Review

Problems involving fractions may be straightforward calculation questions, or they may be word problems.

Typically, they ask you to add, subtract, multiply, divide, or compare fractions.

Working with Fractions

A fraction is a part of something.

> **Example:**
> Let's say that a pizza was cut into 8 equal slices and you ate 3 of them. The fraction $\frac{3}{8}$ tells you what part of the pizza you ate. The following pizza shows this: 3 of the 8 pieces (the ones you ate) are shaded.

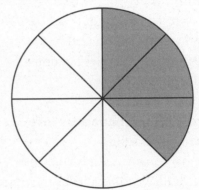

Three Kinds of Fractions

Proper fraction: The top number is less than the bottom number:
$$\frac{1}{2}, \frac{2}{3}, \frac{4}{9}, \frac{8}{13}$$
The value of a proper fraction is less than 1.

Improper fraction: The top number is greater than or equal to the bottom number:
$$\frac{3}{2}, \frac{5}{3}, \frac{14}{9}, \frac{12}{12}$$
The value of an improper fraction is 1 or more.

Mixed number: A whole number and a fraction are combined into one mixed number:
$$3\frac{1}{2}, 4\frac{2}{3}, 12\frac{3}{4}, 24\frac{3}{4}$$
The value of a mixed number is more than 1: It is the sum of the whole number plus the fraction.

Changing Improper Fractions into Mixed or Whole Numbers

It's easier to add and subtract fractions that are mixed numbers rather than improper fractions. To change an improper fraction, say $\frac{13}{2}$, into a mixed number, follow these steps:

1. Divide the bottom number (2) into the top number (13) to get the whole number portion (6) of the mixed number:

$$2\overline{)13} \quad \begin{array}{r} 6 \\ \underline{12} \\ 1 \end{array}$$

2. Write the remainder of the division (1) over the old bottom number (2): $\quad 6\frac{1}{2}$

3. Check: Change the mixed number back into an improper fraction (see steps that follow).

Changing Mixed Numbers into Improper Fractions

It is impossible to multiply and divide mixed fractions, so you have to be able to turn mixed fractions into improper fractions. To change a mixed number, say $2\frac{3}{4}$, into an improper fraction, follow these steps:

1. Multiply the whole number (2) by the bottom number (4): $\quad 2 \times 4 = 8$

2. Add the result (8) to the top number (3): $\quad 8 + 3 = 11$

3. Put the total (11) over the bottom number (4): $\quad \frac{11}{4}$

4. Check: Reverse the process by changing the improper fraction into a mixed number. If you get back the number you started with, your answer is right.

Reducing Fractions

Reducing a fraction means writing it in *lowest terms*; that is, with the smallest numbers possible. For instance, 50¢ is $\frac{50}{100}$ of a dollar, or $\frac{1}{2}$ of a dollar. Reducing a fraction does not change its value.

Follow these steps to reduce a fraction:

1. Find a whole number that divides evenly into both numbers that make up the fraction.

2. Divide that number into the top of the fraction, and replace the top of the fraction with the quotient (the answer you got when you divided).

3. Do the same thing to the bottom number.

4. Repeat steps 1–3 until you can't find a number that divides evenly into both numbers of the fraction.

For example, let's reduce $\frac{8}{24}$. We could do it in two steps $\frac{8 \div 4}{24 \div 4} = \frac{2}{6}$; then $\frac{2 \div 2}{6 \div 2} = \frac{1}{3}$. Or we could do it in a single step $\frac{8 \div 8}{24 \div 8} = \frac{1}{3}$.

Shortcut: When the top and bottom numbers both end in zeros, cross out the same number of zeros in both numbers to begin the reducing process. For example $\frac{300}{4,000}$ reduces to $\frac{3}{40}$ when you cross out two zeros in both numbers.

Whenever you do arithmetic with fractions, reduce your answer. On a multiple-choice test, don't panic if your answer isn't listed. Try to reduce it and then compare it to the choices.

Reduce these fractions to lowest terms.

_____ **5.** $\frac{3}{12}$

_____ **6.** $\frac{14}{35}$

_____ **7.** $\frac{27}{72}$

Equivalent Fractions

Sometimes you need to make **equivalent fractions** to solve problems. Equivalent fractions have the same value but are written differently. There are two ways to find equivalent fractions: dividing and multiplying. When dividing the numerator and denominator of a fraction by the same number, you are reducing the fraction.

For example, $\frac{1}{2}$ is equivalent to $\frac{4}{8}$, since $\frac{1 \times 4}{2 \times 4} = \frac{4}{8}$. Here, we multiplied both the top and bottom of the fraction $\frac{1}{2}$ by 4 to get an equivalent fraction.

Also, $\frac{12}{36}$ is equivalent to $\frac{4}{12}$, since $\frac{12 \div 3}{36 \div 3} = \frac{4}{12}$. Here, we divided both the top and bottom of the fraction $\frac{12}{36}$ by 3 to get an equivalent fraction.

Finding Equivalent Fractions Using Multiplication

You will need to use equivalent fractions in order to add and subtract fractions. This is actually the opposite of reducing a fraction.

Follow these steps to raise $\frac{2}{3}$ to 24ths:

For example, if you wanted to write $\frac{2}{3}$ as $\frac{something}{24}$, you would follow these steps:

1. First, notice what number the existing bottom number needs to be multiplied by in order to arrive at the new desired bottom number. In this case, if you multiply the bottom number, 3, by 8, then the product will be the new desired bottom number, 24. This means that you will multiply both the top and bottom numbers of your fraction by 8. *Hint:* If it's not obvious to you that 8 is the answer here, you can always divide the desired bottom number (24) by the original bottom number (3) to get your answer.
2. Multiply both the top and bottom of $\frac{2}{3}$ by 8 to get $\frac{16}{24}$.
3. Check: Reduce the new fraction to see if you get back the original one: $\frac{16 \div 8}{24 \div 8} = \frac{2}{3}$

Write these fractions as equivalent fractions with the given denominators:

_____ 8. $\frac{5}{12} = \frac{}{24}$

_____ 9. $\frac{2}{9} = \frac{}{27}$

_____ 10. $\frac{2}{5} = \frac{}{500}$

Adding Fractions

You might remember that when adding and subtracting fractions the bottom number in both fractions must be the same number. When adding and subtracting fractions, the bottom number will stay the same, and only the top numbers will be added or subtracted.

If the fractions have the same bottom numbers, just add the top numbers together and write the total over the bottom number.

Examples:

$\frac{2}{9} + \frac{4}{9} = \frac{2+4}{9} = \frac{6}{9}$ Reduce the sum: $\frac{2}{3}$.

$\frac{5}{8} + \frac{7}{8} = \frac{12}{8}$ Change the sum to a mixed number: $1\frac{4}{8}$; then reduce: $1\frac{1}{2}$.

There are a few extra steps to add mixed numbers with the same bottom numbers, say, $2\frac{3}{5} + 1\frac{4}{5}$:

1. Add the fractions: $\frac{3}{5} + \frac{4}{5} = \frac{7}{5}$
2. Change the improper fraction into a mixed number: $\frac{7}{5} = 1\frac{2}{5}$
3. Add the whole numbers: $2 + 1 = 3$
4. Add the results of steps 2 and 3: $1\frac{2}{5} + 3 = 4\frac{2}{5}$

Finding the Least Common Denominator

If the fractions you want to add don't have the same bottom number, you will have to raise some or all of the fractions to higher terms so that they all have the same bottom number, called the **common denomi-**

nator. All of the original bottom numbers divide evenly into the common denominator. If it is the smallest number that they all divide evenly into, it is called the **least common denominator (LCD).**

Here are a few tips for finding the LCD, the smallest number that all the bottom numbers evenly divide into:

- See if all the bottom numbers divide evenly into the biggest bottom number.
- Inspect multiples of the largest bottom number until you find a number that all the other bottom numbers evenly divide into.
- When all else fails, multiply all the bottom numbers together.

Example: $\frac{2}{3} + \frac{4}{5}$

1. Find the LCD. Multiply the bottom numbers: $\qquad 3 \times 5 = 15$
2. Write each fraction with a denominator of 15:

$$\frac{2}{3} = \frac{10}{15}$$
$$+ \frac{4}{5} = \frac{12}{15}$$

3. Add the top numbers together and keep the bottom number the same: $\qquad \frac{22}{15}$

Try these addition problems:

_____ **11.** $\frac{4}{5} + \frac{1}{6}$

_____ **12.** $\frac{7}{8} + \frac{2}{3} + \frac{3}{4}$

_____ **13.** $4\frac{1}{3} + 2\frac{3}{4} + \frac{1}{6}$

Subtracting Fractions

If the fractions have the same bottom numbers, just subtract the top numbers and write the difference over the bottom number.

Example: $\frac{4}{9} - \frac{3}{9} = \frac{4-3}{9} = \frac{1}{9}$

If the fractions you want to subtract don't have the same bottom number, you will have to raise some or all of the fractions to equivalent fractions so that they all have the same bottom number, or LCD. If you forgot how to find the LCD, just read the section on adding fractions with different bottom numbers.

Example: $\frac{5}{6} - \frac{3}{4}$

1. Change each fraction to equivalent fractions with denominators of 12 because 12 is the LCD, the smallest number that 6 and 4 both divide into evenly:

$$\frac{5}{6} = \frac{10}{12}$$
$$- \frac{3}{4} = \frac{9}{12}$$

2. Subtract the top numbers and keep the bottom number the same: $\qquad \frac{1}{12}$

Subtracting mixed numbers with the same bottom number is similar to adding mixed numbers.

Example: $4\frac{3}{5} - 1\frac{2}{5}$

1. Subtract the fractions: $\qquad \frac{3}{5} - \frac{2}{5} = \frac{1}{5}$
2. Subtract the whole numbers: $\qquad 4 - 1 = 3$
3. Add the results of steps 1 and 2: $\qquad \frac{1}{5} + 3 = 3\frac{1}{5}$

Sometimes, there is an extra "borrowing" step when you subtract mixed numbers with the same bottom numbers, say, $7\frac{3}{5} - 2\frac{4}{5}$:

1. You can't subtract the fractions the way they are because $\frac{4}{5}$ is bigger than $\frac{3}{5}$. So you borrow 1 from the 7, making it 6, and change that 1 to $\frac{5}{5}$ because 5 is the bottom number: $\qquad 7\frac{3}{5} = 6\frac{5}{5} + \frac{3}{5}$
2. Add the numbers from step 1: $\qquad 6\frac{5}{5} + \frac{3}{5} = 6\frac{8}{5}$
3. Now you have a different version of the original problem: $\qquad 6\frac{8}{5} - 2\frac{4}{5}$

4. Subtract the fractional parts
of the two mixed numbers: $\frac{8}{5} - \frac{4}{5} = \frac{4}{5}$

5. Subtract the whole number
parts of the two mixed numbers: $6 - 2 = 4$

6. Add the results of the last two
steps together: $4 + \frac{4}{5} = 4\frac{4}{5}$

Try these subtraction problems:

_____ **14.** $\frac{4}{5} - \frac{2}{3}$

_____ **15.** $\frac{7}{8} - \frac{1}{4} - \frac{1}{2}$

_____ **16.** $4\frac{1}{3} - 2\frac{3}{4}$

Now let's put what you have learned about adding and subtracting fractions to work in some real-life problems.

_____ **17.** Visiting nurse Alan drove $3\frac{1}{2}$ miles to the office to check his assignments for the day. Then he drove $4\frac{3}{4}$ miles to his first patient. When he left there, he drove 2 miles to his next patient. Then he drove $3\frac{2}{3}$ miles back to the office for a meeting. Finally, he drove $3\frac{1}{2}$ miles home. How many miles did he travel in total?
a. $17\frac{5}{12}$ miles
b. $16\frac{5}{12}$ miles
c. $15\frac{7}{12}$ miles
d. $15\frac{5}{12}$ miles
e. $13\frac{11}{12}$ miles

_____ **18.** Before leaving the hospital, the ambulance driver noted that the mileage gauge on Ambulance 2 registered $4{,}357\frac{4}{10}$ miles. When he arrived at the scene of the accident, the mileage gauge then registered $4{,}400\frac{1}{10}$ miles. How many miles did he drive from the hospital to the accident?
a. $42\frac{3}{10}$ miles
b. $42\frac{7}{10}$ miles
c. $43\frac{7}{10}$ miles
d. $47\frac{2}{10}$ miles

Multiplying Fractions

Multiplying fractions is actually easier than adding them. All you do is multiply the top numbers and then multiply the bottom numbers.

Examples: $\frac{2}{3} \times \frac{5}{7} = \frac{2 \times 5}{3 \times 7} = \frac{10}{21}$

$\frac{1}{2} \times \frac{3}{5} \times \frac{7}{4} = \frac{1 \times 3 \times 7}{2 \times 5 \times 4} = \frac{21}{40}$

Sometimes, you can *cancel* before multiplying. Canceling is a shortcut that makes the multiplication go faster because you're multiplying with smaller numbers. It's very similar to reducing: If there is a number that divides evenly into a top number and bottom number, do that division before multiplying. If you forget to cancel, you will still get the right answer, but you will have to reduce it.

Example: $\frac{5}{6} \times \frac{9}{20}$

1. Cancel the 6 and the 9 by dividing 3 into both of them: $6 \div 3 = 2$ and $9 \div 3 = 3$. Cross out the 6 and the 9: $\quad \frac{5}{\overset{}{\underset{2}{6}}} \times \frac{\overset{3}{9}}{20}$

2. Cancel the 5 and the 20 by dividing 5 into both of them: $5 \div 5 = 1$ and $20 \div 5 = 4$. Cross out the 5 and the 20: $\quad \frac{\overset{1}{5}}{\underset{2}{6}} \times \frac{\overset{3}{9}}{\underset{4}{20}}$

3. Multiply across the new top numbers and the new bottom numbers: $\quad \frac{1 \times 3}{2 \times 4} = \frac{3}{8}$

Try these multiplication problems:

_____ **19.** $\frac{1}{5} \times \frac{2}{3}$

_____ **20.** $\frac{2}{3} \times \frac{4}{7} \times \frac{3}{5}$

_____ **21.** $\frac{3}{4} \times \frac{8}{9}$

To multiply a fraction by a whole number, first rewrite the whole number as a fraction with a bottom number of 1.

Example: $5 \times \frac{2}{3} = \frac{5}{1} \times \frac{2}{3} = \frac{10}{3}$ (Optional: Convert $\frac{10}{3}$ to a mixed number, $3\frac{1}{3}$.)

To multiply with mixed numbers, it's easier to change them to improper fractions before multiplying.

Example: $4\frac{2}{3} \times 5\frac{1}{2}$

1. Convert $4\frac{2}{3}$ to an improper fraction: $\qquad 4\frac{2}{3} = \frac{4 \times 3 + 2}{3} = \frac{14}{3}$

2. Convert $5\frac{1}{2}$ to an improper fraction: $\qquad 5\frac{1}{2} = \frac{5 \times 2 + 1}{2} = \frac{11}{2}$

3. Cancel and multiply the fractions: $\qquad \frac{\overset{7}{\cancel{14}}}{3} \times \frac{11}{\underset{1}{\cancel{2}}} = \frac{77}{3}$

4. Optional: Convert the improper fraction to a mixed number: $\qquad \frac{77}{3} = 25\frac{2}{3}$

Now try these multiplication problems with mixed numbers and whole numbers:

_____ **22.** $4\frac{1}{3} \times \frac{2}{5}$

_____ **23.** $2\frac{1}{2} \times 6$

_____ **24.** $3\frac{3}{4} \times 4\frac{2}{5}$

Here are a few more real-life problems to test your skills:

_____ **25.** Bobby's two-year-old sister weighs $33\frac{1}{3}$ pounds. Bobby's weight is $2\frac{2}{5}$ times the weight of his sister. How much does Bobby weigh?
   a. 120 pounds
   b. 80 pounds
   c. 200 pounds
   d. 66 pounds
   e. 145 pounds

_____ **26.** If Henry spent $\frac{3}{4}$ of a 40-hour work week learning to use new laboratory equipment, how many hours did he spend in training?
   a. $7\frac{1}{2}$ hours
   b. 10 hours
   c. 20 hours
   d. 25 hours
   e. 30 hours

_____ **27.** Technician Chin makes $14.00 an hour. When she works more than 8 hours a day, she gets overtime pay of $1\frac{1}{2}$ times her regular hourly wage for the extra hours. How much did she earn for working 11 hours in one day?
   a. $77
   b. $154
   c. $175
   d. $210
   e. $231

Dividing Fractions

Dividing fractions is a lot easier than you might imagine. To divide one fraction by a second fraction, follow these three steps:

Example: $\frac{1}{2} \div \frac{3}{5}$

1. Find the *reciprocal* of the second fraction (that means flip the top and bottom numbers). $\frac{5}{3}$
2. Next, change the division sign to a multiplication sign. $\frac{1}{2} \times \frac{5}{3}$
3. Now multiply the first fraction by the reciprocal of the second fraction. $\frac{1}{2} \times \frac{5}{3} = \frac{1 \times 5}{2 \times 3} = \frac{5}{6}$

To divide a fraction by a whole number, first change the whole number to a fraction by putting it over 1. Then follow the division steps above.

Example: $\frac{3}{5} \div 2 = \frac{3}{5} \div \frac{2}{1} = \frac{3}{5} \times \frac{1}{2} = \frac{3 \times 1}{5 \times 2} = \frac{3}{10}$

When the division problem has a mixed number, convert it to an improper fraction and then divide as usual.

Example: $2\frac{3}{4} \div \frac{1}{6}$

1. Convert $2\frac{3}{4}$ to an improper fraction: $2\frac{3}{4} = \frac{2 \times 4 + 3}{4} = \frac{11}{4}$
2. Divide $\frac{11}{4}$ by $\frac{1}{6}$: $\frac{11}{4} \div \frac{1}{6} = \frac{11}{4} \times \frac{6}{1}$
3. Flip $\frac{1}{6}$ to $\frac{6}{1}$, change ÷ to ×, cancel, and multiply: $\frac{11}{\underset{2}{4}} \times \frac{\overset{3}{6}}{1} = \frac{11 \times 3}{2 \times 1} = \frac{33}{2}$

Here are a few division problems to try.

_____ **28.** $\frac{1}{3} \div \frac{2}{3}$

_____ **29.** $2\frac{3}{4} \div \frac{1}{2}$

_____ **30.** $\frac{3}{5} \div 3$

_____ **31.** $4\frac{5}{6} \div 7\frac{2}{3}$

Let's wrap this up with some real-life problems.

_____ **32.** Annika uses $140\frac{1}{4}$ ounces of flour to bake loaves of cinnamon bread for a hospital fund-raiser. Each loaf takes $12\frac{3}{4}$ ounces of flour. How many loaves did she bake?
   a. 11 loaves
   b. 12 loaves
   c. 13 loaves
   d. 14 loaves
   e. 15 loaves

_____ **33.** How many $2\frac{1}{2}$-pound chunks of cheese can be cut from a single 20-pound piece of cheese?
   a. 2 chunks
   b. 4 chunks
   c. 6 chunks
   d. 8 chunks
   e. 10 chunks

_____ **34.** Ms. Goldbaum earned $36.75 for working $3\frac{1}{2}$ hours. What was her hourly wage?
   a. $10.00
   b. $10.50
   c. $10.75
   d. $12.00
   e. $12.25

Decimals

What Is a Decimal?

A decimal is a number that can be represented by a special kind of fraction. This special kind of fraction involves powers of the number 10: 10; 100; 1,000; etc. You use decimals every day when you deal with money—$10.35 is a decimal that represents 10 dollars and 35 cents. The decimal point separates the dollars from the cents. Because there are 100 cents in one dollar, 1 cent is $\frac{1}{100}$ of a dollar, or $0.01.

Each decimal digit to the right of the decimal point has a name:

Examples: $0.1 = 1$ tenth $= \frac{1}{10}$
$0.02 = 2$ hundredths $= \frac{2}{100}$
$0.003 = 3$ thousandths $= \frac{3}{1,000}$
$0.0004 = 4$ ten-thousandths $= \frac{4}{10,000}$

When you add zeros after the rightmost decimal place, you don't change the value of the decimal. For example, 6.17 is the same as all of these:

6.170
6.1700
6.17000000000000000

If there are digits on both sides of the decimal point (like 10.35), the number is called a **mixed decimal**. If there are digits only to the right of the decimal point (like 0.53), the number is called a decimal. A whole number (like 15) is understood to have a decimal point at its right (15.). Thus, 15 is the same as 15.0, 15.00, 15.000, and so on.

Changing Fractions to Decimals

Sometimes it is necessary to change fractions to decimals. The fraction bar that separates the top and bottom numbers in a fraction stands for division, so to change a fraction to a decimal, divide the bottom number into the top number. Once you have set up your division problem, you will need to put a decimal point and a few zeros on the right of the top number, which is inside the division box. When you divide, bring the decimal point up into your answer.

Example: Change $\frac{3}{4}$ to a decimal.

1. Add a decimal point and two zeros to the top number (3):   3.00
2. Divide the bottom number (4) into 3.00:

$$\begin{array}{r} .75 \\ 4\overline{)3.00} \\ \underline{2\ 8} \\ 20 \\ \underline{20} \\ 0 \end{array}$$

3. The quotient (result of the division) is the answer: 0.75

Some fractions may require you to add many decimal zeros in order for the division to come out evenly. In fact, when you convert a fraction like $\frac{2}{3}$ to a decimal, you can keep adding decimal zeros to the top number forever because the division will never come out evenly. As you divide 3 into 2, you will keep getting 6's:

$$2 \div 3 = 0.6666666666 \text{ etc.}$$

This is called a *repeating decimal* and it can be written as $.\overline{666}$ or as $.66\frac{2}{3}$. You can approximate it as 0.67, 0.667, 0.6667, and so on. When a bar is written above a digit or digits in a repeating decimal, it is those numbers that repeat (for example, $0.\overline{42}$ means 0.42424242 . . . and $5.68\overline{374}$ measn 5.68374374374 . . .).

Changing Decimals to Fractions

It is also important to be able to change a decimal to a fraction. First, determine what place the *last digit* of the decimal holds. For example, the last digit can be in the tenths place, like 4.7; in the hundredths place, like 0.93; in the thousandths place, like 1.005; and so on. Once you have determined the place of the last digit of the decimal, write that in the denominator of a fraction. Next write the digits of the decimal as the top number in that fraction.

Example: 0.018

1. Three places to the right of the decimal means *thousandths,* so write 1,000 as the bottom number: $\overline{1,000}$
2. Write 18 as the top of the fraction: $\frac{18}{}$
3. Reduce by dividing 2 into the top and bottom numbers: $\frac{18 \div 2}{1,000 \div 2} = \frac{9}{500}$

Change these decimals or mixed decimals to fractions:

_____ **35.** 0.0125

_____ **36.** 3.48

_____ **37.** 123.456

Comparing Decimals

Because decimals are easier to compare when they have the same number of digits after the decimal point, tack zeros onto the end of the shorter decimals. Then all you have to do is compare the numbers as if the decimal points weren't there:

Example: Compare 0.08 and 0.1

1. Tack one zero at the end of 0.1: .10
2. To compare 0.10 to 0.08, just compare 10 to 8.
3. Since 10 is larger than 8, 0.1 is larger than 0.08.

Adding and Subtracting Decimals

To add or subtract decimals, line them up so their decimal points are aligned. You may want to tack on zeros at the end of shorter decimals so you can keep all your digits lined up evenly. Remember, if a number doesn't have a decimal point, then put one at the right end of the number.

Example: 1.23 + 57 + 0.038

1. Line up the numbers like this:

$$
\begin{array}{r}
1.230 \\
57.000 \\
+\ 0.038 \\
\hline
\end{array}
$$

2. Add:

$$
\begin{array}{r}
\hline
58.268
\end{array}
$$

Example: 1.23 − 0.038

1. Line up the numbers like this:

$$
\begin{array}{r}
1.230 \\
-\ 0.038 \\
\hline
\end{array}
$$

2. Subtract:

$$
\begin{array}{r}
1.192
\end{array}
$$

Try these addition and subtraction problems:

_____ **38.** 905 + 0.02 + 3.075

_____ **39.** 3.48 − 2.573

_____ **40.** 123.456 − 122

_____ **41.** James drove 3.7 miles to his physical therapist's office. He then walked 1.6 miles on the treadmill to strengthen his legs. He got back into the car, drove 2.75 miles to his radiology appointment, and then drove 2 miles back home. How many miles did he drive in total?
a. 8.05 miles
b. 8.45 miles
c. 8.8 miles
d. 10 miles
e. 10.05 miles

_____ **42.** The average number of emergency room visits at City Hospital fell from 486.4 per week to 402.5 per week. By how many emergency room visits per week did the average fall?

   a. 73.9 visits
   b. 83 visits
   c. 83.1 visits
   d. 83.9 visits
   e. 84.9 visits

Multiplying Decimals

To multiply decimals, ignore the decimal points and just multiply the numbers. Then count the total number of decimal digits (the digits to the *right* of the decimal point) in the numbers you are multiplying. Count off that number of digits in your answer beginning at the right side and put the decimal point to the *left* of those digits.

   Example: 215.7 × 2.4

1. Multiply 2,157 times 24:

$$\begin{array}{r} 2{,}157 \\ \times\ 24 \\ \hline 8628 \\ 4314 \\ \hline 51768 \end{array}$$

2. Because there are a total of two decimal digits in 215.7 and 2.4, count off two places from the right in 51,768, placing the decimal point to the *left* of the last two digits: 517.68

If your answer doesn't have enough digits, tack zeros on to the left of the answer.

   Example: 0.03 × 0.006

1. Multiply 3 times 6:   3 ×6 = 18
2. You need five decimal digits in your answer, so tack on three zeros: 00018
3. Put the decimal point at the front of the number (which is five digits in from the right):   0.00018

You can practice multiplying decimals with these:

_____ **43.** 0.05 × 0.6

_____ **44.** 0.053 × 6.4

_____ **45.** 38.1 × 0.0184

_____ **46.** Joe earns $42.65 per hour as an occupational therapist. Last week, he worked 12.75 hours. How much money did he earn that week?
   a. $518.00
   b. $518.50
   c. $525.00
   d. $536.50
   e. $543.79

47. Nuts cost $3.50 per pound.
Approximately how much will 4.25
pounds of nuts cost?
a. $12.25
b. $12.50
c. $12.88
d. $14.50
e. $14.88

Dividing Decimals

Before we learn how to divide a decimal by a decimal,
let's begin with dividing a decimal by a whole number.

To divide a decimal by a whole number, set up
the division $(8\overline{).256})$ and immediately bring the decimal point straight up into the answer $(8\overline{)1256})$. Then
divide as you would normally divide whole numbers:

Example:
$$\begin{array}{r} .032 \\ 8\overline{)1256} \\ \underline{0} \\ 25 \\ \underline{24} \\ 16 \\ \underline{16} \\ 0 \end{array}$$

When dividing *by* a decimal, there is one extra
step involved. First, set up your problem in a division
box. Then, working with the decimal you're dividing
by (the one on the outside of the box), move the decimal point to the right end of the number so it's now a
whole number. Count the number of places you had
to move the decimal to the right in order to create that
whole number, and move the decimal of the number
inside the division box the same number of spaces to
the right. Now the problem will look like you are dividing by a whole number.

Example: $0.06\overline{)1.218}$

1. Because there are two decimal
digits in 0.06, move the decimal
point two places to the right in
both numbers and move the
decimal point straight up into
the answer:
2. Divide using the new
numbers:

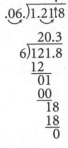

$$\begin{array}{r} 20.3 \\ 6\overline{)121.8} \\ \underline{12} \\ 01 \\ \underline{00} \\ 18 \\ \underline{18} \\ 0 \end{array}$$

Under certain conditions, you have to tack on
zeros to the right of the last decimal digit in the number you are dividing into:

- if there aren't enough digits for you to move the
decimal point to the right
- if the answer doesn't come out evenly when you
do the division
- if you are dividing a whole number by a decimal. Then you will have to tack on the decimal
point as well as some zeros.

Try your skills on these division problems:

48. $7\overline{)9.8}$

49. $0.0004\overline{)0.0512}$

50. $0.05\overline{)28.6}$

51. $0.14\overline{)196}$

_____ **52.** If James Worthington drove the mobile blood bank unit 92.4 miles in 2.1 hours, what was his average speed in miles per hour?
- **a.** 41 miles per hour
- **b.** 44 miles per hour
- **c.** 90. miles per hour
- **d.** 94.5 miles per hour

_____ **53.** Mary Sanders walked a total of 18.6 miles in four days. On average, how many miles did she walk each day?
- **a.** 4.15 miles
- **b.** 4.60 miles
- **c.** 4.65 miles
- **d.** 22.60 miles
- **e.** 74.40 miles

Percents

What Is a Percent?

A percent is a special kind of fraction with a *denominator* that is always 100. For example, 17% is the same as $\frac{17}{100}$. Literally, the word *percent* means *per 100 parts*. The root *cent* means 100: A *century* is 100 years; there are 100 *cents* in a dollar, etc. Thus, 17% means 17 parts out of 100. Because fractions can also be expressed as decimals, 17% is also equivalent to 0.17, which is 17 hundredths.

You come into contact with percents every day. Sales tax, interest, and discounts are just a few common examples.

If you're shaky on fractions, you may want to review the fraction section before reading further.

Changing a Decimal to a Percent and Vice Versa

To change a decimal to a percent, move the decimal point two places to the right and tack on a percent sign (%) at the end. If the decimal point moves to the very right of the number, you don't have to write the decimal point. If there aren't enough places to move the decimal point, add zeros on the right before moving the decimal point.

Examples:
0.035 will become 3.5%
2 will become 200%
0.7 will become 70%

Try changing these decimals to percents:

_____ **54.** 0.45

_____ **55.** 0.008

_____ **56.** 0.169

To change a percent to a decimal, drop off the percent sign and move the decimal point two places to the left. If there aren't enough places to move the decimal point, add zeros on the left before moving the decimal point.

Examples:
345% will become 3.45
$26\frac{3}{4}$% will become 0.2675
0.6% will become 0.006

Now, change these percents to decimals:

_____ **57.** 12%

_____ **58.** $87\frac{1}{2}$%

_____ **59.** 250%

Changing a Fraction to a Percent and Vice Versa

To change a fraction to a percent, there are two techniques. Each is illustrated by changing the fraction $\frac{1}{4}$ to a percent:

Technique 1:   Multiply the fraction by 100%.
Multiply $\frac{1}{4}$ by 100%:

$$\frac{1}{\underset{1}{\cancel{4}}} \times \frac{\overset{25}{\cancel{100}}\%}{1} = 25\%$$

Technique 2:   Divide the fraction's bottom number into the top number; then move the decimal point two places to the right and tack on a percent sign (%).
Divide 4 into 1 and move the decimal point two places to the right:

$$4\overline{)1.00}^{\;.25}$$

$$0.25 = 25\%$$

Example: Change 4% to a fraction.

1. Remove the % and write the fraction 4 over 100:

$$\frac{4}{100}$$

2. Reduce:

$$\frac{4 \div 4}{100 \div 4} = \frac{1}{25}$$

Here's a more complicated example: Change $16\frac{2}{3}\%$ to a fraction.

1. Remove the % and write the fraction $16\frac{2}{3}$ over 100:

$$\frac{16\frac{2}{3}}{100}$$

2. Since a fraction means "top number divided by bottom number," rewrite the fraction as a division problem:

$$16\frac{2}{3} \div 100$$

3. Change the mixed number $(16\frac{2}{3})$ to an improper fraction $(\frac{50}{3})$:

$$\frac{50}{3} \div \frac{100}{1}$$

4. Flip the second fraction $(\frac{100}{1})$ and multiply:

$$\frac{\overset{1}{\cancel{50}}}{3} \times \frac{1}{\underset{2}{\cancel{100}}} = \frac{1}{6}$$

Try changing these fractions to percents:

_____ **60.** $\frac{1}{8}$

_____ **61.** $\frac{13}{25}$

_____ **62.** $\frac{7}{12}$

Now change these percents to fractions:

_____ **63.** 95%

_____ **64.** $37\frac{1}{2}\%$

_____ **65.** 125%

To change a percent to a fraction, remove the percent sign and write the number over 100. Then reduce if possible.

Sometimes it is more convenient to work with a percentage as a fraction or a decimal. Rather than having to *calculate* the equivalent fraction or decimal, it is a good idea to memorize all of the conversions in the following table. Not only will this increase your efficiency on the math test, but it will also be practical for real-life situations.

CONVERSION TABLE		
DECIMAL	**%**	**FRACTION**
0.25	25%	$\frac{1}{4}$
0.50	50%	$\frac{1}{2}$
0.75	75%	$\frac{3}{4}$
0.10	10%	$\frac{1}{10}$
0.20	20%	$\frac{1}{5}$
0.40	40%	$\frac{2}{5}$
0.60	60%	$\frac{3}{5}$
0.80	80%	$\frac{4}{5}$
$0.33\overline{3}$	$33\frac{1}{3}\%$	$\frac{1}{3}$
$0.66\overline{6}$	$66\frac{2}{3}\%$	$\frac{2}{3}$

Percent Word Problems

Word problems involving percents come in three main varieties:

- Find a percent of a whole.
  Example: What is 30% of 40?
- Find what percent one number is of another number.
  Example: 12 is what percent of 40?
- Find the whole when the percent of it is given.
  Example: 12 is 30% of what number?

While each variety has its own approach, there is a single shortcut formula you can use to solve each of these:

$$\frac{is}{of} = \frac{\%}{100}$$

The *is* is the number that usually follows or is just before the word *is* in the question.

The *of* is the number that usually follows the word *of* in the question.

The **%** is the number that is in front of the **%** or *percent* in the question.

Or you may think of the shortcut formula as:

$$\frac{part}{whole} = \frac{\%}{100}$$

To solve each of the three varieties, we're going to use the fact that the **cross products** are equal. The cross products are the products of the numbers diagonally across from each other. Remembering that *product* means *multiply*, here's how to create the cross products for the percent shortcut:

$$\frac{part}{whole} = \frac{\%}{100}$$

$$part \times 100 = whole \times \%$$

Here's how to use the shortcut with cross products:

- Find a percent of a whole.
  What is 30% of 40?
  30 is the % and 40 is
  the *of* number: $\frac{is}{40} = \frac{30}{100}$
  Cross multiply and solve
  for *is*: $is \times 100 = 40 \times 30$
      $is \times 100 = 1{,}200$
      $\mathbf{12} \times 100 = 1{,}200$

Thus, **12** *is* 30% of 40.

- Find what percent one number is of another number.
  12 is what percent of 40?
  12 is the *is* number and 40
  is the *of* number: $\frac{12}{40} = \frac{\%}{100}$
  Cross multiply and solve
  for %: $12 \times 100 = 40 \times \mathbf{\%}$
      $1{,}200 = 40 \times \mathbf{\%}$
      $1{,}200 = 40 \times \mathbf{30}$

Thus, 12 is **30%** of 40.

- Find the whole when the percent of it is given.

12 is 30% of what number?

12 is the *is* number and 30 is the %:

$$\frac{12}{of} = \frac{30}{100}$$

Cross multiply and solve for the *of* number:

$$12 \times 100 = of \times 30$$
$$1{,}200 = of \times 30$$
$$1{,}200 = 40 \times 30$$

Thus, 12 is 30% *of* **40**.

Find a percent of a whole:

_____ **66.** 1% of 25

_____ **67.** 18.2% of 50

_____ **68.** $44\frac{1}{2}$% of 600

_____ **69.** 125% of 60

Find the percent that one number is of another number:

_____ **70.** 10 is what % of 20?

_____ **71.** 4 is what % of 12?

_____ **72.** 12 is what % of 4?

Find the whole when the percent of it is given:

_____ **73.** 15% of what number is 15?

_____ **74.** $37\frac{1}{2}$% of what number is 3?

_____ **75.** 200% of what number is 20?

Calculating Percent Increase and Percent Decrease

Sometimes you'll need to calculate the percent of increase or percent of decrease of something. To do this type of calculation, use the following formula:

$$\text{Percent of change} = \frac{amount\ of\ change}{original\ amount}$$

The *amount of change* is the difference between the original and new values (found by subtracting them). If something has increased in value, then the *original value* will be the lower value. But if something has decreased in value, then the *original value* will be the higher value. Once you have created this fraction, you will just turn it into a percent by using one of the methods discussed earlier in this chapter.

> **Example:** If a merchant puts the store's $20 hats on sale for $15, by what percent does the merchant decrease the selling price?

$$\text{Percent of change} = \frac{amount\ of\ change}{original\ amount}$$

$$\text{Percent of change} = \frac{20 - 15}{20}$$

$$\text{Percent of change} = \frac{5}{20} = \frac{1}{4} = 0.25 = 25\%$$

Thus, the selling price is decreased by 25%.

The interesting thing about percents is that if the same merchant were to raise $15 T-shirts to $20, that would *not* be a 25% increase, even though going from $20 to $15 was a 25% decrease. This is because the $5 change in price is now being compared to an original price of $15, instead of being compared to an original price of $20. Look at how this changes the outcome:

$$\text{Percent of change} = \frac{amount\ of\ change}{original\ amount}$$

Percent of change $= \frac{20-15}{15}$

Percent of change $= \frac{5}{15} = \frac{1}{3} = 0.\overline{33} = 33\frac{1}{3}\%$

Thus the selling price in this example would be increased by $33\frac{1}{3}\%$.

Now try your percent skills on some real-life problems:

_____ **76.** 15% of a 220-member nursing staff took vacation. How many nurses took vacation last week?
   a. 5 nurses
   b. 22 nurses
   c. 33 nurses
   d. 15 nurses
   e. 100 nurses

_____ **77.** Forty percent of General Hospital's medical technologists are women. If there are 80 female medical technologists, how many medical technologists are male?
   a. 32
   b. 112
   c. 120
   d. 160
   e. 200

_____ **78.** Of the 840 biopsies performed last month, 42 were positive. What percent of the biopsies were positive?
   a. 0.5%
   b. 2%
   c. 5%
   d. 20%
   e. 50%

_____ **79.** Sam's Shoe Store put all of its merchandise on sale for 20% off. If Jason saved $10 by purchasing one pair of shoes during the sale, what was the original price of the shoes before the sale?
   a. $12
   b. $20
   c. $40
   d. $50
   e. $70

Averages

An **average**, also called an arithmetic mean, is a measure of center that *typifies* a group of numbers. You come into contact with averages on a regular basis: your bowling average, the average grade on a test, the average number of hours you work per week.

To calculate an average, add up the number of items being averaged and divide by the number of items.

Example: What is the average of 6, 10, and 20?

Solution: Add the three numbers together and divide by 3: $\frac{6+10+20}{3} = 12$

Shortcut

Here's a neat shortcut for some average problems.

- Look at the numbers being averaged. If they are equally spaced, like 5, 10, 15, 20, and 25, then the average is the number in the middle, or 15 in this case.
- If there are an even number of such numbers, say 10, 20, 30, and 40, then there is no middle number. In this case, the average is halfway between the two middle numbers. In this case, the average is halfway between 20 and 30, or 25.

■ If the numbers are almost evenly spaced, you can probably estimate the average without going to the trouble of actually computing it. For example, the average of 10, 20, and 32 is just a little more than 20, the middle number.

Try these average questions:

_____ **80.** Bob's bowling scores for the last five games were 180, 182, 184, 186, and 188. What was his average bowling score?
   a. 182
   b. 183
   c. 184
   d. 185
   e. 186

_____ **81.** Ambulance driver Conroy averaged 30 miles per hour for the two hours he drove in town and 60 miles per hour for the two hours he drove on the highway. What was his average speed in miles per hour?
   a. 18 miles per hour
   b. $22\frac{1}{2}$ miles per hour
   c. 45 miles per hour
   d. 60 miles per hour
   e. 90 miles per hour

_____ **82.** There are 10 females and 20 males in the first aid course. If the females achieved an average score of 85 and the males achieved an average score of 95, what was the class average? (Hint: Don't fall for the trap of taking the average of 85 and 95; there are more 95s being averaged than 85s, so the average is closer to 95.)
   a. $90\frac{2}{3}$
   b. $91\frac{2}{3}$
   c. 92
   d. $92\frac{2}{3}$
   e. 95

Working with Length and Time Units

The United States uses the *English system* to measure length; however, most other countries use the *metric system*, which is also prevalent in scientific use in the United States. The English system requires knowing many different equivalences, but you're probably used to dealing with these equivalences on a daily basis. Mathematically, however, it's simpler to work in metric units because their equivalences are all multiples of 10. The meter is the basic unit of length, with all other length units defined in terms of the meter.

Length Conversions

Math questions on standardized tests, especially geometry word problems, may require conversions within a particular system. An easy way to convert from one unit of measurement to another is to multiply by an equivalence ratio. A *ratio* is one number divided by another, and an *equivalence ratio* is when one unit of measurement (such as 1 foot), is placed over (or under) another unit of measurement (such as 12 inches) that has the same value. Such ratios don't change the value of the unit of measurement because each ratio is equivalent to 1.

ENGLISH SYSTEM	
UNIT	**EQUIVALENCE**
foot (ft.)	1 ft. = 12 in.
yard (yd.)	1 yd. = 3 ft. 1 yd. = 36 in.
mile (mi.)	1 mi. = 5,280 ft. 1 mi. = 1,760 yds.

METRIC SYSTEM	
UNIT	**EQUIVALENCE**
meter (m)	Basic unit A giant step is about 1 meter long.
centimeter (cm)	100 cm = 1 m Your index finger is about 1 cm wide.
millimeter (mm)	10 mm = 1 cm; 1,000 mm = 1 m Your fingernail is about 1 mm thick.
kilometer (km)	1 km = 1,000 m Five city blocks are about 1 km long.

ENGLISH SYSTEM	
TO CONVERT BETWEEN	**MULTIPLY BY THIS RATIO**
inches and feet	$\frac{12 \text{ in.}}{1 \text{ ft.}}$ or $\frac{1 \text{ ft.}}{12 \text{ in.}}$
inches and yards	$\frac{36 \text{ in.}}{1 \text{ yd.}}$ or $\frac{1 \text{ yd.}}{36 \text{ in.}}$
feet and yards	$\frac{3 \text{ ft.}}{1 \text{ yd.}}$ or $\frac{1 \text{ yd.}}{3 \text{ ft.}}$
feet and miles	$\frac{5,280 \text{ ft.}}{1 \text{ mi.}}$ or $\frac{1 \text{ mi.}}{5,280 \text{ ft.}}$
yards and miles	$\frac{1,760 \text{ yds.}}{1 \text{ mi.}}$ or $\frac{1 \text{ mi.}}{1,760 \text{ yds.}}$

METRIC SYSTEM	
TO CONVERT BETWEEN	**MULTIPLY BY THIS RATIO**
millimeters and centimeters	$\frac{10 \text{ mm}}{1 \text{ cm}}$ or $\frac{1 \text{ cm}}{10 \text{ mm}}$
meters and millimeters	$\frac{1,000 \text{ mm}}{1 \text{ m}}$ or $\frac{1 \text{ m}}{1,000 \text{ mm}}$
meters and centimeters	$\frac{100 \text{ cm}}{1 \text{ m}}$ or $\frac{1 \text{ m}}{100 \text{ cm}}$
meters and kilometers	$\frac{1,000 \text{ m}}{1 \text{ km}}$ or $\frac{1 \text{ km}}{1,000 \text{ m}}$

Example: Convert 3 yards into feet.

Multiply 3 yards by the ratio $\frac{3 \text{ ft.}}{1 \text{ yd.}}$. Notice that we chose $\frac{3 \text{ ft.}}{1 \text{ yd.}}$ rather than $\frac{1 \text{ yd.}}{3 \text{ ft.}}$ because the yards in the bottom of the equivalence ratio cancel with the yards on top during the multiplication:

$$3 \text{ yds.} \times \frac{3 \text{ ft.}}{1 \text{ yd.}} = \frac{3 \text{ yds.} \times 3 \text{ ft.}}{1 \text{ yd.}} = \textbf{9 ft.}$$

Example: Convert 31 inches into feet and inches.

1. First, multiply 31 inches by the ratio $\frac{1 \text{ ft.}}{12 \text{ in.}}$:

$$31 \text{ in.} \times \frac{1 \text{ ft.}}{12 \text{ in.}} =$$
$$\frac{31 \text{ in.} \times 1 \text{ ft.}}{12 \text{ in.}} = \frac{31}{12} \text{ ft.} = 2\frac{7}{12} \text{ ft.}$$

2. Then change the $\frac{7}{12}$ portion of $2\frac{7}{12}$ ft. to inches:

$$\frac{7 \text{ ft.}}{12} \times \frac{12 \text{ in.}}{1 \text{ ft.}} =$$
$$\frac{7 \text{ ft.} \times 12 \text{ in.}}{12 \times 1 \text{ ft.}} = 7 \text{ } in.$$

3. Thus, 31 inches is equivalent to both $2\frac{7}{12}$ **ft.** and **2 feet 7 inches.**

Convert as indicated.

83. 2 ft. = _____ in.

84. 3 cm = _____ mm

85. 16 m = _____ cm

86. 294 cm = _____ m

Addition and Subtraction with Length Units

In the health field, you will need to be able to combine numbers that contain different units of measurement. In the following example, finding the perimeter, or distance around the outside of the figure, will require adding lengths of different units.

Example: Find the perimeter of the figure below.

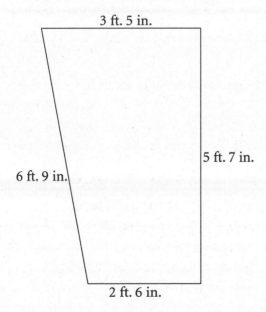

3 ft. 5 in.

5 ft. 7 in.

6 ft. 9 in.

2 ft. 6 in.

To add the lengths, add each column of length units separately:

$$
\begin{array}{rr}
5 \text{ ft.} & 7 \text{ in.} \\
2 \text{ ft.} & 6 \text{ in.} \\
6 \text{ ft.} & 9 \text{ in.} \\
+\ 3 \text{ ft.} & 5 \text{ in.} \\
\hline
\mathbf{16 \text{ ft.}} & \mathbf{27 \text{ in.}}
\end{array}
$$

Since 27 inches is more than 1 foot, the total of **16 ft. 27 in.** must be simplified:

Convert 27 inches to feet and inches:

$$27 \text{ in.} \times \frac{1 \text{ ft.}}{12 \text{ in.}} = \frac{27}{12} \text{ ft.} = 2\frac{3}{12} \text{ ft.} = 2 \text{ ft. 3 in.}$$

Add:
$$
\begin{array}{r}
16 \text{ ft.} \\
+\ 2 \text{ ft. 3 in.} \\
\hline
\mathbf{18 \text{ ft. 3 in.}}
\end{array}
$$
Thus, the perimeter is **18 feet 3 inches.**

Finding the length of a line segment may require subtracting lengths of different units.

Example: Find the length of line segment *AB* below.

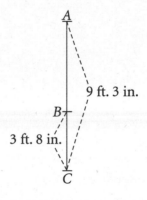

A

9 ft. 3 in.

B

3 ft. 8 in.

C

To subtract the lengths, subtract each column of length units separately, starting with the rightmost column.

$$9 \text{ ft. } 3 \text{ in.}$$
$$- 3 \text{ ft. } 8 \text{ in.}$$

Warning: You can't subtract 8 inches from 3 inches because 8 is larger than 3! As in regular subtraction, you have to *borrow* 1 from the column on the left. However, borrowing 1 ft. is the same as borrowing 12 inches; adding the borrowed 12 inches to the 3 inches gives 15 inches. Thus:

$$\overset{8}{\cancel{9}} \text{ ft. } \overset{12\ \ 15}{\cancel{3}} \text{ in.}$$
$$- 3 \text{ ft. } 8 \text{ in.}$$
$$\overline{\mathbf{5 \text{ ft. } 7 \text{ in.}}}$$

Thus, the length of $\overline{AB}$ is **5 feet 7 inches**.

Add and simplify.

87.   5 ft. 3 in.
         + 2 ft. 9 in.

88.   7 km 220 m
           4 km 180 m
         + 9 km 770 m

Subtract and simplify.

89.   4 ft. 1 in.
         − 2 ft. 9 in.

90.   14 cm 2 mm
         − 6 cm 4 mm

Time Conversions

Word problems involving time typically ask you to determine how long something takes. You might have to add together the amount of time several activities take in order to determine the total amount of time the entire process takes or calculate the elapsed time from the start to the finish of a particular activity.

Adding and subtracting time units is a lot like adding and subtracting length units. You have to make sure that you are adding hours to hours, minutes to minutes, and seconds to seconds. If the given information is in different time units, then you'll have to convert to a common time unit before you can proceed. Use the following conversion ratios:

- **To convert minutes to hours:** $\frac{1 \text{ hour}}{60 \text{ minutes}}$
- **To convert hours to minutes:** $\frac{60 \text{ minutes}}{1 \text{ hour}}$
- **To convert seconds to minutes:** $\frac{1 \text{ minute}}{60 \text{ seconds}}$
- **To convert minutes to seconds:** $\frac{60 \text{ seconds}}{1 \text{ minute}}$

Example: Convert $2\frac{1}{4}$ hours to seconds.

1. Convert hours to minutes: $2\frac{1}{4} \cancel{\text{ hr.}} \times \frac{60 \text{ min.}}{1 \cancel{\text{ hr.}}} = 135 \text{ min.}$

2. Convert minutes to seconds: $135 \cancel{\text{ min.}} \frac{60 \text{ sec.}}{1 \cancel{\text{ min.}}} = 8{,}100 \text{ sec.}$

The hours and minutes cancel, giving an answer in seconds.

Calculating Elapsed Time

Calculating elapsed time when you're given the starting and ending time can be a bit tricky, depending on the starting and ending time. If the starting and ending times are both A.M. or both P.M. of the same day, you can calculate the elapsed time by simply subtracting the starting time from the ending time. However, you may have to "regroup," or "borrow."

Example: Radiology Associates opens at 6:45 A.M. and closes for lunch at 11:35 A.M. How long are they open in the morning?

1. Set up the subtraction:

$$\begin{array}{r} {}^{10}\;{}^{9} \\ \cancel{11}{:}\cancel{35} \\ -\;6{:}45 \\ \hline 4{:}50 \end{array}$$

2. You can't subtract 45 minutes from 35 minutes, so you have to "borrow" 1 hour from the 11 hours. Borrowing 1 hour from 11 hours is equivalent to borrowing 60 minutes. Thus, you're actually subtracting 45 minutes from 95 minutes (that is, 35 + 60 minutes).

Radiology Associates is open for 4 hours 50 minutes in the morning.

If the starting time is A.M. and ending time is P.M. of the same day, you have to calculate the elapsed time in two steps and then add the step results together. Calculate the elapsed morning time by subtracting the starting time from noon. The elapsed afternoon time is equivalent to the ending time. So you add the elapsed morning time and the elapsed afternoon time to get the total elapsed time.

Example: If Radiology Associates opens at 7:15 A.M. and closes at 5:30 P.M., how long are they open?

1. Subtract the starting time from noon: (You'll have to "borrow" 60 minutes from 12.)

$$\begin{array}{r} {}^{1}\;{}^{5}\;{}^{6}\;{}^{10} \\ \cancel{12}{:}\cancel{00} \\ -\;7{:}15 \\ \hline 4{:}45 \end{array}$$

Radiology Associates is open for 4 hours 45 minutes in the morning.

2. Radiology Associates closes at 5:30 P.M. Thus, they're open for 5 hours 30 minutes in the afternoon.

3. Add the results together:

$$\begin{array}{r} 4{:}45 \\ +\;5{:}30 \\ \hline 9{:}75 \end{array}$$

4. The sum of 9 hours 75 minutes needs to be adjusted because 75 minutes is more than one hour. There's a "carry" of 1 hour: The 75 minutes is equivalent to 1 hour 15 minutes. Thus, 9 hours 75 minutes is the same as 10 hours 15 minutes.

You follow the same procedure when the starting time is P.M. of one day and the ending time is A.M. of the next day. Calculate the elapsed P.M. time by subtracting the starting time from midnight. Then add the elapsed A.M. time, which is equivalent to the ending time.

If the starting and ending times are on different days, you calculate the elapsed time in three steps: elapsed time on the starting day, elapsed time on the ending day, and the time of the intervening days. Then you add the results of the three steps together.

Example: Each week, Radiology Associates turns their computers on at 6:45 A.M. on Monday and turns them off for the weekend at 5:30 P.M. on Friday. How long are the computers on, in hours?

1. Starting day, Monday

a. For the A.M. hours, subtract the starting time from noon:

$$\begin{array}{r} \overset{5}{}\overset{\cancel{1}\ \cancel{6}\ 10}{12:00} \\ -\ 6:45 \\ \hline 5:15 \end{array}$$

b. For the P.M. hours, there are 12 hours from noon until midnight.

c. Add the A.M. and P.M. hours to get the total hours on the starting day:

$$\begin{array}{r} 5:15 \\ +\ 12:00 \\ \hline 17:15 \end{array}$$

On Monday, 17 hours 15 minutes elapse.

2. Ending day, Friday

a. For the A.M. hours, there are 12 hours from midnight until noon: $\quad$ 12:00

b. For the P.M. hours, the ending time is the elapsed time: $\quad +\ 5:30$

c. Add the A.M. and P.M. hours to get the total hours on the ending day: $\quad$ 17:30

On Friday, 17 hours 30 minutes elapse.

3. The intervening days: Tuesday, Wednesday, and Thursday

3 days × 24 hours per day = 72 hours

4. Add the results of steps 1–3 together:

$$\begin{array}{r} 17:15 \\ 17:30 \\ +\ 72:00 \\ \hline 106:45 \end{array}$$

The total elapsed time is 106 hours 45 minutes.

5. Since the question asks for the amount of time the computers are on in hours, the 45 minutes portion of the answer must be converted to a fraction of an hour:

45 minutes $\times\ \frac{1\ \text{hour}}{60\ \text{minutes}} = \frac{3}{4}$ hour

Thus, the computers were on for a total of $106\frac{3}{4}$ hours.

Now try these time problems:

_____ **91.** Jan ran three tests in the lab that each required 45 minutes. If she then ran a final test and all four tests required a total of $3\frac{1}{4}$ hours, how long did the final test take?

a. $\frac{1}{2}$ hour

b. $\frac{2}{3}$ hour

c. $\frac{3}{4}$ hour

d. 1 hour

e. $1\frac{1}{4}$ hours

_____ **92.** The staff at a hospital started to use a radiology room at 8:15 A.M. The room was used for 6 hours 15 minutes. What time did the staff finish using the radiology room?

a. 8:15 P.M.

b. 1:45 P.M.

c. 2:15 P.M.

d. 3:30 P.M.

e. 2:30 P.M.

_____ **93.** Clara cultured a particular virus at 2:30 P.M. on Monday and stored the culture in the refrigerator until 11:30 A.M. on Wednesday. How long was the culture in the refrigerator?

a. 3 hours

b. 21 hours

c. 27 hours

d. 45 hours

e. 69 hours

Algebra

Popular topics for algebra questions on health occupations exams include:

- solving equations
- positive and negative numbers
- algebraic expressions

What Is Algebra?

Algebra is the mathematics that lets us use equations with numbers and symbols in order to model mathematical relationships. These symbols, called *unknowns* or *variables*, are letters of the alphabet that are used to represent numbers.

For example, let's say you are asked to find out what number, when added to 3, gives you a total of 5. Using algebra, you could express the problem as $x + 3 = 5$. The variable x represents the number you are trying to find.

Here's another example, but this one uses only variables. To find the distance traveled, multiply the rate of travel (speed) by the amount of time traveled: $d = r \times t$. The variable d stands for *distance*, r stands for *rate*, and t stands for *time*.

In algebra, the variables may take on different values. In other words, they *vary*, and that's why they're called *variables*.

Operations

Algebra uses the same operations as arithmetic: addition, subtraction, multiplication, and division. In arithmetic, we might say $3 + 4 = 7$, while in algebra, we would talk about two numbers whose values we don't know that add up to 7, or $x + y = 7$. Here's how each operation translates to algebra:

ALGEBRAIC OPERATIONS	
The sum of 2 numbers	$a + b$
The difference of 2 numbers	$a - b$
The product of 2 numbers	$a \times b$ or $a \cdot b$ or ab
The quotient of 2 numbers	$\frac{a}{b}$

Equations

An equation is a mathematical sentence stating that two quantities are equal. For example:

$$2x = 10$$
$$x + 5 = 8$$

The idea is to find a replacement for the unknown that will make the sentence true. You solve equations *for* the unknown variable. For example, in the equation $2x = 10$, $x = 5$ because $2 \times 5 = 10$. In the second example, $x = 3$ because $3 + 5 = 8$.

Sometimes you can solve an equation by inspection, as with the previous examples. Other equations may be more complicated and require a step-by-step solution, for example:

$$\frac{n + 2}{4} + 1 = 3$$

The general approach is to consider an equation like a balance scale, with both sides equally balanced. Essentially, whatever you do to one side, you must also do to the other side to maintain the balance. Thus, if you were to add 2 to the left side, you would also have to add 2 to the right side.

Let's apply this *balance* concept to our previous complicated equation. Remembering that we want to solve it for n, we must somehow rearrange it so the n is isolated on one side of the equation. Its value will then be on the other side. Looking at the equation, you can see that n has been increased by 2 and then divided by 4 and ultimately added to 1. Therefore, we will undo these operations to isolate n.

Begin by subtracting 1 from both sides of the equation:

$$\frac{n+2}{4} + 1 = 3$$
$$\underline{ -1 -1}$$
$$\frac{n+2}{4} = 2$$

Next, multiply both sides by 4:

$$4 \times \frac{n+2}{4} = 2 \times 4$$
$$n + 2 = 8$$

Finally, subtract 2 from both sides: $\underline{ -2 -2}$

This isolates n and solves the equation: $n = 6$

Notice that each operation in the original equation was undone by using the inverse operation. That is, addition was undone by subtraction, and division was undone by multiplication. In general, each operation can be undone by its *inverse*.

ALGEBRAIC INVERSES			
OPERATION	INVERSE	OPERATION	INVERSE
Addition	Subtraction	Subtraction	Addition
Multiplication	Division	Division	Multiplication
Square	Square Root	Square Root	Square

After you solve an equation, check your work by substituting the answer back into the original equation to make sure it balances. Let's see what happens when we substitute 6 in for n:

$$\frac{6+2}{4} + 1 = 3 \ ?$$
$$\frac{8}{4} + 1 = 3 \ ?$$
$$2 + 1 = 3 \ ?$$
$$3 = 3 \ ✓$$

Solve each equation:

_____ **94.** $x + 5 = 12$

_____ **95.** $5x - 4 = 26$

_____ **96.** $\frac{1}{4}x = 7$

Positive and Negative Numbers

Positive and negative numbers, also known as *signed* numbers, are best shown as points along the number line:

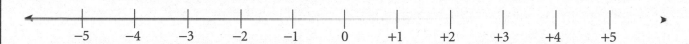

Numbers to the left of 0 are *negative* and those to the right of 0 are *positive*. Zero is neither negative nor positive. If a number is written without a sign, it is assumed to be *positive*. Notice that when you are on the negative side of the number line, bigger numbers have smaller values. For example, −5 is *less than* −2. You come into contact with negative numbers more often than you might think; for example, very cold temperatures are recorded as negative numbers.

As you move to the right along the number line, the numbers get larger. Mathematically, to indicate that one number, say 4, is *greater than* another number, say −2, the *greater than* sign (>) is used:

$$4 > -2$$

On the other hand, to say that −2 is *less than* 4, we use the *less than* sign (<):

$$-2 < 4$$

Arithmetic with Positive and Negative Numbers

The table on the next page illustrates the rules for doing arithmetic with signed numbers. Notice that when a negative number follows an operation (as it does in the second example that follows), it is often enclosed in parentheses to avoid confusion.

When more than one arithmetic operation appears, you must know the correct sequence in which to perform the operations. For example, do you know what to do first to calculate 2 + 3 × 4? You're right if you said, "Multiply first." The correct answer is 14. If you add first, you'll get the wrong answer of 20! The correct sequence of operations is:

1. **Parentheses**
2. **Exponents**
3. **Multiplication** or **Division**
   (whichever comes first when reading left to right)
4. **Addition** or **Subtraction**
   (whichever comes first when reading left to right)

This sequence of steps is often memorized by using the mnemonic **PEMDAS**, which some people like to remember with the expression "**P**lease **E**xcuse **M**y **D**ear **A**unt **S**ally."

Even when signed numbers appear in an equation, the step-by-step process works exactly as it does for positive numbers. You just have to remember the arithmetic rules for negative numbers. For example, let's solve $-14x + 2 = 5$.

1. Subtract 2 from both sides:

$$
\begin{array}{rcr}
-14x & + 2 & = -5 \\
 & -2 & -2 \\
\hline
\dfrac{-14x}{-14} & & = \dfrac{-7}{-14}
\end{array}
$$

2. Divide both sides by -14: $\qquad x \qquad = \dfrac{1}{2}$

EXAMPLE

ADDITION

If both numbers have the same sign, just add them. The answer has the same sign as the numbers being added.	$3 + 5 = 8$ $-3 + (-5) = -8$
If both numbers have different signs, subtract the smaller number from the larger. The answer has the same sign as the larger number.	$-3 + 5 = 2$ $3 + (-5) = -2$
If both numbers are the same but have opposite signs, the sum is zero.	$3 + (-3) = 0$

SUBTRACTION

Change the subtraction sign to addition and also change the sign of the number being subtracted. Add as above.	$3 - 5 = 3 + (-5) = -2$ $-3 - 5 = -3 + (-5) = -8$ $-3 - (-5) = -3 + 5 = 2$
If both numbers are the same, the difference is zero.	$5 - 5 = 0$ $-6 - (-6) = 0$

MULTIPLICATION

Multiply the numbers together. If both numbers have the same sign, the answer is positive; otherwise, it is negative.	$3 \times 5 = 15$ $-3 \times (-5) = 15$ $-3 \times 5 = -15$ $3 \times (-5) = -15$
If one number (or both) is zero, the answer is zero.	$3 \times 0 = 0$

DIVISION

Divide the numbers. If both numbers have the same sign, the answer is positive; otherwise, it is negative.	$15 \div 3 = 5$ $-15 \div (-3) = 5$ $15 \div (-3) = -5$ $-15 \div 3 = -5$
If the number to be divided (or the top number of a fraction) is zero, the answer is zero. You cannot divide by zero; thus, the bottom number of a fraction cannot be zero.	$3 \div 0$ is undefined. $0 \div 3 = 0$

Algebraic Expressions

An algebraic expression is a group of numbers, unknowns, and arithmetic operations, like $3x - 2y$. This one may be translated as, "three times some number minus two times another number." To *evaluate* an algebraic expression, replace each variable with its value. For example, if $x = 5$ and $y = 4$, we would evaluate $3x - 2y$ as follows:

$$3(5) - 2(4) = 15 - 8 = 7$$

Even when signed numbers appear in an equation, the step-by-step solution works exactly as it does for positive numbers.

For example, let's solve $3x - 2y$ for $x = -5$ and $y = -8$.

1. Replace x with -5 and y with -8:
   $3(-5) - 2(-8)$
2. Perform the multiplication:
   $-15 - (-16)$
3. Turn the subtraction into an addition problem and complete:
   $-15 + 16 = 1$

Now try these problems with signed numbers.

_____ **97.** $-8x - 7 = 65$

_____ **98.** $-3x + 6 = -18$

_____ **99.** $-\frac{x}{4} + 3 = -7$

Evaluate these expressions.

_____ **100.** $4a + 3b$; $a = 2$ and $b = -1$

_____ **101.** $3mn - 4m + 2n$; $m = 3$ and $n = -3$

_____ **102.** $-2x - \frac{1}{2}y + 4z$; $x = 5$, $y = -4$, and $z = 6$

_____ **103.** The volume of a cylinder is given by the formula $V = \pi r^2 h$, where r is the radius of the base and h is the height of the cylinder. What is the volume of a cylinder with a base radius of 3 and height of 4? (Leave π in your answer.)

Squares and Square Roots

It's not uncommon to see squares and square roots on standardized math tests, especially on questions that involve right triangles.

To find the **square** of a number, multiply that number by itself. For example, the square of 4 is 16, because $4 \times 4 = 16$. Mathematically, this is expressed as:

$$4^2 = 16$$

4 squared equals 16.

To find the **square root** of a number, ask yourself, "What number times itself equals the given number?" For example, the square root of 16 is 4 because $4 \times 4 = 16$. Mathematically, this is expressed as:

$$\sqrt{16} = 4$$

The square root of 16 is 4.

Because certain squares and square roots tend to appear more often than others on standardized tests, the best course is to memorize the most common ones.

COMMON SQUARES AND SQUARE ROOTS					
SQUARES			**SQUARE ROOTS**		
$1^2 = 1$	$7^2 = 49$	$13^2 = 169$	$\sqrt{1} = 1$	$\sqrt{49} = 7$	$\sqrt{169} = 13$
$2^2 = 4$	$8^2 = 64$	$14^2 = 196$	$\sqrt{4} = 2$	$\sqrt{64} = 8$	$\sqrt{196} = 14$
$3^2 = 9$	$9^2 = 81$	$15^2 = 225$	$\sqrt{9} = 3$	$\sqrt{81} = 9$	$\sqrt{225} = 15$
$4^2 = 16$	$10^2 = 100$	$16^2 = 256$	$\sqrt{16} = 4$	$\sqrt{100} = 10$	$\sqrt{256} = 16$
$5^2 = 25$	$11^2 = 121$	$20^2 = 400$	$\sqrt{25} = 5$	$\sqrt{121} = 11$	$\sqrt{400} = 20$
$6^2 = 36$	$12^2 = 144$	$25^2 = 625$	$\sqrt{36} = 6$	$\sqrt{144} = 12$	$\sqrt{625} = 25$

You can multiply and divide square roots, but you cannot add or subtract them:

$$\sqrt{a} + \sqrt{b} \neq \sqrt{a+b} \qquad \sqrt{a} \times \sqrt{b} = \sqrt{a \times b}$$
$$\sqrt{a} - \sqrt{b} \neq \sqrt{a-b} \qquad \sqrt{\frac{a}{b}} = \frac{\sqrt{a}}{\sqrt{b}}$$

Use the previous rules to solve these problems in squares and square roots.

_____ **104.** $\sqrt{4} \times \sqrt{9} = ?$

_____ **105.** $\sqrt{\frac{16}{49}} = ?$

_____ **106.** $\sqrt{400} - \sqrt{64} = ?$

Parentheses and the Distributive Property

Another skill you'll need when working with algebraic equations is how to handle parentheses. When there is a number directly to the left or the right of parentheses, that means the items inside the parentheses are being multiplied by that number. The **distributive property** helps us to get rid of parentheses by allowing us to multiply the numbers on the inside by the number on the outside. It works like this:

$$5(y - 7 + 3w) = 5(y) - 5(7) + 5(3w)$$
$$= 5y - 35 + 15w$$
$$(11k - 13r)2 = 11k(2) - 13r(2) = 22k - 26r$$

It is a little more difficult to distribute a signed number, because you have to remember that the negative sign must be used in each step of multiplication:

$$-8(2 - 6h) = (-8)(2) - (-8)(6h) = -16 - (-48h)$$
$$= -16 + 48h$$

How to Solve an Equation

Example: $5 - 2(3x + 1) = 7x - 8$

1. Remove parentheses by distribution: $\qquad 5 - 6x - 2 = 7x - 8$

2. If there are like terms on the same side of the equals sign, combine them: $\quad 3 - 6x = 7x - 8$

3. Decide where you want all of the x terms. Put all the x terms on one side by addition and subtraction:

$$\underline{+\,6x = +\,6x}$$
$$3 = 13x - 8$$

4. Get all the constants on the other side by addition and subtraction:

$$3 = 13x - 8$$
$$\underline{+\,8 = \qquad +\,8}$$
$$11 = 13x$$

5. Solve for x:

$$\frac{11}{13} = \frac{\cancel{13}x}{\cancel{13}}$$
$$\frac{11}{13} = x$$

_____ **107.** $3(x + 5) = -9$

_____ **108.** $-2 - 4(7 - x) = 6x$

Geometry

Geometry questions cover points, lines, planes, angles, triangles, rectangles, squares, and circles. You may be asked to determine the area or perimeter of a particular shape, the measure of an angle, the length of a line, and so forth.

Points, Lines, and Planes
What Is a Point?

A point has position but no size or dimension. It is usually represented by a dot named with an uppercase letter:

•*A*

What Is a Line?

A line consists of an infinite number of points that extend endlessly in both directions.

A line can be named in two ways:

1. by a letter at one end (typically in lowercase): *l*

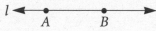

2. by two points on the line: $\overleftrightarrow{AB}$ or $\overleftrightarrow{BA}$

The following terminology is frequently used on math tests:

- Points are **collinear** if they lie on the same line. Points *J*, *U*, *D*, and *I* are collinear.

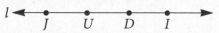

- A **line segment** is a section of a line with two endpoints. The line segment below is indicated as $\overline{AB}$.

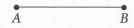

- The **midpoint** is a point on a line segment that divides it into two line segments of equal length. *M* is the midpoint of line segment *AB*.

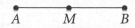

- Two line segments of the same length are said to be **congruent**. Congruent line segments are indicated by the same mark on each line segment.

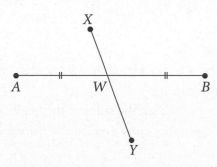

- A line segment (or line) that divides another line segment into two congruent line segments is said to **bisect** it. $\overline{XY}$ bisects $\overline{AB}$ since $\overline{AW}$ is congruent to $\overline{BW}$. (Congruency is shown by drawing hash marks of equal number through each segment, as can be seen here.)

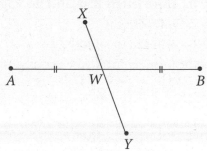

- A **ray** is a section of a line that has one endpoint. The ray below is indicated as $\overrightarrow{AB}$.

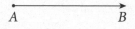

What Is a Plane?

A plane is like a flat surface with no thickness. Although a plane extends endlessly in all directions, it is usually represented by a four-sided figure and named by an uppercase letter in a corner of the plane: *K*.

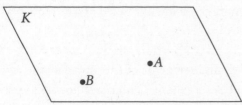

Points are *coplanar* if they lie on the same plane. Points *A* and *B* are coplanar.

Angles

An angle is formed when two lines, segments, or rays meet at a point:

The lines are called the **sides** of the angle, and the point where they meet is called the **vertex** of the angle.

The symbol used to indicate an angle is ∠.

There are three ways to name an angle:

- by the letter that labels the vertex: ∠*B*
- by the three letters that label the angle: ∠*ABC* or ∠*CBA*, with the vertex letter in the middle
- by the number inside the vertex: ∠1

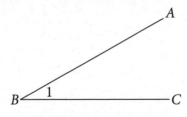

An angle's size is based on the opening between its sides. Size is measured in **degrees** (°). The smaller the angle, the fewer degrees it has. Angles are classified by size. Notice how the arc shows which of two angles is indicated:

Acute angle: less than 90°

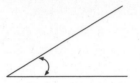

Right angle: exactly 90°

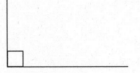

The little box indicates a right angle. A right angle is formed by two perpendicular lines.

Straight angle: exactly 180°

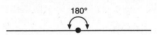

Obtuse angle: more than 90° and less than 180°

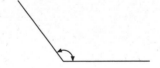

Special Angle Pairs

- **Congruent angles:** two angles that have the same degree measure.

Congruent angles are marked the same way.

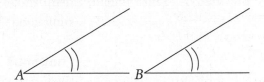

The symbol ≅ is used to indicate that two angles are congruent: ∠A ≅ ∠B.

- **Complementary angles:** two angles whose sum is 90°.

∠ABD and ∠DBC are **complementary** angles.

∠ABD is the **complement** of ∠DBC, and vice versa.

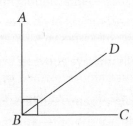

- **Supplementary angles:** two angles whose sum is 180°.

∠ABD and ∠DBC are **supplementary** angles.

∠ABD is the **supplement** of ∠DBC, and vice versa.

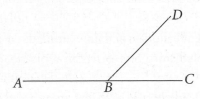

Hook: To prevent confusing complementary and supplementary:
C comes before S in the alphabet, and 90 comes before 180.

> Complementary: 90°
> Supplementary: 180°

- **Vertical angles:** two angles that are opposite each other when two lines cross.

Two sets of vertical angles are formed:
> ∠1 and ∠4
> ∠2 and ∠3

Vertical angles are congruent which means ∠1 ≅ ∠4 and ∠2 ≅ ∠3.

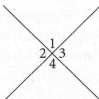

- When two lines cross, the **adjacent** angles (angles that are next to each other) are supplementary and combine to make a straight angle of 180°. The sum of all four angles is 360°.

Angle-pair problems tend to ask for an angle's complement or supplement.

Example: If the measure of ∠2 = 70°, what are the measures of the other three angles?

1. ∠2 ≅ ∠3 because they're vertical angles. Therefore, ∠3 = **70°**.
2. ∠1 and ∠2 are adjacent angles and therefore supplementary.
   Thus, ∠1 = **110°** (180° − 70° = 110°).
3. ∠1 ≅ ∠4 because they're also vertical angles.

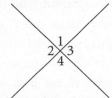

Therefore, ∠4 = **110°**.

Check: Add the angles to be sure their sum is 360°.

To solve geometry problems more easily, draw a picture if one is not provided. Try to draw the picture to scale. As the problem presents information about the size of an angle or line segment, label the corresponding part of your picture to reflect the given information. As you begin to find the missing information, label your picture accordingly.

These word problems require you to find the measures of angles.

_____ **109.** In order to paint the second story of his house, Alex leaned a ladder against the side of his house, making an acute angle of 58° with the ground. Find the size of the obtuse angle the ladder made with the ground.

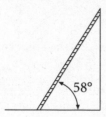

_____ **110.** Confusion Corner is an appropriately named intersection that confuses drivers unfamiliar with the area. Referring to the following street plan, find the size of the marked angle.

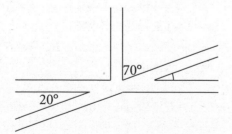

Special Line Pairs
Parallel Lines

Parallel lines lie in the same plane and don't cross at any point.

The arrowheads on the lines indicate that they are parallel. The symbol || is used to indicate that two lines are parallel: $l \parallel m$.

When two parallel lines are crossed by another line, two groups of four angles each are formed. One group consists of $\angle 1$, $\angle 2$, $\angle 3$, and $\angle 4$; the other group contains $\angle 5$, $\angle 6$, $\angle 7$, and $\angle 8$.

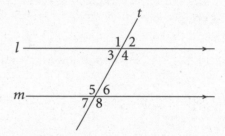

These angles have special relationships. The easiest way to remember these relationships is to recall that all the obtuse angles formed are congruent to each other, and all the acute angles formed are also congruent:

- The four obtuse angles are congruent: $\angle 1 \cong \angle 4 \cong \angle 5 \cong \angle 8$.
- The four acute angles are congruent: $\angle 2 \cong \angle 3 \cong \angle 6 \cong \angle 7$.
- The sum of any one acute angle and any one obtuse angle is 180° because the acute angles lie on the same line as the obtuse angles.

Don't be fooled into thinking two lines are parallel just because they look parallel. Either the lines must be marked with similar arrowheads or there must be an angle pair as just described.

Perpendicular Lines

Perpendicular lines lie in the same plane and cross to form four right angles.

The little box where the lines cross indicates a right angle. Because vertical angles are equal and the sum of all four angles is 360°, each of the four angles is a right angle. However, only one little box is needed to indicate this.

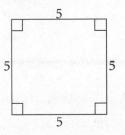

The symbol ⊥ is used to indicate that two lines are perpendicular: $\overleftrightarrow{AB} \perp \overleftrightarrow{CD}$.

Don't be fooled into thinking two lines are perpendicular just because they look perpendicular. The problem must indicate the presence of a right angle (by stating that an angle measures 90° or by the little right angle box in a corresponding diagram), or you must be able to prove the presence of a 90° angle.

Determine the measure of the marked angles.

_____ **111.**

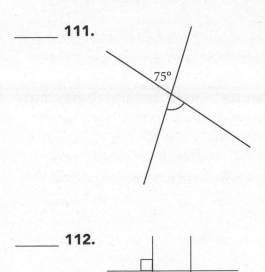

_____ **112.**

Polygons

A polygon is a closed, one-dimensional (flat) figure formed by three or more connected line segments that don't cross each other. Familiarize yourself with the following polygons; they are the four most common polygons appearing on standardized tests—and in life.

Triangle

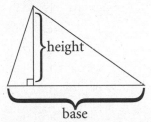

Three-sided polygon; the height is always the *perpendicular* line drawn from the base of the triangle to the opposite vertex.

Square

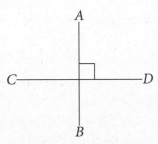

Four-sided polygon with four right angles; all sides are congruent (equal), and each pair of opposite sides is parallel.

Rectangle

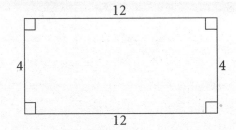

Four-sided polygon with four right angles; each pair of opposite sides is parallel and congruent.

Parallelogram

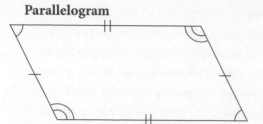

Four-sided polygon; opposite sides are both parallel and congruent, and opposite angles are also congruent.

Perimeter

Perimeter is the distance around a polygon. The word *perimeter* is derived from *peri*, which means around (as in *peri*scope and *peri*pheral vision), and *meter*, which means *measure*. Thus *perimeter* is the *measure around* something. There are many everyday applications of perimeter. For instance, a carpenter measures the perimeter of a room to determine how many feet of ceiling molding she needs. A farmer measures the perimeter of a field to determine how many feet of fencing he needs to surround it.

Perimeter is measured in length units, like feet, yards, inches, meters, and so on. It is usually represented by the letter *P*.

> To find the perimeter of a polygon, add the lengths of the sides.

Example: Find the perimeter of the polygon:

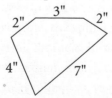

Write down the length of each side and add:

$$\begin{array}{r} 3 \text{ inches} \\ 2 \text{ inches} \\ 7 \text{ inches} \\ 4 \text{ inches} \\ + \ 2 \text{ inches} \\ \hline 18 \text{ inches} \end{array}$$

The perimeter *P* is 18 inches.

Find the perimeters for these word problems:

_____ **113.**

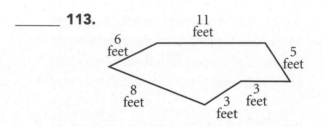

_____ **114.**

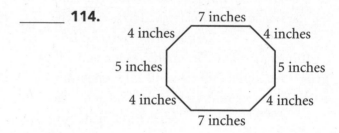

Area

Area is the amount of space taken by a figure's surface. Area is measured in square units.

For instance, a square that is 1 unit on all sides covers *1 square unit*. If the unit of measurement for each side is feet, for example, then the area is measured in *square feet*; other possibilities are units like square inches, square miles, square meters, and so on.

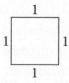

You could measure the area of any figure by counting the number of square units the figure occupies. The first two figures are easy to measure because the square units fit into them evenly, while the following two figures are more difficult to measure because the square units don't fit into them evenly.

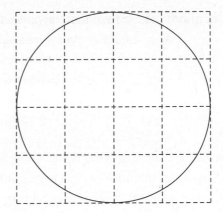

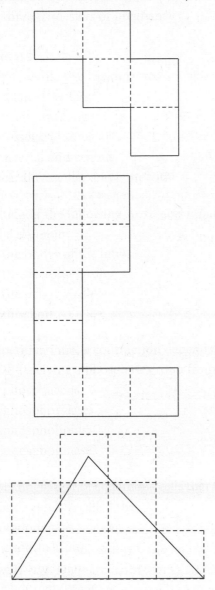

Because it's not always practical to measure a particular figure's area by counting the number of square units it occupies, an area formula is used. As each figure is discussed, you'll learn its area formula. Although there are perimeter formulas as well, you don't really need them as long as you understand that this perimeter is just the sum of the lengths of the sides. (The only perimeter formula you will need to learn is the one for circles, which is called circumference and will be introduced later.)

Triangles

A triangle is a polygon with three sides, like those shown here:

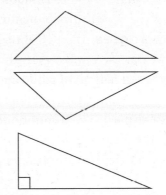

The symbol used to indicate a triangle is Δ. Each vertex—the point at which two lines meet—is named by a capital letter. The triangle is named by the three letters at the vertices, usually in alphabetical order: ΔABC.

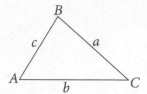

There are two ways to refer to a side of a triangle:

- by the letters at each end of the side: AB
- by the letter—typically a lowercase letter—next to the side: c

  (Notice that the name of the side is the same as the name of the angle opposite it, except the angle's name is a capital letter and the side's name is a lowercase letter.)

There are two ways to refer to an angle of a triangle:

- by the letter at the vertex: ∠A
- by the triangle's three letters, with that angle's vertex letter in the middle: ∠BAC or ∠CAB

Types of Triangles

Triangles can be classified in two ways: by the sizes of their angles or by the lengths of their sides.

Equilateral Triangle

- Three congruent angles, each 60°
- Three congruent sides

Hook to help you remember: The word *equilateral* comes from *equi*, meaning *equal*, and *lat*, meaning *side*. Thus, *all equal sides*.

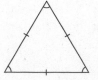

Isosceles Triangle

- 2 congruent angles, called *base angles*; the third angle is the *vertex angle*.
- Sides opposite the base angles are congruent.
- An equilateral triangle is also isosceles.

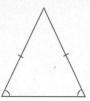

Right Triangle

- 1 right angle (90°), the largest angle in the triangle
- The side opposite the right angle is the *hypotenuse*, the longest side of the triangle. (**Hook:** The word *hypotenuse* reminds us of *hippopotamus*, a very large animal.)

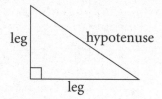

- The other two sides are called *legs*.

Area of a Triangle

To find the area of a triangle, use this formula:

$$A = \frac{1}{2}(bh)$$

Although any side of a triangle may be called its **base**, it's often easiest to use the side on the bottom. To use another side, rotate the page and view the triangle from another perspective.

A triangle's **height** is always the perpendicular line drawn from the angle opposite the base to the base. Depending on the triangle, the height may be inside, outside, or on the triangle. Notice the height of the second triangle: We extended the base to draw the height perpendicular to the base. The third triangle is a **right** triangle: One leg is used as the base and the other leg is its height, since the two legs form a 90° angle.

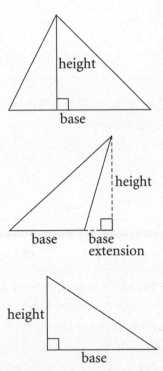

height
base

height
base   base extension

height
base

Hook: Think of a triangle as being half a rectangle. The area of that triangle is half the area of the rectangle.

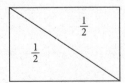

$\frac{1}{2}$
$\frac{1}{2}$

Example: Find the area of a triangle with a 2-inch base and a 3-inch height.

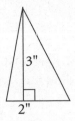

3"
2"

1. Draw the triangle as close to scale as you can.
2. Label the size of the base and height.
3. Write the area formula; then substitute the base and height numbers into it: $A = \frac{1}{2}(bh)$
4. The area of the triangle is **3 square inches.**

$$A = \frac{1}{2}(2 \times 3)$$
$$= \frac{1}{2} \times 6$$
$$A = 3$$

Find the area of the triangles.

_____ **115.**

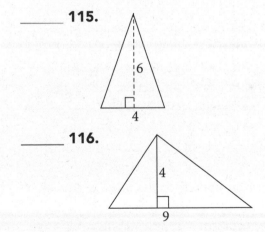

6
4

_____ **116.**

4
9

Triangle Rules

The following rules tend to appear more frequently on standardized tests than other rules. A typical test question follows each rule.

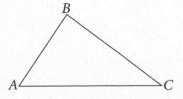

B
A   C

The sum of the angles in a triangle is 180°:
∠A + ∠B + ∠C = 180°

Example: One base angle of an isosceles triangle is 30°. Find the vertex angle.

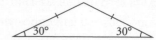

1. Draw a picture of an isosceles triangle. Drawing it to scale helps: Since it is an isosceles triangle, draw both base angles the same size (as close to 30° as you can) and make sure the sides opposite them are the same length. Label one base angle as 30°.
2. Since the base angles are congruent, label the other base angle as 30°.
3. There are two steps needed to find the vertex angle:
   ■ Add the two base angles together:
   30° + 30° = 60°
   ■ The sum of all three angles is 180°. To find the vertex angle, subtract the sum of the two base angles (60°) from 180°:
   180° − 60° = **120°**

Thus, the vertex angle is **120°**.

Check: Add all three angles together to make sure their sum is 180°:
30° + 30° + 120° = 180° ✔

The longest side of a triangle is opposite the largest angle. This rule implies that the second-longest side is opposite the second-largest angle, and the shortest side is opposite the shortest angle.

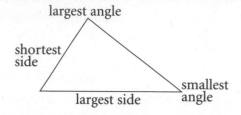

Example: In the triangle shown below, which side is the shortest?

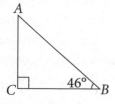

1. Determine the size of ∠A, the missing angle, by adding the two known angles and then subtracting their sum from 180°:
   90° + 46° = 136°.
   Thus, ∠A is 44°. 180° − 136° = 44°
2. Since ∠A is the smallest angle, side BC, which is opposite ∠A, is the shortest side.

Find the missing angles.

_____ **117.**

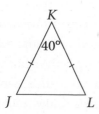

_____118.

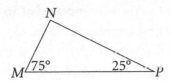

The Pythagorean Theorem

The Pythagorean theorem is a special rule about side lengths that applies only to *right* triangles. It states that the sum of the squares of the legs of a right triangle is equal to the square of the hypotenuse. The following formula shows how this is normally represented. (It is standard to label the hypotenuse as *c* and the legs as *a* and *b*, but a right triangle doesn't have to be labeled that way.)

> The *Pythagorean theorem:*
> $$a^2 + b^2 = c^2$$
> (*c* is the hypotenuse)

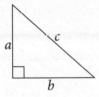

Example: What is the length of the missing side of the preceding triangle?

1. We find the length of the missing side by using the Pythagorean theorem:

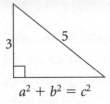

$$a^2 + b^2 = c^2$$

2. Side *c* is the hypotenuse because it is the side opposite the right triangle. Substitute the given sides for two of the letters: $a = 3$ and $c = 5$

$$3^2 + b^2 = 5^2$$
$$9 + b^2 = 25$$

3. To solve this equation, subtract 9 from both sides:

$$\frac{-9 \quad -9}{b^2 = 16}$$

4. Then, take the square root of both sides.
Thus, the missing side has a length of **4** units:

$$\sqrt{b^2} = \sqrt{16}$$

$$b = 4$$

Simplifying Radicals

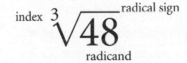

You often have to simplify square roots of numbers that are not perfect squares. Let's talk about how to simplify radicals of non-perfect squares. This will help you simplify square roots when applying the Pythagorean theorem.

A radical is in **simplified** form if there is no perfect square factor of the radicand, or number within the square root symbol.

In order to simplify a square root with a non-perfect square, rewrite the radicand as the product of two numbers, making sure that one of the numbers is a perfect square. (A perfect square is a number whose square root is a whole number.) Once the radicand is written as the product of a perfect square and a non-perfect square, the simplified radicand will be rewritten as the product of the square roots of the perfect square times the remaining non-perfect square, which is still in the radical sign.

Example: Simplify $\sqrt{50}$.

$$\sqrt{50} = \sqrt{25 \times 2} = \sqrt{25} \times \sqrt{2} = 5\sqrt{2}$$

Now simplify these radicals:

_____ **119.** $\sqrt{242}$

_____ **120.** $\sqrt{75}$

Perimeter of Right Triangles

Find the perimeter of the right triangle.

1. Use the Pythagorean theorem to find the length of the missing side. Let $a = 6$ and $c = 20$. We find the value of b.

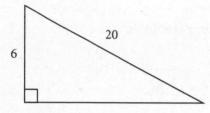

$a^2 + b^2 = c^2$
$6^2 + b^2 = 20^2$
$36 + b^2 = 400$
$b^2 = 364$
$b = \sqrt{364}$
$b = \sqrt{4} \times \sqrt{91}$
$b = 2\sqrt{91}$

2. Now, find the perimeter of the triangle. Add the length of all three sides. Add the whole numbers together. The radical term is not combined with the whole numbers because of the radicals. You can only add or subtract radical terms that have the same radical part.

$P = 6 + 20 + \sqrt{91}$
   $= 26 + 2\sqrt{91}$

The perimeter is $26 + 2\sqrt{91}$ units.

Find the perimeter and area of each triangle. **Hint:** Use the Pythagorean theorem.

_____ **121.**

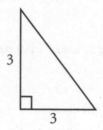

_____ **122.**

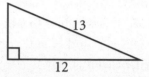

_____ **123.** Irene is fishing at the edge of a 40-foot-wide river, directly across from her friend Sam, who is fishing at the edge of the other side. Sam's friend Arthur is fishing 30 feet down the river from Sam. How far is Irene from Arthur?

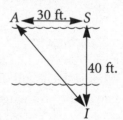

Quadrilaterals

A quadrilateral is a four-sided polygon. Following are three quadrilaterals that are most likely to appear on standardized tests (and in life):

Rectangle

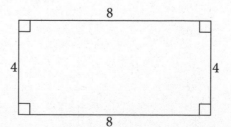

Square

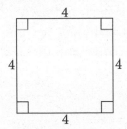

These quadrilaterals have something in common besides having four sides:

- Opposite sides are the same size and parallel.
- Opposite angles are congruent.

However, each quadrilateral has its own distinguishing characteristics:

Parallelogram

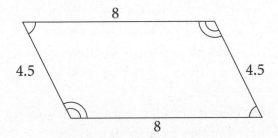

QUADRILATERALS			
	RECTANGLE	**SQUARE**	**PARALLELOGRAM**
SIDES	Adjacent sides are not necessarily the same length.	All four sides are the same size.	Adjacent sides are not necessarily the same length.
ANGLES	All the angles are right angles.	All the angles are right angles.	The opposite angles are the same size, but they don't have to be right angles. (A rectangle leaning to one side is a parallelogram.)

Rhombus

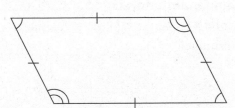

Four-sided polygon with two pairs of opposite and parallel sides, two pairs of opposite and congruent angles, and four congruent sides.

Trapezoid

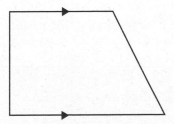

Four-sided polygon with exactly one pair of opposite parallel sides.

Isosceles Trapezoid

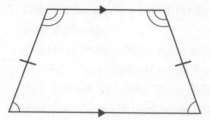

Trapezoid whose nonparallel sides (called legs) are congruent. The two obtuse angles are congruent and the two acute angles are congruent.

The naming conventions for quadrilaterals are similar to those for triangles:

- The figure is named by the letters at its four consecutive corners, usually in alphabetic order: rectangle *ABCD*.
- A side is named by the letters at its ends: side *AB*.
- An angle is named by its vertex letter: $\angle A$.

The sum of the angles of a quadrilateral is 360°: $\angle A + \angle B + \angle C + \angle D = 360°$

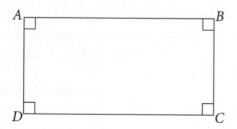

Perimeter of Quadrilaterals

To find the perimeter of a quadrilateral, follow this simple rule:

$$P = \text{Sum of all four sides}$$

Shortcut: Take advantage of the fact that the opposite sides of a rectangle and a parallelogram are equal: Just add two adjacent sides and double the sum. Similarly, multiply one side of a square by four.

Sometimes perimeter formulas are necessary if you are given the perimeter of a shape and need to work backward to solve for one of the side lengths. The formulas for the area of a rectangle and the area of a square look like this:

$$\text{Perimeter of square} = 4s$$
$$(\text{where } s = \text{side length})$$
$$\text{Perimeter of rectangle/parallelogram} =$$
$$2l + 2w \text{ (where } l = \text{length and } w = \text{width})$$

Here are some word problems on perimeters of quadrilaterals:

_____ **124.** What is the length of a side of a square room whose perimeter is 58 feet?
- **a.** 8 feet
- **b.** 14 feet
- **c.** 14.5 feet
- **d.** 29 feet
- **e.** 232 feet

_____ **125.** Find the dimensions of a rectangle with a perimeter of 16 feet and whose long side is three times its short side.
- **a.** 4 ft. by 4 ft.
- **b.** 4 ft. by 12 ft.
- **c.** 3 ft. by 5 ft.
- **d.** 2 ft. by 6 ft.
- **e.** 2 ft. by 8 ft.

Area of Certain Quadrilaterals

To find the area of a rectangle, square, or parallelogram, use this formula:

$$A = bh$$

The **base** is the size of one of the sides. It is easiest if you call the side on the bottom the base, but any side can be a base. The **height** (or **altitude**) is the length of the perpendicular line drawn from the base to the side opposite it. The height of a rectangle and a square is the same as the size of its non-base side.

Rectangle

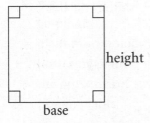

Square

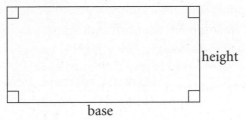

Caution: A parallelogram's height is not the same as the length connecting the base to its opposite side (called the *slant height*), but the size of a perpendicular line drawn from the base to the side opposite it.

Example: Find the area of a rectangle with a base of 4 meters and a height of 3 meters.

1. Draw the rectangle as close to scale as possible.
2. Label the size of the base and height.
3. Write the area formula; then substitute the base and height numbers into it: $A = bh$
$A = 4 \times 3 = 12$
Thus, the area is **12 square meters**.

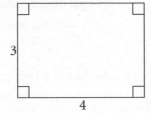

Now try some area word problems:

_____ **126.** Tristan is laying 12-inch-by-18-inch tiles on the laboratory floor. If the lab measures 15 feet by 18 feet, how many tiles does Tristan need, assuming there's no waste? (Hint: Do *all* your work in either feet or inches.)
  a. 12 tiles
  b. 120 tiles
  c. 180 tiles
  d. 216 tiles
  e. 270 tiles

_____ **127.** A rectangular operating room has an area of 63 square meters. Its width is 7 meters. What is the length of the operating room?
  a. 70 meters
  b. 9 meters
  c. 18 meters
  d. 49 meters
  e. 7 meters

Circles

We can all recognize a circle when we see one, but its definition is a bit technical. A **circle** is a set of points that are all the same distance from a given point called the **center**. The distance from the center point to the outside of the circle is called the **radius**. The **diameter** is twice the length of the radius; it passes through the center of the circle.

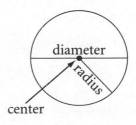

Circumference

The **circumference** (*C*) of a circle is the distance around the circle (it is the perimeter of the circle). To determine the circumference of a circle, use either of these two equivalent formulas:

$$C = 2\pi r$$
$$\text{or}$$
$$C = \pi d$$

- *r* is the radius
- *d* is the diameter
- π is approximately equal (denoted by the symbol $\approx$) to 3.14 or $\frac{22}{7}$

Note: Math often uses letters of the Greek alphabet, like π (pi). Perhaps that's what makes math seem like Greek to some people! In the case of the circle, you can use π as a hook to recognize a circle question: A *pie* is shaped like a circle.

Example: Find the circumference of a circle whose radius is 7 inches.

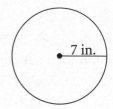

7 in.

1. Draw this circle and write the radius version of the circumference formula (because you're given the radius): $C = 2\pi r$
2. Substitute 7 for the radius: $C = 2(\pi)7$
3. On a multiple-choice test, look at the answer choices to determine whether to leave π in your answer or substitute the value of π in the formula.

If the answer choices don't include π, substitute $\frac{22}{7}$ or 3.14 for π and multiply:

$$C = 2 \times \frac{22}{7} \times 7;$$
$$C \approx \mathbf{44}$$
$$C = 2 \times 3.14 \times 7;$$
$$C \approx \mathbf{43.96}$$

If the answer choices include π, just multiply:

$$C = 2 \times \pi \times 7;$$
$$C = \mathbf{14\pi}$$

All the answers—**44 inches, 43.96 inches,** and **14π inches**—are considered correct.

Example: What is the diameter of a circle with a circumference of 62.8 centimeters? Use 3.14 for π.

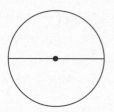

1. Draw a circle with its diameter and write the diameter version of the circumference formula (because you're asked to find the diameter):
   $C = \pi d$
2. Substitute 62.8 for the circumference, 3.14 for π, and solve the equation:
   $$62.8 = 3.14d$$
   $$\frac{62.8}{3.14} = \frac{31.4d}{3.14} \text{ (divide both sides by 3.14)}$$
   $$20 = d$$
   So the diameter is equal to 20 centimeters.

These word problems require you to find the circumference:

_____ **128.** What is the circumference of a circular room whose diameter is 15 feet?
   a. 7.5π ft.
   b. 15π ft.
   c. 30π ft.
   d. 45π ft.
   e. 225π ft.

_____ **129.** What is the approximate circumference of a round tower whose radius is $3\frac{2}{11}$ feet?
  a. 10 ft.
  b. 20 ft.
  c. 33 ft.
  d. 40 ft.
  e. 48 ft.

_____ **130.** Find the circumference of a water pipe whose radius is 1.2 inches.
  a. 1.2π in.
  b. 1.44π in.
  c. 2.4π in.
  d. 12π in.
  e. 24π in.

Area of Circles

The **area** of a circle is the space its surface occupies. To determine the area of a circle, use this formula:

$$A = \pi r^2$$

Hook: To avoid confusing the area and circumference formulas, just remember that *area* is always measured in *square* units, like 12 *square yards* of carpeting. Thus, the *area* formula is the one with the *squared* term in it.

  Example: Find the area of the circle below, rounded to the nearest tenth:

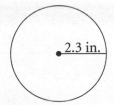
2.3 in.

1. Write the area formula: $A = \pi r^2$
2. Substitute 2.3 for the radius: $A = \pi \times 2.3^2$
3. On a multiple-choice test, look at the answer choices to determine whether to use π or an approximate *value of* π (decimal or fraction) in the formula.

If the answers don't include π, use 3.14 for π (because the radius is a decimal): $A = 3.14 \times 2.3 \times 2.3$ $A = 16.6$
If the answers include π, multiply and round: $A = \pi \times 2.3 \times 2.3$ $A = 5.3\pi$

Both answers—**16.6 square inches** and **5.3π square inches**—are correct.

  Example: What is the diameter of a circle with an area of 9π square centimeters?

1. Draw a circle with its diameter (to help you remember that the question asks for the diameter); then write the area formula: $A = \pi r^2$
2. Substitute 9π for the area and solve the equation: $9\pi = \pi r^2$ $9 = r^2$

Since the radius is 3 centimeters, the diameter is **6 centimeters**. $3 = r$

Try these word problems on the area of a circle:

_____ **131.** What is the area in square inches of the bottom of a beaker with a diameter of 6 inches?
  a. 6π square inches
  b. 9π square inches
  c. 12π square inches
  d. 18π square inches
  e. 36π square inches

_____ **132.** A hospital serves the residents living within a 12-mile radius of the hospital. What is the approximate area, in square miles, of the region served by the hospital?
  a. 144 square miles
  b. 452 square miles
  c. 24 square miles
  d. 48 square miles
  e. 113 square miles

_____ **133.** If a circular parking lot covers an area of 2,826 square feet, what is the size of its radius? (Use 3.14 for π.)

a. 30 ft.
b. 60 ft.
c. 90 ft.
d. 450 ft.
e. 900 ft.

Answers to Math Problems

Word Problems

1. a.
2. e.
3. b.
4. e.

Fractions

5. $\frac{1}{4}$
6. $\frac{2}{5}$
7. $\frac{3}{8}$
8. 10
9. 6
10. 200
11. $\frac{29}{30}$
12. $\frac{55}{24}$ or $2\frac{7}{24}$
13. $7\frac{1}{4}$
14. $\frac{2}{15}$
15. $\frac{1}{8}$
16. $\frac{19}{12}$ or $1\frac{7}{12}$
17. a.
18. b.
19. $\frac{2}{15}$
20. $\frac{8}{35}$
21. $\frac{2}{3}$
22. $\frac{26}{15}$ or $1\frac{11}{15}$
23. 15
24. $\frac{33}{2}$ or $16\frac{1}{2}$
25. b.
26. e.
27. c.
28. $\frac{1}{2}$

29. $5\frac{1}{2}$

30. $\frac{1}{5}$

31. $\frac{29}{46}$

32. a.

33. d.

34. b.

Decimals

35. $\frac{1}{80}$

36. $3\frac{12}{25}$

37. $123\frac{456}{1,000}$ or $123\frac{57}{125}$

38. 908.095

39. 0.907

40. 1.456

41. b.

42. d.

43. 0.03

44. 0.3392

45. 0.70104

46. e.

47. e.

48. 1.4

49. 128

50. 572

51. 1,400

52. b.

53. c.

Percents

54. 45%

55. 0.8%

56. 16.9%

57. 0.12

58. 0.875

59. 2.5

60. 12.5% or $12\frac{1}{2}$%

61. 52%

62. $58.\overline{3}$% or $58\frac{1}{3}$%

63. $\frac{19}{20}$

64. $\frac{3}{8}$

65. $\frac{5}{4}$ or $1\frac{1}{4}$

66. $\frac{1}{4}$ or 0.25

67. 9.1

68. 267

69. 75

70. 50%

71. $33\frac{1}{3}$%

72. 300%

73. 100

74. 8

75. 10

76. c.

77. c.

78. c.

79. d.

Averages
80. c.
81. c.
82. b.

Length and Time
83. 24
84. 30
85. 1,600
86. 2.94
87. 8 ft.
88. 21 km 170 m
89. 1 ft. 4 in.
90. 7 cm 8 mm
91. d.
92. e.
93. d.

Algebra
94. $x = 7$
95. $x = 6$
96. 28
97. $x = -9$
98. 8
99. 40
100. 5
101. -45
102. 16
103. 36π
104. 6
105. $\frac{4}{7}$
106. 12
107. $x = -8$
108. $x = -15$

Geometry
109. 122°
110. 20°
111. 75°
112. 91° (The horizontal lines are not parallel.)
113. 36 feet
114. 40 inches
115. 12 square units
116. 18 square units
117. $\angle J = \angle L = 70°$
118. $\angle N = 80°$
119. $11\sqrt{2}$
120. $5\sqrt{3}$
121. Perimeter = $6 + 3\sqrt{2}$ units
   Area = 4.5 square units
122. Perimeter = 30 units
   Area = 30 square units
123. 50 feet
124. c.
125. d.
126. c.
127. b.
128. b.
129. b.
130. c.
131. b.
132. b.
133. a.

7 ▶ BIOLOGY REVIEW

CHAPTER SUMMARY
This chapter reviews the key biology concepts tested by health occupations entrance exams. After surveying the important concepts and testing yourself with the sample questions in this chapter, you will know where to concentrate further studies.

Biology Review: Important Concepts

I. General Introduction

A. Description of How Health Occupations Entrance Exams Test Biology
Health occupations entrance exams do not measure scientific knowledge in the same way. The natural sciences section of the Health Occupations Aptitude Exam (HOAE) is made up of approximately 65 multiple-choice questions, which can include biology questions. Other entrance exams, like the Health Occupations Basic Entrance Test (HOBET), require only that you can read and understand college-level scientific material and identify key scientific concepts. It does not contain a separate test section on biology.

The following subject areas are important for you to know for your entrance exam: cell biology, heredity, human structure and function, bacteria and viruses, and plants.

B. How to Use This Chapter
This chapter includes major biology concepts you will encounter on the exam. There is also a section on other content areas that will be helpful to you in taking the test: the scientific method, the origin of life, a brief description of taxonomic classification systems, and the social behavior of animals. The general discussions in this

chapter, lists of terms and concepts, and "You Should Review" sections are meant to guide you in your studies—*they are not exhaustive* and must be supplemented with a good college textbook, a reliable medical dictionary and dictionary of biology, and a fair amount of general reading on the subject.

After each main subject heading in this chapter, you will find several sample questions that represent the content and level of difficulty of the questions that will appear on the test. You should first read through the outline and try to answer the sample questions, and then make notes on those areas in which you need more work. After that, you will want to go to your source material and review all subject areas, with special emphasis on those areas where you feel least confident.

Allow yourself plenty of time to prepare before the exam. Remember that thorough preparation is the most important factor in test-taking success. By studying and taking practice tests, you become familiar with subject areas and typical test questions, boosting your ability to do your best on the exam.

II. Main Topics

A. Cell Biology
1. Definition of a Cell
The cell is the structural and functional unit of life. **The cell theory**, generally credited to Schleiden (1838) and Schwann (1839), maintains that

- All living things are made up of cells and the products formed by cells.
- Cells are the basic units of structure and function.
- All cells arise from preexisting cells.

2. Two Types of Cells
a. Prokaryotic Cells
Prokaryotic cells: cells found only in bacteria and archaea. These cells lack a true nucleus and other subcellular structures called organelles.

b. Eukaryotic Cells
Eukaryotic cells: cells found in all organisms except bacteria and archaea. These cells contain organelles, including a nucleus.

3. Organization of a Cell
Cells contain specialized structures, and each serves a specific purpose.

Nucleus: The membrane-enclosed organelle that houses the genetic material in eukaryotic cells. Prokaryotic cells do not have a nucleus.

Organelle: A specialized compartment within a cell that is designed to perform a specific function. Only eukaryotes possess organelles.

Cell membrane: A primarily phospholipid boundary that separates the cell interior from its exterior. Found in all types of cells.

Cytoplasm: The material inside the cell membrane of a cell but outside of the nucleus. In eukaryotes, the cytoplasm includes the organelles (except the nucleus) and the liquid that surrounds them. In prokaryotes, the cytoplasm includes everything inside the cell membrane.

Chromosome: A long threadlike structure carrying genes in a linear sequence, consisting of DNA and protein. Human beings possess 46 chromosomes. In eukaryotes, chromosomes are found in the nucleus. The chromosome in prokaryotes forms a circular coil known as a plasmid.

Ribosomes: Responsible for protein assembly. The ribosome receives messenger RNA (mRNA) and translates it into proteins. Found in all types of cells.

Cell wall: A semirigid outer layer that lies outside the cell membrane. It gives structural support and protection to the cell. Cell walls are found in plant, bacterial, fungal, and algal cells.

Mitochondria: The "power plant" of the cell. The mitochondria are responsible for generating most of the cell's energy (in the form of ATP). Found in eukaryotes.

Chloroplasts: The organelle responsible for photosynthesis. Chloroplasts contain machinery that allows them to extract energy from light and convert it to ATP or to convert carbon dioxide to sugars, releasing oxygen.

Golgi apparatus: The organelle responsible for packaging and processing complex macromolecules before they are shipped to other parts of the cell. Found in eukaryotes.

Lysosomes: Organelles found primarily in animal cells and in some plant cells as well. Lysosomes are compartments that envelop and destroy waste materials within the cell.

Vacuoles: Compartments in the cell that store and isolate various items depending on a cell's needs. These organelles are found primarily in plant cells, but may also be observed in other organisms.

Cilia: Finger-like projections found in eukaryotes that primarily serve as sensors for the cell. In more complex organisms, cilia along multiple cells can also be used to transport small particles—for example, to sweep particles out of the trachea.

Flagella: Similar to cilia, flagella are tail-like structures that protrude from the cell and are used to control the motion of the cell. Found in prokaryotes and eukaryotes.

Centrioles: Found in animal cells, these organelles aid in the process of cell division.

	PROKARYOTES	EUKARYOTES	
	BACTERIA AND ARCHAEA	PLANTS	ANIMALS
Nucleus		✔	✔
Organelle		✔	✔
Cell membrane	✔	✔	✔
Cytoplasm	✔	✔	✔
Chromosome(s)	✔	✔	✔
Ribosomes	✔	✔	✔
Cell wall	✔	✔	
Mitochondria		✔	✔
Chloroplasts		✔	
Endoplasmic reticulum		✔	✔
Golgi apparatus		✔	✔
Lysosomes		✔	✔
Vacuoles		✔	✔
Cilia			✔
Flagella	✔		✔
Centrioles		✔	✔

4. Energy Transformation in a Cell
a. General Discussion of Energy

The two concepts most basic to science are **matter** and **energy**.

> **Matter:** anything that has mass and takes up space (volume)
>
> **Energy:** the capacity to do work

There are two types of energy: **kinetic** and **potential**.

> **Kinetic energy:** the energy an object possesses due to its motion
>
> **Potential energy:** the energy stored in a system (e.g., in the chemical bonds of ATP or in a compressed spring)

b. Thermodynamics

> **Thermodynamics:** the physics of what is and is not possible with regard to energy.
>
> > **First law of thermodynamics:** Energy can be transferred and transformed, but it cannot be created or destroyed (conservation of energy).
> >
> > **Second law of thermodynamics:** Every energy transfer or transformation results in the release of heat from the system to the rest of the universe.

c. Cell Metabolism

> **Cell metabolism:** energy management by a cell. Many metabolic reactions occur within a cell, aided by enzymes.
>
> **Bioenergetics:** the study of how organisms manage energy, including heat production and transfer; and regulation of body temperature (endothermy and ectothermy).
>
> **Metabolism:** the totality of chemical reactions that take place in an organism.
>
> **Anabolism:** the metabolic synthesis of proteins, fats, etc., from simpler molecules; requires energy in the form of adenosine triphosphate (ATP).

> **Catabolism:** the metabolic breakdown of molecules (for example, respiration).
>
> **Cellular respiration:** a catabolic pathway for the production of ATP, in which oxygen is sometimes consumed along with an organic fuel (food). At other times, the process proceeds without atmospheric oxygen, but this is less efficient.
>
> - **Anaerobic pathway of cellular respiration:** Food (especially carbohydrates) is partially oxidized and chemical energy is released; however, atmospheric oxygen is not involved in the process.
> - **Aerobic pathway of cellular respiration:** Food is completely oxidized to carbon dioxide and water, and chemical energy is released; atmospheric oxygen is involved in the process. The Krebs cycle, electron-transport chain, and oxidative phosphorylation are important concepts here.
>
> **Photosynthesis:** conversion of light energy into chemical energy, on which, directly or indirectly, all living things depend. Photosynthesis occurs in plants, algae, and certain prokaryotes.

d. Enzymology

> **Enzymology:** the study of the speed of the transformation of energy in a cell; enzymes are biological catalysts that accelerate the rate of a reaction without themselves being consumed by that reaction.

e. Movement of Molecules

Small molecules are steadily transported across the cell membrane. Types of transport include **diffusion** and **passive transport**; **osmosis** (a special case of passive transport); and **active transport**.

5. Cell Reproduction
a. General Discussion of Cell Reproduction

All cells arise from other cells. The basis of all biological reproduction is cell division. A single, intact chain of life extends backward from today to the first bacteria on Earth.

Prokaryotes often reproduce by binary fission, or division into identical halves. Eukaryotes have much more complicated genomes, and therefore, the process of reproduction is more complex.

b. The Cell Cycle

The cell cycle describes the entire reproductive life cycle of a cell and occurs in an orderly sequence. The cell cycle can be divided into interphase, where most time is spent, and M phase, where cell mitosis (division) occurs. Each of these phases can be divided into smaller components. When not dividing or preparing to divide, the cell exists in a resting state, known as G0 phase. G0 phase follows cell division.

c. Interphase

Interphase is the time when the cell grows, takes in nutrients, and copies its DNA. It can be divided into three shorter phases.

G1 phase: The point in the cell life cycle where most cell growth occurs, organelles are synthesized, and nutrients are collected. Only when certain safeguards are met will the cell move on to the next phase. The boundary between the G1 and S phases is called the restriction point because the safeguards here can restrict abnormal cells from dividing.

S phase: Chromosomes are replicated. During this phase, minimal RNA transcription takes place.

G2 phase: The last phase before mitosis. Critical machinery is manufactured within the cell to enable cell division to occur. At the end of G2 phase, M phase begins.

d. M phase

It is during M phase that division of the nucleus and cytoplasm occurs (replication of the chromosomes was completed during the S phase of interphase).

Mitosis: division of the nucleus; distribution of nuclear materials, particularly

chromosomes. For descriptive purposes, mitosis is divided into phases: prophase, metaphase, anaphase, and telophase.

Prophase: DNA fibers (chromatin) condense into chromosomes, the nuclear envelope breaks down, and spindles begin to form at the poles of the cell.

Metaphase: Chromosomes align at the center of the cell.

Anaphase: Chromosomes split, and sister chromatids separate to opposite poles of the cell.

Telophase: Nuclear envelopes re-form around separated sister chromatids.

Cytokinesis: Division of the cytoplasm into two identical daughter cells, which occurs during the telophase stage of mitosis.

e. Control of Cell Division

A certain timing and rate of division are necessary to normal growth. Cell division can be interfered with by lack of nutrients, poisons, lack of growth factors (for example, platelet-derived growth factor or PDGF), cell size, and density.

f. When Things Go Wrong

In abnormal cell division (e.g., cancer), cells do not heed the restriction point; they may divide excessively, invading surrounding tissue. If given enough nutrients, they may divide "forever" (see "immortal" or HeLa cells); or abnormal cells may stop dividing at any point in the cell cycle, not just at the restriction point.

You Should Review

- the structure and function of prokaryotic and eukaryotic cells; comparison of the two
- the composition, structure, and function of organelles: nucleus (chromosomes and nucleolus); ribosomes; rough endoplasmic reticulum; smooth endoplasmic reticulum; Golgi apparatus; lysosomes; peroxisomes; central vacuole in plants; mitochondria; chloroplasts in plants and some protists; cytoskeleton; cell wall in

plants, fungi, and some protists; glycocalyx in animals; and intercellular junctions
- cell membrane structure and function
- major features of bioorganic molecules; makeup of amino acids; genetic code (codons) for amino acids
- why compartmental organization is important in eukaryotic cells and an understanding of the way in which the various compartments inter-relate—i.e., how organelles "cooperate"
- biological membranes and the importance of their selective permeability; the fluid mosaic model of cell membrane structure; structure and function of lipids, proteins, and carbohydrates
- differences between organelles of cells found in organisms in the various kingdoms. (For more on classification of living organisms, see page 183.)
- properties of energy
- heat production and transfer mechanisms in various species; regulation of body temperature
- ATP: structure and hydrolysis; how it performs; regeneration from ADP and phosphate; metabolic disequilibrium; ATP synthases
- metabolic map—the catabolic and anabolic pathways
- control of metabolism: feedback inhibition
- how body size affects metabolic rate
- enzymes (most of which are proteins): six major groups (oxidoreductases, transferases, hydrolases, lyases, isomerases, ligases) and the ways in which the various classes work; molecular structure; how enzymes function as biological catalysts; types and shapes of active sites; response to environmental conditions; enzyme inhibitors
- coenzymes, especially vitamins: classifications and functions
- cellular respiration
- basic mechanisms of prokaryotic and eukaryotic cell reproduction
- the cell cycle

- how cell division is controlled
- main features of abnormal cell division
- the following terms and concepts (among others): genome, haploid nucleus, diploid nucleus, chromatin, chromosome, centriole, atrophy, karyolysis, nucleic acid (especially DNA and RNA), pyrimidines (cytosine, thymine, uracil), purines (guanine and adenine), nucleotide, transcription, translation, meiosis (do not confuse with mitosis), basal metabolic rate

Questions

1. Most of a cell membrane's specific functions are controlled by
   a. lipids.
   b. proteins.
   c. plasma.
   d. nitrogen.

2. The basic method by which chloroplasts and mitochondria generate ATP is
   a. oxidation.
   b. photorespiration.
   c. respiration.
   d. chemiosmosis.

3. Which of the following regions exists just outside the nuclear membrane of most animal cells?
   a. the centrosome
   b. the equatorial plane
   c. the organelle
   d. the pellicle

4. The decay of a leaf after it falls from a tree indicates an increase in its
   a. ecological efficiency.
   b. entropy.
   c. metabolic disequilibrium.
   d. estivation.

5. The sodium-potassium pump is an example of
  a. passive transport.
  b. active transport.
  c. osmosis.
  d. diffusion.

6. Phagocytosis is a form of
  a. hydrolysis.
  b. exocytosis.
  c. glycolysis.
  d. endocytosis.

7. Which of the following is found in both plant and animal cells?
  a. chloroplasts
  b. centrioles
  c. flagella
  d. ribosomes

8. Which of the following is the electron acceptor in fermentation?
  a. pyridoxine
  b. pyruvate
  c. pyrimidine
  d. pyrrole

9. The small spherical bodies within a cell where proteins are assembled according to genetic instructions are called
  a. mitochondria.
  b. ribosomes.
  c. Golgi apparatus.
  d. lysosomes.

10. The resting or G0 phase of a cell happens after
  a. anaphase.
  b. interphase.
  c. cell division.
  d. G2 phase.

Answers

1. b. Although a cell membrane's main fabric is made of lipids, its specific functions are largely determined by proteins.

2. d. Chemiosmosis is the term used for this process. It is important to cellular work, including ATP synthesis.

3. a. The centrosome (also called the microtubule-organizing center) is found in all eukaryotic cells and is important during cell division.

4. b. Entropy (symbol S) is the quantitative measure of a system's disorder or randomness. As systems—whether houses, people, leaves, or stars—break down and undergo irreversible changes, making less energy available to them, their entropy increases.

5. b. In active transport, the cell provides energy to move substances across a membrane. The sodium-potassium pump is an example of active transport. The sodium-potassium pump uses the energy of ATP to move potassium ions into a cell and sodium ions out of a cell.

6. d. Phagocytosis and pinocytosis are both forms of endocytosis, the process by which materials enter a cell without passing through the cell membrane.

7. d. Chloroplasts are found in plant cells, but not animal cells. Flagella and centrioles are found in animal cells, but not plant cells. Ribosomes are found in both plant and animal cells.

8. b. Pyruvate is the correct answer. Under anaerobic conditions, like fermentation, it is converted to lactate or ethanol.

9. b. The ribosome is the site of protein synthesis.

10. c. A cell enters the resting or G0 phase when it is not dividing or preparing to divide, which occurs after cell division.

B. Heredity

1. Pre-Mendelian Concepts

Before Mendel's discoveries, theories included averages or blending of colors like the mixing of paints; physical characteristics carried only by the male; characteristics carried by blood; small human grown large; pangenesis; and others.

2. Mendelian Inheritance

a. Mendel's Experiments

Gregor Mendel, the father of classical genetics, was an Austrian monk who, in a small monastery, tended a little garden and did experiments on garden peas, which have great variety. He allowed pure strains (one with purple flowers, one with white) to either self-pollinate or cross-pollinate, strictly controlling the parentage. Cross-pollinated breeds (hybrids) of purple and white flowers showed all purple flowers in the first generation. But when the second generation self-pollinated, the white trait reappeared. Through his work, the theory of dominant and recessive traits was formed.

b. Mendel's Major Discoveries

Mendel found that no averages or blendings take place; instead, particular characteristics are retained, which are either dominant or recessive. Today, we know the mechanisms: genes and chromosomes, made up of DNA.

3. Chromosomal Genetics

Not all of a eukaryotic cell's genes are located on nuclear chromosomes—some are found in cytoplasmic organelles.

a. Genes and Chromosomes

Gene: a discrete heritable unit of information located on the chromosomes and made up of DNA

Chromosome: a long threadlike structure carrying genes in a linear sequence, found in the nucleus of eukaryotic cells, consisting of DNA (which stores or contains genetic information) and protein. Human beings possess 46 chromosomes; the ovum and sperm each contain 23, of which 22 are autosomes and one is a sex chromosome.

Chromatin: the substance that composes eukaryotic chromosomes, consisting mostly of proteins, DNA, and RNA

Chromatid: a threadlike strand formed as a chromosome condenses during the early stages of cell division

Character (or trait): a heritable feature; for each character, an organism inherits two genes

Genome: all the genes contained in a single set of chromosomes; an organism's genetic material

Autosome: a chromosome not directly involved in determining sex

Alleles: alternative versions of a gene, one from each parent. The existence of alleles explains why there is variation in inherited traits. An expressed trait is determined by two alleles. A dominant allele is fully expressed in the organism's appearance; a recessive allele has no noticeable effect unless two recessive alleles are inherited, in which case, the recessive trait will be expressed. For some traits, there is incomplete dominance.

Phenotype: an organism's appearance; its observable, physical and physiological traits; often depends on environment as well as genes

Genotype: an organism's genetic makeup (which is not always apparent), its genetic composition; the combination of alleles it possesses

b. Punnett Square

A **Punnett square** is a convenient tool for determining possible genotypes and phenotypes when two organisms with known genotypes are crossed. For example, if two blue flowers with a heterozygous genotype—one dominant blue allele (B) and one recessive white allele (b)—are crossed, the offspring can have one of three genotypes with the following probabilities: BB (25%), Bb (50%), or bb (25%). There is a 75% chance the offspring will carry a blue phenotype.

	B	b
B	BB	Bb
b	Bb	bb

c. DNA and RNA

DNA (deoxyribonucleic acid): a double-stranded, helical nucleic acid molecule capable of replicating. DNA makes up the genetic material of most living organisms and plays a central role in determining heredity.

RNA (ribonucleic acid): a single-stranded nucleic acid molecule involved in protein synthesis, the structure of which is specified by DNA. Messenger RNA (mRNA) is responsible for carrying the genetic code transcribed from DNA to specialized sites within a cell (ribosomes) where the information is translated into amino acids, the building blocks of proteins.

4. Molecular and Human Genetics
a. Molecular Genetics

Molecular genetics is a specialized type of molecular biology, concerned with the analysis of genes.

b. Human Genetics

Because human beings are much more complex organisms than the ones Mendel studied, and because experimental breeding of humans is socially unacceptable, study of human genetics must be done by analyzing the results of matings that have already occurred. This is done by examining the pedigree of the subjects involved—the interrelationships of parents and children across generations—and constructing a pedigree chart to study both past and future. Through the study of pedi-

grees, one can analyze genetic traits, from harmless (such as eye color and texture of hair) to harmful or lethal (such as the diseases discussed in the next section). Various tests for genetic defects are also useful in the study of human genetics.

5. Treatment of Genetic Diseases and Genetic Engineering
a. Genetic Diseases

Although most harmful alleles are recessive, some genetic combinations can lead to lethal conditions. Examples are Huntington's disease, Tay-Sachs disease, sickle-cell anemia, and cystic fibrosis, as well as sex-linked disorders such as hemophilia. The likelihood of two carriers of the same harmful allele mating is increased in consanguineous ("same blood") mating—i.e., mating between two close relatives (for example, siblings or first cousins). However, consanguineous mating can also lead to concentration of favorable alleles.

In addition to simple Mendelian disorders, there are multifactorial disorders, resulting from effects of harmful alleles along with environmental factors—for example, heart disease, diabetes, cancer, alcoholism, schizophrenia, and bipolar disorder.

Genetic engineering (discussed next) may be important in the treatment of some genetic diseases. Already, genetic screening and counseling is being undertaken in many hospitals, using tests along with family history to compute the odds for getting certain hereditary diseases. Trait recognition in fetuses is now possible through various tests, such as amniocentesis and chorionic villi sampling. Likewise, newborns can be screened for genetic disorders, most of which are untreatable, but a few of which—for example, phenylketonuria—can be treated.

b. Genetic Engineering

Begun in the 1970s, genetic engineering is the manipulation of genes—that is, inserting new genes into DNA, removing existing genes, or changing part of a gene. Here are a few examples of genetic engineering in practice:

- The gene for human insulin has been added to a common bacterium, so that the bacterium produces insulin; bacteria is grown in tanks and the insulin is then removed for treatment of diabetes.
- Human protein (hormones, enzymes, and other biological chemicals) made in the same manner can be used to treat hemophilia, multiple sclerosis, and other previously untreatable diseases.
- New genes can be introduced into farm animals to make them larger, or into plants to make them disease- or insect-resistant.

Scientists have set up regulatory and ethics committees to regulate genetic engineering because of the worry that the process might create dangerous new life forms.

You Should Review

- Mendel's experiments with garden peas—self-pollination and cross-pollination; dominant and recessive characteristics
- the genetic basis of variation among individuals in a population
- how to use probability to determine inherited characteristics; the statistical nature of inheritance or inheritance as a game of chance; the rule of multiplication and the rule of addition
- the testcross: breeding of a recessive homozygote with an organism of dominant phenotype but unknown genotype
- inheritance patterns based on dominant and recessive alleles
- the "particulate model"—that is, parents pass on discrete heritable units
- aneuploidy (chromosomal aberration); also, polyploidy (triploidy and tetraploidy), deletion, duplication, inversion, and translocation
- genomic imprinting

- mutation
- the Punnett square: a grid representing all possible genotypic combinations in the second generation produced by a male (gametes listed horizontally) and a female (gametes listed vertically) of the first generation
- the process of hybridization
- Mendel's Law of Segregation (named after the sorting of alleles into separate gametes)
- Mendel's Law of Independent Assortment
- segregation of genes during gamete production
- recessively inherited disorders and dominantly inherited disorders; multifactorial disorders
- Thomas Hunt Morgan's experiments with *Drosophila melanogaster* (the fruit fly)
- genetic mapping
- the process of transcribing DNA to mRNA
- discovery of the double helix by Rosalind Franklin, James Watson, and Francis Crick and what the discovery has meant to the study of genetics
- processes of DNA replication and DNA repair
- process of protein synthesis
- the genetic code
- the basics of genetic engineering
- recombinant DNA and gene cloning
- the following terms and concepts (among others): homozygous and heterozygous; genotypic ratio; protein synthesis; transcription; translation; linked genes; crossing over; Barr body; karyotype; complete dominance, incomplete dominance, and codominance; pleiotropy; epistasis; quantitative characters; polygenetic inheritance; norm of reaction; gene sequencing; pedigree chart

Questions

11. The probabilities for all possible outcomes of an event must add up to
    a. 0.1.
    b. 1.
    c. 10.
    d. 100.

12. When a red snapdragon is crossed with a white one, all the F1 hybrids have pink flowers. This is an example of
  a. inheritance of acquired characteristics.
  b. the blending theory of inheritance.
  c. incomplete dominance.
  d. codominance.

13. While doing his experiments on garden peas, Gregor Mendel was unaware of the
  a. laws of probability.
  b. statistical nature of inheritance.
  c. existence of particulate inheritance.
  d. role of chromosomes in inheritance.

14. Which of the following is NOT a feature of Mendel's Law of Segregation?
  a. The variation in inherited characters is caused by alternative versions of heritable factors.
  b. For each character, an organism inherits two heritable factors, one from each parent.
  c. The two heritable factors for each character segregate during gamete production.
  d. When heritable factors cannot segregate, they must be linked together and then passed on.

15. Sometimes, a gene at one locus (site) on the chromosome suppresses the phenotypic expression of a gene at a different locus. This is called
  a. epistasis.
  b. meiosis.
  c. carrier recognition.
  d. consanguinity.

16. In a species of rabbit, black fur (B) is dominant to brown fur (b). Which of the following could be the genotype of a rabbit with brown fur?
  a. Bb or bb
  b. Bb or BB
  c. bb only
  d. BB only

17. When, in the 1960s, molecular biologists performed a series of experiments that showed the amino acid translations of each of the codons of nucleic acids, they
  a. created a model for most later genetic studies.
  b. called into question an important Mendelian law.
  c. cracked the code of life.
  d. established the first link between practical and applied genetics.

18. Lethal recessive mutations are perpetuated by the reproduction of carriers with normal
  a. genotypes.
  b. Barr bodies.
  c. linked genes.
  d. phenotypes.

19. In helping determine whether a genetic disorder is present in a fetus, which of the following is an alternative to amniocentesis?
  a. chorionic villi sampling
  b. carrier recognition testing
  c. RFLP analysis
  d. use of labeled DNA probes

20. The symptoms of sickle-cell anemia occur due to one abnormal gene causing several different traits. Which type of genetic inheritance causes sickle-cell anemia?
  a. pleiotropy
  b. codominance
  c. polygenetic inheritance
  d. incomplete dominance

Answers

11. b. The probabilities for all possible outcomes of an event, added together, must equal 1. For example, in the toss of a two-headed coin, the probability of tossing tails is $\frac{1}{2}$ and of tossing heads $\frac{1}{2}$; in the throw of a six-sided die, the probability of rolling the number 3 is $\frac{1}{6}$, and the probability of rolling a number other than 3 is $\frac{5}{6}$.

12. c. Incomplete dominance is the correct answer. Characteristics acquired during an individual's lifetime (choice **a**)—for example, increased muscle mass in a runner's legs due to running—are not genetically controlled and are therefore not heritable. The blending theory of inheritance (choice **b**) is discredited by Mendel's experiments with garden peas. The blending theory would predict only pink offspring from this crossing, whereas the reality is that the red or white traits can appear in the next generation—that is, one can predict a phenotypic ratio of 1 red to 2 pink to 1 white. Codominance (choice **d**) arises when both alleles in a heterozygous organism are dominant and shown in the phenotype.

13. d. Until 1918, most biologists dismissed the importance of chromosomes in inheritance. Mendel died in 1884.

14. d. The discovery of linked heritable factors (now called genes) did not occur until after Mendel's death. The discovery was made by Bateson and Punnett of Cambridge University in 1906.

15. a. Epistasis (Greek for *standing still on*) is the correct answer.

16. c. The recessive trait, brown fur, will be expressed only if both alleles for brown fur are present. A species of the rabbit with brown fur must have two recessive alleles, which is the genotype bb.

17. c. Cracking the genetic code was one of the most important steps taken in the field of molecular biology. Marshall Nirenberg, of the National Institutes of Health, deciphered the first codon in 1961.

18. d. Unlike lethal dominant alleles, lethal recessive alleles are masked in the heterozygous carriers.

19. a. Chorionic villi sampling is the suctioning off of a small amount of fetal tissue from the villi of the embryonic membrane. It yields more rapid results than amniocentesis, but its risks are comparable.

20. a. Pleiotropy is a type of inheritance where one gene results in several different traits. The gene responsible for sickle-cell anemia causes abnormal red blood cells, which in turn cause anemia, blockage in blood vessels, damage to the kidneys, and other symptoms of the disease.

C. Structure and Function of Human Systems

1. Integumentary System

a. Definition and Structure

The integument is the outermost covering of the body and is its largest organ. It consists of the epidermis (thinner, outermost layer) and dermis (thicker, innermost layer). It also includes specialized structures, the hair, and nails. Within the layers, there are also other structures. Beneath the skin is the subcutaneous tissue.

b. Function

The integumentary system has the following functions:

- In cooperation with the immune system, it provides protection for the body from injury, dehydration, and invasion by harmful agents such as bacteria.

- As a sense organ, it provides sensitivity to pain, temperature, and pressure.
- It aids in the regulation of body temperature.

2. Skeletal System
a. Definition and Structure

The skeleton is the chief structural system which, along with the skin, provides form and shape to the body. Comprised of 206 bones in adults, along with cartilage and ligaments, the skeletal system is rigid, yet flexible because of joints; the bones form levers that are moved by muscles.

There are two types of tissue that make up bone:

1. **Cortical, or compact bone** is strong and dense. It makes up the hard outer portion of bone that supports the skeletal system.
2. **Cancellous, or trabecular bone** is spongy. It has a high surface area, contains many blood vessels, and makes up the inner portion of bones.

There are five types of bone:

1. **Long** bones are longer than they are wide—for example, the femur, humerus, tibia, and fibula.
2. **Flat** bones form long, flat plates—for example, the cranium and pelvis.
3. **Short** bones are cube-shaped—for example, the bones of the wrist and ankle.
4. **Sesamoid** bones are embedded in the tendons—for example, the patella (kneecap).
5. **Irregular** bones are bones that do not fit into the aforementioned types—for example, the vertebrae of the spine.

b. Function

The skeletal system has the following functions:

- It provides mechanical support.
- It protects vulnerable organs within the body.
- Along with the muscular system, it makes body movement possible.
- It stores calcium in the bones, which contain marrow for production of red and white blood cells and platelets.

3. Muscular System
a. Definition and Structure

The muscular system is made up of muscle tissue in sheets or bundles of cells. Muscles can only contract—relaxation is passive—and are attached to the skeleton, generally in pairs that work against each other. There are three major types:

- **voluntary (skeletal):** can be controlled by conscious thought—for example, the biceps.
- **involuntary (visceral, smooth):** cannot be controlled by the will—for example, the walls of the esophagus.
- **cardiac (heart muscles):** specialized and particular to the heart, contract involuntarily, and are regulated by nervous system intervention.

b. Function

Along with the skeletal system, the muscular system is responsible for flexibility, movement, and tension.

4. Circulatory System
a. Definition and Structure

The circulatory system consists of the cardiovascular and lymphatic systems: the heart; blood vessels (tubes through which blood is carried to and from the heart, including arteries, arterioles, capillaries, venules, and veins); blood; lymphatic vessels and sinuses; and lymph.

b. Function

The circulatory system distributes blood and associated chemicals throughout the body and underlies all functions within the human body.

5. Immune System
a. Definition and Structure

The immune system is the body's protective mechanism. It consists of the lymphatic system; the white cells of the blood and bone marrow; the thymus gland; and the outer fortress, the skin. There are two types of immunity, inherited (natural or innate) and acquired (active and passive).

The basic characteristics of the immune system include the following concepts:

- **Specificity:** the immune system's capacity to recognize and get rid of antigens—harmful pathogens and molecules—by producing lymphocytes and antibodies (specific proteins). An antigen (literally meaning "antibody-generating") can include anything "foreign" to the body, such as the molecules of viruses, bacteria, fungi, protozoans, parasitic worms, pollen, insect poison, and, unfortunately, tissue that has been transplanted from another person.
- **Diversity:** the immune system's capacity to respond to literally millions of invaders, due to the great variety of lymphocytes keyed to particular antigen markers.
- **Self/nonself recognition:** the immune system's ability to distinguish its own body's molecules ("self") from antigens ("nonself").
- **Memory:** the immunological system's capacity to remember formerly encountered antigens and react more quickly when exposed again—called acquired immunity. There are two kinds of acquired immunity: active, as a response by the individual's own immune system, either naturally or artificially acquired as through vaccines; and passive, as a response by antibodies transferred from one person to another—for example, a mother's passing antibodies to the fetus or the artificial introduction of antibodies from an immune animal or human.

b. Function

The immune system protects the body from infection (invasion by pathologic agents—microorganisms or viruses), diseases, and injury-causing agents.

6. Respiratory System
a. Definition and Structure

The respiratory system consists of the organs responsible for the exchange of gases between body and atmosphere—the lungs (its center), the nose, pharynx, larynx, trachea, bronchi, and diaphragm.

b. Function

The respiratory system functions to take in oxygen and eliminate carbon dioxide.

7. Digestive (or Gastrointestinal) System
a. Definition and Structure

The digestive system includes the gastrointestinal tract (or alimentary canal), a tube with two openings; the mouth and anus, for intake of food and elimination of waste; as well as accessory structures and organs such as teeth, tongue, liver, pancreas, and gallbladder.

b. Function

The digestive system's function is to break down food for energy, reabsorb water and nutrients, and eliminate waste.

8. Renal System
a. Definition and Structure

The renal system consists of

- two kidneys: compact, bean-shaped organs through which blood is cycled for removal of nitrogenous waste and other substances
- the nephrons or excretory tubules contained within the kidneys
- the blood vessels that serve the kidneys

- the structures that carry waste, in the form of urine, out of the body (ureters, bladder, urethra). Urine is 95% water and 5% solids in solution, including organic constituents (urea, uric acid, creatinine) and inorganic constituents (mainly salts of sodium and potassium).

b. Function
The renal system removes nitrogenous waste or toxic byproducts from the blood and maintains homeostasis of blood and body fluids.

9. Nervous System
a. Definition and Structure
The nervous system is one of two coordinating systems. (The other is the endocrine system, with which the nervous system interacts and cooperates.) It is made up of the nerves, brain, and sense organs for sight, sound, smell, taste, and touch. The nervous system is divided into two parts:

- the **central nervous system:** the brain and spinal cord
- the **peripheral nervous system:** the rest of the neural network—the cervical, thoracic, lumbar, and sacral nerves that branch from the spine

The brain is the nervous system's main control center and consists of three parts:

- the cerebral hemispheres, which are responsible for higher functions, such as speech and hearing
- the cerebellum, which is responsible for subconscious activities and some balance functions
- the brain stem, which is responsible for necessary functions such as breathing and circulation

The cells of the nervous system consist of neurons and supporting cells.

b. Function
The nervous system controls the flow of information in the body between the sensory and motor cells and organs.

10. Endocrine System
a. Definition and Structure
The endocrine system is the internal system of chemical communication, involving

- **Hormones:** substances that regulate growth or functioning of a specific tissue or organ in a distant part of the body—for example, insulin, sex hormones, corticosteroids, adrenaline, thyroxine, and growth hormone
- the ductless glands that secrete hormones directly into the interstitial spaces: the pituitary, adrenal, thyroid, parathyroid, ovary, testis, placenta, and part of the pancreas
- the molecular receptors on or in target cells that respond to hormones

b. Function
In concert with the nervous system, the endocrine system affects internal regulation and maintains homeostasis. Hormones affect the rate of metabolism and metabolism of specific substances, growth and developmental processes, development and functioning of reproductive organs and sexual characteristics, development of higher nervous functions (for example, personality), and the ability of the body to handle stress and resist disease.

11. Reproductive System
a. Definition and Structure
Reproduction is the method by which new individuals are created from existing ones. In humans, this involves two sets of organs, the internal reproductive organs and the external genitalia. Reproduction involves the fusion of two haploid gametes—the female ovum and the male spermatozoon—to form a diploid zygote.

The male reproductive system is made up of

- the external genitalia: the scrotum and penis
- the internal reproductive organs: the gonads (testes) and hormones, accessory glands, and a set of ducts that carry sperm and glandular secretions

The female reproductive system is made up of

- the external genitalia: the clitoris and two sets of labia
- the internal system: the fallopian tubes, ovaries, uterus, vagina, and related organs. The ovaries contain thousands of eggs. During a female's fertile years, an egg is released by one of the ovaries into the fallopian tube about once a month. If fertilization occurs, the egg attaches to the wall of the uterus and grows into a fetus.

b. Function

The reproductive system functions to create new individuals from existing ones and propagate the species.

c. Fertilization, Descriptive Embryology, and Developmental Mechanics

Fertilization (syngamy): the union of male and female gametes to form a zygote, in human sexual reproduction. Each gamete contains half the correct number of chromosomes; together, they form a full complement.

Embryology: the science that studies the development of the human embryo

The development of the embryo occurs roughly in the second through eighth week after fertilization. During the first week, the zygote is formed and enters the uterus, where implantation occurs. In the second through eighth weeks, the embryo develops and begins to show human form. The development of the embryo occurs in the following stages:

- **Cleavage:** zygote divides to form the blastula
- **Gastrulation:** cells become arranged into three primary germ layers
- **Organogenesis or organogeny:** further cell division and differentiation results in the formation of organs

At nine weeks, we refer to the growing organism as a fetus. From the third to the ninth month, the fetus develops until it possesses all the organs necessary for life outside the womb.

You Should Review

- the structure of the skin, including sweat pores; temperature receptors; pain receptors; papillary region; hair and hair follicles; sebaceous glands; arrector pili; Meissner's corpuscle; stratum corneum; stratum granulosum; Malpighian layer; sweat glands and sweat ducts; blood capillaries; the Pacinian corpuscles (pressure receptors); sensory nerves; adipose (fat) tissue
- the way the skin functions in the immune system
- the main parts of the skeleton and a little about their individual functions, including the cranium and its parts, as well as the mandible, sternum, clavicle, rib cage, vertebrae, carpals, metacarpals, phalanges, femur, patella, tibia, fibula, metatarsals, tarsals, phalanges, scapula, humerus, iliac crest, ulna, radius, pelvis, coccyx, and ischium
- the structure and function of the synovial joints: the ball-and-socket, ellipsoidal, gliding, hinged, pivot, saddle, sutures/immovable joints
- the way bones, muscle, and cartilage work together to support weight and enable movement
- axial versus appendicular skeletal components
- the location, size, and shape of the main muscle groups, their action, origin, insertion, and innervation (You needn't memorize all—there are about 700 of them!)
- the structure and action of a voluntary muscle: the tendon, epimysium, bundle of muscle fibers, nucleus, single muscle fiber, and myofibril (light

band, dark band, sarcomere unit containing contractile proteins); flexor versus extensor muscles

- the structure and action of an involuntary muscle; location is in the skin, around hair follicles, and in the internal organs (digestive tract, respiratory tract, urogenital tract, and circulatory system); the way an involuntary muscle is supplied by the autonomic nervous system; its composition of fusiform or spindle-shaped cells without striations
- the structure and function of the cardiac muscle: for example, Purkinje fibers; intercalated discs; pacemaker channels; that it is striated but involuntary; action of the vagus nerve to produce bradycardia; action of cholinergic stimulation to increase blood pressure and heart rate
- the structures of the heart; how the cardiac muscle works; how blood circulates; names of major blood vessels and lymphatic vessels
- the makeup of blood: (1) plasma—90% water; also contains fibrinogen (plasma protein to help clotting), inorganic ions, dissolved gases (e.g., oxygen and carbon dioxide), organic nutrients (amino acids and fats), hormones, antibodies, enzymes, and waste materials (e.g., uric acid and urea); (2) erythrocytes (red blood cells); (3) leukocytes and phagocytes (white blood cells); and (4) platelets. You should become familiar with what each type of blood cell does.
- the makeup of lymph (called tissue fluid in the intercellular spaces): alkaline, colorless (or yellowish or milky), and consisting mostly of water; also contains (1) proteins (serum albumin, serum globulin, serum fibrinogen); (2) salts; and (3) organic substances (urea, creatinine, neutral fats, glucose). You should become familiar with what each component contributes.
- general facts about blood groups, blood banks, tissue and organ transplants
- general facts about blood types/antigens (e.g., ABO, Rh factor) and blood transfusion; why blood typing is important

- some common blood disorders: for example, various kinds of anemia, hemophilia, leukemia, polycythemia, or thrombosis
- basics of homeostasis: acids, bases, normal blood pH, fluid and electrolyte balance
- the basic characteristics of the immune system
- characteristics and importance of B cells and T cells (the two main classes of lymphocytes) and their antigen receptors; the central role of T cells—cytotoxic or killer T cells and helper T cells
- the molecular basis of antigen-antibody specificity
- the nature of antibodies (a class of proteins called immunoglobulins or Igs—includes IgM, IgG, IgA, IgD, and IgE) and how they work in the human body
- the cellular basis for specificity and diversity
- the humoral response and activation of B cells; T-dependent and T-independent antigens
- the main immune disorders—autoimmune diseases, immunodeficiency, especially acquired immunodeficiency syndrome (AIDS) and human immunodeficiency virus (HIV)—and their treatment
- the following terms and concepts related to the immune system (among others): humoral immunity, cell-mediated immunity, effector cells, plasma cells, clonal selection, primary and secondary immune responses, memory cells, self-tolerance, cytokines (e.g., interleukin-1 and -2), interferon
- the organs of respiration (especially the lungs) and their specific structures and functions
- how breathing is controlled (nerves in the breathing center)
- gas exchange in humans
- the following terms and concepts related to the respiratory system (among others): oxygen transport and carbon dioxide transport, negative pressure breathing, tidal volume, volume capacity, residual volume

- major structures of the digestive system and the function of each: oral cavity, esophagus, diaphragm, liver, gallbladder, stomach, pancreas, spleen, large intestine (colon), small intestine, cecum, sigmoid colon, appendix, rectum, anus. The alimentary canal and accessory organs—the salivary glands (saliva, salivary amylase), pancreas, liver, and gallbladder—and their functions
- the various sphincters and the mechanism of peristalsis
- the function and composition of gastric juices (e.g., pepsin/pepsinogen, hydrochloric acid), zymogens, gastrin, acid chyme
- hormones and enzymes involved in the digestive process
- how digestive secretions are regulated
- absorption and distribution of nutrients—the villi, microvilli, lacteal, chylomicrons, lipoproteins, capillaries, and hepatic portal vein leading to the liver
- the process of elimination of waste
- the structure and function of the renal system, especially the kidneys (collecting duct, cortex, medulla, glomeruli, Bowman's capsule, loop of Henle, and others) and the renin-angiotensin-aldosterone axis
- renal fluid composition
- concepts of pressure gradients, diffusion, osmosis, active transport, filtration, concentration, diuresis
- the nervous system and functions of its main parts—for example, the spinal cord and its regions (cervical, thoracic, lumbar, sacral); and nerves (ulnar, median, radial, cauda equina, sciatic, femoral, saphenous, vagus)
- the brain and functions of main parts—frontal lobe, temporal lobe, parietal lobe, occipital lobe, cerebellum, brain stem
- the various areas of control in the brain—for example, the voluntary motor area, frontal lobe, speech center, olfactory area, somatic sensory area, visual area, cerebellum, auditory area
- the cells of the nervous system, (i.e., the neurons and supporting cells)
- neurons—cell body, dendrites, axons, Schwann cells, myelin sheath (covers the axons of nerve cells, composed of lipids and proteins), synaptic terminals, synapses. The three kinds of neurons: sensory neurons, motor neurons, and interneurons
- supporting cells (glial cells—meaning "glue cells")—for example, in the central nervous system, astrocytes (which contribute to the blood-brain barrier) and oligodendrocytes; in the peripheral nervous system, Schwann cells
- how electrical signals are transmitted along a neuron
- the origin of electrical membrane potential
- the endocrine glands: hypophysis/pituitary, parathyroid, thyroid, suprarenal/adrenal glands, islet of Langerhans in the pancreas, and gonads (ovaries/testes)
- the hormones (chemical signals transmitted throughout the body via the circulatory system; act upon body structures more or less distant) and their target cells
- the three general classes of hormones based on chemical structure: (1) steroid hormones, including sex hormones; (2) amino acid derivatives, generally from tyrosine, which include epinephrine/adrenaline, the "fight-or-flight" hormone; and (3) peptides, the most diverse class, which includes insulin
- the hormone receptors
- the male and female reproductive structures and functions
- the hormonal control of human reproduction: (1) in males, androgens, especially testosterone; (2) in females, the menstrual cycle, which can be described by changes in either the uterus or ovary: the uterine cycle consists of the menstrual flow, proliferative, and secretory phases,

while the ovarian cycle consists of the follicular phase, ovulation, and luteal phase; hormones, in particular estrogen, progesterone, and oxytocin

- spermatogenesis and oogenesis
- the main aspects of fertilization, embryo formation, and development from zygote to fetus
- the three trimesters of pregnancy

Questions

21. What are the two major systems making up the circulatory system?
  a. heart and lung
  b. vessel and sinus
  c. arterial and venous
  d. cardiovascular and lymphatic

22. Which of the following structures is part of the axial skeleton?
  a. the bones of the limbs
  b. the pectoral girdle
  c. the pelvic girdle
  d. the skull

23. Repetitive muscle contraction depends upon ADP receiving a phosphate group from
  a. phosphagens.
  b. phosphorylases.
  c. phospholipids.
  d. phosphokinase.

24. The inner layer of squamous cells that lines the blood vessels is called the
  a. endoderm.
  b. endothelium.
  c. endometrium.
  d. endomembrane.

25. Which of the following aspects of the immune system is responsible for the rejection of organ transplants?
  a. phagocytosis
  b. the formation of antibodies
  c. the major histocompatibility complex
  d. the activation of B cells

26. The enzyme that hydrolyzes protein in the digestive system is called
  a. erepsin.
  b. steapsin.
  c. ptyalin.
  d. pepsin.

27. Which of the following is NOT a primary function of the integumentary system?
  a. protecting the body from bacteria
  b. sensing pressure and pain
  c. regulation of body temperature
  d. providing mechanical support

28. Which of the following is a disorder of body fluids common in renal disease?
  a. acidocytosis
  b. phagocytosis
  c. acidosis
  d. polyposis

29. Which disorder occurs due to a breakdown in the body's ability to recognize self and nonself?
  a. cystic fibrosis
  b. hemophilia
  c. rheumatoid arthritis
  d. hepatitis B

30. The area of the brain that integrates endocrine and neural functions is the
  a. hippocampus.
  b. gyrus.
  c. hypothalamus.
  d. pons.

31. LH and FSH are both
  a. pituitary gonadotropins.
  b. placental hormones.
  c. steroids.
  d. androgens.

32. Which of the following structures is partially responsible for the fact that a mother does not reject the embryo as a foreign body, as she would a tissue or organ graft?
  a. the endometrium
  b. the erythroblast
  c. the placenta
  d. the trophoblast

Answers

21. d. The cardiovascular and lymphatic systems make up the circulatory system. They both deliver fluids (blood and lymph, respectively) and their associated materials throughout the body. The arterial and venous systems are the divisions of the cardiovascular system, and vessels and sinuses are the conduits of the lymphatic system.

22. d. The vertebrate frame has two parts, the axial skeleton and the appendicular skeleton. The skull, vertebral column, and rib cage make up the axial skeleton. The other answer choices make up the appendicular skeleton.

23. a. Phosphagens are high-energy phosphate compounds, found in animal tissues, that supply a phosphate group to ADP to make ATP. Phosphorylases (choice **b**) are the enzymes that add the phosphate groups from phosphagens to ADP, but phosphorylases do not themselves supply the phosphate groups.

24. b. Endothelium is the correct answer. The other choices relate to systems other than the human circulatory system.

25. c. The major histocompatibility complex is part of the cell-mediated response system. Choice **a**, phagocytosis, is involved in the inflammatory response; choices **b** and **d** are part of the humoral immune response system.

26. d. Pepsin is the chief enzyme found in gastric juice and is responsible for hydrolyzing protein. Choices **a**, **b**, and **c** are enzymes present in intestinal juice, pancreatic juice, and saliva, respectively.

27. d. The primary functions of the integumentary system include protecting the body from bacteria; sensing temperature, pressure, and pain; and regulating the body's temperature. Providing mechanical support is a main function of the skeletal system.

28. c. Acidosis is the excess acidity of body fluids found in renal disease and diabetes.

29. c. An autoimmune disorder is a disorder where the immune system fails to distinguish between self and nonself and attacks the body's own tissues. Rheumatoid arthritis is an autoimmune disorder.

30. c. The hypothalamus initiates endocrine signals after receiving information about the environment from the peripheral nerves and other parts of the brain.

31. a. LH (luteinizing hormone) and FSH (follicle-stimulating hormone) are pituitary gonadotropins, hormones whose levels affect oogenesis and spermatogenesis.

32. d. The trophoblast is a barrier that prevents the embryo from coming into contact with maternal tissue.

D. Viruses, Bacteria, and Archaea
1. Definitions
a. Viruses

Viruses: the simplest of all genetic systems, infectious particles the largest of which can barely be seen with a light microscope

Viruses hover between life and nonlife, being either very complex molecules or very simple life forms. They lack the structure and most of the equipment of cells, and they lack enzymes for metabolism; they are merely aggregates of nucleic acids and proteins—cores of nucleic acid packaged in protein coats called *capsids*. Some also bear an outer envelope of proteins and lipids. Viruses are parasites of animals, plants, and some bacteria, and can only metabolize and reproduce within a living host cell. The discovery of viruses began with the German scientist Adolf Mayer in 1883; however, most of the research on viruses has been done in the last 30 years.

> **Structure:** nucleic acid coated with a shell of protein called a capsid, and sometimes a membranous envelope (shell of protein and lipids) coating the capsid. The envelope may help the virus enter the host cell. Whereas other genes are made of double-stranded DNA, viral genomes may consist of double-stranded or single-stranded DNA (DNA viruses), or double-stranded or single-stranded RNA (RNA viruses).

b. Bacteria and Archaea

> **Bacteria and Archaea:** unicellular organisms—prokaryotes   with no true nucleus

Bacteria are classified into two groups, gram-positive and gram-negative, based on differences in cell wall composition detected by Gram's staining. Gram-negative bacteria are more dangerous to other life forms than gram-positive bacteria. Bacteria are extremely adaptable with regard to their physiological adjustment to changes in the environment. They are the principal decomposers of most ecosystems. Bacteria were discovered by the Dutch maker of microscopes, Antonie van Leeuwenhoek (1632–1723).

Archaea may be descendants of the earliest forms of life. Many species are adapted to life in harsh conditions, such as extremely hot, acidic, or salty environments, and can use a variety of energy sources, including sulfur, methane, ammonia, and sunlight.

2. Structure, Shapes, Metabolism, and Life Cycle of Bacteria and Archaea
a. Structure

The bacterial and archaeal genome is mainly a single, circular, double-stranded DNA molecule (plasmid). Prokaryotes lack membrane-enclosed organelles. (See Section A, page 156, for more detail.)

b. Shapes and Metabolic Requirements

Bacteria and archaea are initially grouped according to:

- **Shape.** They can be placed in three groups: cocci, with a spherical shape; bacilli, with a rod-like shape; and spirilla, with a spiral shape.
- **Metabolic requirements.** They are further classified by how they get their energy and nutrients, such as whether they require oxygen.
  - **Aerobes** require oxygen.
  - **Anaerobes** do not require oxygen.

Bacteria and archaea have greater metabolic diversity than all eukaryotes combined. With regard to procurement of energy and carbon, they fall into four categories:

- **Photoautotrophs** harness light energy for synthesis of organic compounds from carbon dioxide—for example, cyanobacteria (formerly called blue-green algae).
- **Photoheterotrophs** use light to generate ATP but can get carbon only in organic form. (i.e., not from CO_2)
- **Chemoautotrophs** obtain energy by oxidizing inorganic substances, although they need only CO_2 as source of carbon—for example, *Sulfobolus*, which oxidizes sulfur.
- **Chemoheterotrophs** use organic molecules for both energy and carbon—the majority of bacteria are in this category.

Bacteria and archaea also vary in the effect oxygen has on metabolism (obligate aerobes, facultative anaerobes, obligate anaerobes), and in nitrogen metabolism.

c. Life Cycle

In their life cycle, bacteria and archaea do not undergo mitosis or meiosis, although they may undergo genetic recombination by three mechanisms: transformation, conjugation, and transduction. Instead, they reproduce by binary fission, each daughter cell receiving a copy of the single parental chromosome. Bacteria and archaea are exceptionally resistant to environmental destruction; some cannot even be killed by boiling water, and endospores may remain dormant for centuries. Unchecked by unfavorable environmental conditions, their growth is exponential. Generation times are usually one to three hours, but some species may double every 20 minutes.

3. Classification of Bacteria and Archaea
a. Bacteria

Bacteria used to be classified as plants; however, prokaryotes and plants have a completely different molecular composition. Instead of cellulose, bacterial walls are composed of peptidoglycan, which consists of polymers of modified sugars cross-linked by short polypeptides that vary according to species. Bacteria are usually classified as one of three domains, in Domain Bacteria.

Bacteria include, among others, actinomycetes (e.g., *Mycobacterium*), chemoautotrophic bacteria (e.g., *Nitrobacter*), cyanobacteria (e.g., *Chroococcus*), endospore-forming bacteria (e.g., *Bacillus*), enteric bacteria (e.g., *Escherichia*), mycoplasmas (e.g., *Mycoplasma*), myxobacteria (e.g., *Myxococcus*), nitrogen-fixing aerobic bacteria (e.g., *Azotobacter*), pseudomonads (e.g., *Pseudomonas*), rickettsias and chlamydias (e.g., *Rickettsia* and *Chlamydia*), and spirochetes (e.g., *Borrelia*).

b. Archaea

Archaea used to be considered a type of bacteria, but have since been placed in their own domain, Domain Archaea. Archaea are considered to be more closely related to eukaryotes (Domain Eukarya, the final domain) than bacteria, even though both archaea and bacteria are prokaryotes. They include methanogens, extreme halophiles, and thermoacidophiles.

4. Diseases
a. Viral Diseases

Not all viruses are disease-causing; many viruses do no apparent harm. Diseases caused by viruses include the common cold, influenza, AIDS, herpes, viral pneumonia, meningitis, hepatitis, polio, and rabies in animals, and tobacco mosaic disease in plants. Types of viruses include adenovirus, arbovirus, herpesvirus, HIV, myxovirus, papillomavirus, picornavirus, poxvirus, retrovirus, and (in plants) the tobacco mosaic virus.

Bacterial viruses are called *bacteriophages* or simply phages and include, among many others, seven that infect *Escherichia coli*.

b. Bacterial Diseases

Approximately half of all human diseases are caused by bacteria; they may be intruders from outside or opportunistic, that is, they live inside the body of a healthy host, becoming destructive only when the host's defenses are weakened. Pathogenic bacteria can disrupt the physiology of the host by growing inside and invading the tissues. Others exude poisons that are one of two types: exotoxins or endotoxins. (See Mechanisms of Infection/Bacteria, page 177.)

Examples of diseases caused by bacteria include pneumonia, caused by the bacterium *Streptococcus pneumoniae*; tuberculosis, caused by the bacterium *Mycobacterium tuberculosis*, which destroys parts of the lung tissue and is spread through inhalation and exhalation; syphilis, caused by the bacterium *Treponema pallidum*; and many others.

5. Mechanisms of Infection

a. Viruses

Lock-and-key fit is the method by which viruses identify their hosts. Some viruses can infect several species, such as the swine flu virus and the rabies virus; some can infect only a single species, for example, the human cold virus and HIV. Some viruses depend on coinfection by other viruses. The host range is the range of host cells a particular type of virus can infect.

- **Lytic cycle:** the reproductive cycle of virulent viruses that ends in the death of the host
- **Lysogenic cycle:** the reproductive cycle of temperate viruses, which coexist with the host rather than killing it
- **Vaccines:** variants or derivatives of pathogenic microbes that help the cell defend against infection (e.g., polio, rubella, measles, and mumps). There is little that can be done to cure a viral infection once it begins, as antibiotics are powerless; however, many new antiviral agents have been developed in recent years.

b. Bacteria

One mechanism of infection is reproducing rapidly and invading tissues. Bacteria that use this mechanism include rickettsias that cause Rocky Mountain spotted fever and typhus, and actinomycetes that cause tuberculosis and leprosy. Others produce toxins of two types:

- **Exotoxins:** proteins secreted by the bacterial cell; examples are *Clostridium botulinum*, which causes the often fatal disease botulism, and *Vibrio cholerae*, which causes cholera
- **Endotoxins:** not secreted by the bacterium, but are merely components of its outer membrane; examples are the various species of *Salmonella* that cause food poisoning, and *Salmonella typhi*, which causes typhoid fever

Many bacteria are harmless or even beneficial; certainly they have had wide-ranging benefits to humankind. From bacteria, we have learned much about metabolism and molecular biology. Methanogens are used for sewage treatment by aerating sewage. Some soil species of pseudomonads are used to decompose pesticides and certain harmful synthetic substances. Bacteria are used to make vitamins, antibiotics, and certain foods—for example, to convert milk to yogurt and some types of cheese.

Whether destructive or beneficial, bacteria do not act alone but form relationships with other bacterial species and organisms from other kingdoms through symbiosis, which means "living together"—if one symbiont is larger than another, it is known as the host. There are three categories of symbiotic relationships:

- **Mutualism:** both symbionts benefit
- **Commensalism:** one symbiont receives benefits while neither harming nor helping the other
- **Parasitism:** one symbiont benefits but harms the host

You Should Review

- the structure and evolutionary origin of viruses
- reproduction mechanism of viruses
- plant viruses and viroids (even simpler pathogens than viruses)
- characteristics of the two kinds of virus, DNA and RNA
- Gram's staining
- metabolic processes of prokaryotes
- nutritional needs of prokaryotes: Some are very specific in their needs (for example, *Lactobacillus* needs all 20 amino acids, several vitamins, and various organic compounds); some are not specific (for example *E. coli* can grow on a medium containing glucose or a substitute for glucose as the only organic component).
- process of nitrogen fixation
- kinds of chemoheterotrophic bacteria—for example, saprophytes (decomposers) and para-

sites; there are no known present-day phagotrophic bacteria

- life cycle of bacteria
- reproductive process of binary fission
- the various diseases caused by viruses and bacteria
- Koch's postulates
- the reproductive cycle of the HIV virus
- the lytic cycle and defense mechanisms of certain bacteria against certain phages (e.g., restriction enzymes)
- the many variations of viral infection among animal viruses, especially viruses with envelopes and viruses with RNA genomes, and the reproductive cycle of each
- retroviruses; reverse transcriptase
- viruses and cancer; tumor viruses: HIV (the AIDS-causing virus)
- the main groups of bacteria and kinds of bacteria in these groups
- sizes of various bacteria, along with motility; capsules; spores; reproduction; colony formation; food, oxygen, and temperature requirements; and activities (enzyme production, toxin production, etc.)

Questions

33. Bacteria and archaea are both classified as
    a. eukaryotes.
    b. prokaryotes.
    c. bacteria.
    d. viruses.

34. Which of the following diseases could be effectively treated with antibiotics?
    a. smallpox
    b. rabies
    c. hepatitis A
    d. typhoid fever

35. The resistant cells some bacteria form to resist environmental destruction are called
    a. endospores.
    b. coenocytes.
    c. coenobia.
    d. endosomes.

36. If one member of an isolated bacterial colony is found to be genetically different from the rest, which of the following is the most likely explanation?
    a. Mitosis has taken place.
    b. Mutation has taken place.
    c. Sexual reproduction has taken place.
    d. Cloning has taken place.

37. Which of the following groups of microorganisms is an example of an obligate anaerobe?
    a. methanogens
    b. cyanobacteria
    c. chemoautotrophs
    d. chemoheterotrophs

38. The ability of certain bacteria to assimilate atmospheric nitrogen into nitrogenous compounds that can be used by plants is called nitrogen
    a. production.
    b. fixation.
    c. cycling.
    d. equilibrium.

39. Which of the following is the main reason that an influenza vaccine is generally only effective for one season?
    a. The virus responsible for influenza constantly mutates.
    b. The antibodies present in the vaccine degrade after a short time.
    c. The influenza virus responds to the vaccine and transforms.
    d. The antigen in the vaccine is weakened by the immune system.

40. Which of the following is a kind of movement of which certain bacteria are capable?
   a. chemotaxis
   b. chemosmosis
   c. chemosynthesis
   d. chemylosis

41. Destruction of bacteria by a lytic agent is called
   a. bacteriogenesis.
   b. bacteriophagia.
   c. bacteremia.
   d. bacteriostasis.

42. The discovery of the virus began with German scientist Adolf Mayer, while he was seeking the cause of
   a. Rocky Mountain spotted fever.
   b. rabies.
   c. tobacco mosaic disease.
   d. fungal blight.

Answers

33. b. Bacteria and archaea are both classified as prokaryotes, as both are single-celled organisms that do not have organelles. Archaea used to be classified as a type of bacteria, but they are now placed in their own domain.

34. d. Antibiotics are effective against bacterial diseases only. Smallpox, rabies, and hepatitis A are all viruses, and so cannot be effectively treated with antibiotics.

35. a. The resistant cells, called endospores, can survive almost anything, including boiling water, lack of nutrients or water, and most poisons.

36. b. Since bacteria reproduce asexually by binary fission, generally in an isolated colony all will be genetically identical. Differences in offspring in an isolated colony can, however, be caused by mutation. Neither mitosis nor sexual reproduction (choices **a** and **c**) take place in bacteria; cloning (choice **d**) produces genetically identical individuals.

37. a. Methanogens produce methane and are obligate or strict anaerobes, found in oxygen-deficient environments such as marshes, swamps, sludge, and the digestive systems of ruminants (such as cows).

38. b. Nitrogen fixation is important to the nutrition of plants and can only be performed by certain bacteria. In terms of nutrition, this ability makes cyanobacteria the most self-sufficient organisms on Earth.

39. a. Vaccines for viruses such as influenza are usually effective for only a short time because the virus mutates. Once the virus mutates, the immune system is unable to recognize the virus and the vaccine's effectiveness is negated.

40. a. The word *chemotaxis* is derived from the Greek *chemeia* (chemistry) + *taxis* (arrangement). Positive chemotaxis is the moving toward a chemical; negative chemotaxis is the moving away from a chemical.

41. b. Bacteriophages are viruses that are parasitic to bacteria. The lytic cycle of a bacteriophage culminates in the death of the host.

42. c. Mayer noted that tobacco mosaic disease was contagious, but he could find no microbe in the infectious sap. He concluded that the causal agent was a bacterium too small to be seen with a microscope. Only later were scientists able to discern the characteristics that set viruses apart from bacteria.

E. Plants

1. Distinction between Plants and Animals

Plants are multicellular eukaryotes, nearly all terrestrial in origin, though some have evolved so that they can live in water. They differ from animals in structure, life cycle, and modes of nutrition, and are the mainstay of most ecosystems on Earth. They draw their energy directly from sunlight and directly or indirectly feed the rest of the creatures on Earth, including animals; without them most ecosystems would simply die. They are autotrophic in nutrition, making food by photosynthesis, or the conversion of light energy into chemical energy, a property they share with algae and certain prokaryotes.

2. Photosynthesis

a. Definition

Photosynthesis: the process by which light energy, captured by the chloroplasts of plants, is converted to chemical energy

b. Process

Plants are equipped with the light-absorbing molecules chlorophyll a and chlorophyll b and certain carotenoid pigments that maximize the collection of solar energy.

3. Cellular Anatomy

The cell walls of plants consist mostly of cellulose, and they store food in the form of starch. See Section A, Cell Biology (page 156), for more on the structure of plant cells.

4. Nutritional Requirements

In order to live, plants require both macronutrients (nutrients required in large quantities), including carbon, oxygen, hydrogen, nitrogen, sulfur, phosphorus, calcium, potassium, and magnesium, and micronutrients (nutrients required in smaller quantities), including iron, chlorine, copper, manganese, zinc, molybdenum, boron, and nickel. Fixed nitrogen is important to all aspects of a plant's life cycle.

5. Structure and Function

Plants are classified as either nonvascular or vascular.

a. Nonvascular Plants

Nonvascular plants have simpler tissues than vascular plants. They are covered by a waxy cuticle to prevent dehydration, require water to reproduce, and lack woody tissue and so do not grow tall but rather grow in mats low to the ground. The nonvascular plants include mosses, liverworts, and hornworts.

b. Vascular Plants

Vascular plants have much more elaborate tissues, including vascular tissue; cells are joined into tubes for transport of nutrients and water throughout. There are two types of vascular tissue: phloem, which transports sugars from leaves to other parts of the plant; and xylem, which transports water and dissolved mineral nutrients from roots to other parts of the plant. Vascular plants are of two types: seedless, including horsetails and ferns, and seed plants. Seed plants in turn fall into two categories:

- **Gymnosperms:** seeds are uncovered; plants achieve fertilization mainly through wind-borne pollen. This category includes conifers and cycads, pines, firs, and spruce.
- **Angiosperms:** flowering plants such as grasses, wildflowers, and hardwood trees; the dominant plant form today (about 235,000 species). Angiosperms have the most advanced structural form: Seeds are enclosed in carpels, and animals and insects are employed for transfer of pollen in order to achieve fertilization. Important structures of flowering plants include the flower, which is the reproductive structure (includes the stamen with its filament and anthers, petals, pistil with its stigma, style, ovary, and sepal); and the fruit, which is the structure formed from the ovary of a flower, usually after ovules have been fertilized, and which protects dormant seeds and aids dispersal.

6. Reproduction and Development

Some plants reproduce sexually; seeded plants hold an egg, which, after the plant matures, is fertilized by pollen from itself or another plant. Others reproduce asexually by cloning; bulbs, feelers, and rhizomes require only one plant; there is no change in the chromosome number; and the offspring is exactly the same genetically as the parent.

You Should Review

- the process of photosynthesis
- plant cellular structure
- main characteristics of nonvascular and vascular plants
- plant morphology and anatomy, especially of flowering plants
- the processes of sexual and asexual reproduction in plants
- division of plants into monoecious plants (have both male and female reproductive organs in the same flower) and dioecious plants (have either male or female reproductive organs in separate flowers)
- symbiotic relationships that exist between certain plants and animals
- the various types of plants cells—for example, parenchyma cells, collenchyma cells, sclerenchyma cells, water-conducting cells, food-conducting cells
- the transport systems of plants
- plant hormones
- the following concepts and terms (among others): autotrophic nutrition; photoautotrophy; light reactions; the Calvin cycle; nitrogen fixation; dermal, vascular, and ground tissue systems; sporophyte and gametophyte

Questions

43. The sticky tip of the carpel of a flower, which receives the pollen, is called the
    a. stigma.
    b. filament.
    c. anther.
    d. style.

44. Plants require the most of which of the following nutrients?
    a. zinc
    b. copper
    c. nickel
    d. sulfur

45. A representation of the most recent evolutionary stage of plants is
    a. the cypress tree.
    b. the orchid.
    c. the ostrich fern.
    d. the liverwort.

46. The European butterwort, sundew, and pitcher plant are examples of plants that are
    a. medicinal.
    b. poisonous.
    c. parasitic.
    d. carnivorous.

47. The term *morphogenesis*, an area particularly important in plant development, refers to the development of an organism's
    a. external form.
    b. reproductive organs.
    c. cytoskeleton.
    d. nutritional uptake system.

48. Which plant hormones are produced in the roots and stimulate cell division during plant growth?
    a. ethylene
    b. gibberellins
    c. abscisic acid
    d. cytokinins

49. Which of the following could be called a plant "antiaging hormone"?
    a. cytokinin
    b. gibberellin
    c. auxin
    d. florigen

50. The major sites of photosynthesis in most plants are the
  a. stems.
  b. seeds.
  c. leaves.
  d. taproots.

51. The least specialized of all plant cells are the
  a. sclerenchyma cells.
  b. water-conducting cells.
  c. food-conducting cells.
  d. parenchyma cells.

52. Angiosperms respond physiologically to day length by flowering. This response is called
  a. the circadian rhythm.
  b. day-neutrality.
  c. photoperiodism.
  d. vernalization.

Answers

43. a. The stigma, located at the carpel, one of the reproductive organs of a flower, receives pollen.

44. d. Plant nutrients are divided into macronutrients, which plants require in relatively large amounts, and micronutrients, which plants require in relatively small amounts. Sulfur is a macronutrient. Zinc, copper, and nickel are micronutrients.

45. b. The orchid is an angiosperm, a type of flowering plant. Flowering plants came into existence about 140 to 125 million years ago. The other choices are considerably older.

46. d. All these plants are carnivorous, supplementing their nutrition (usually in nutrient-poor habitats such as acid bogs) by feeding on insects.

47. a. The term morphogenesis is related to the term morphology, which is the study of the external structure of an organism.

48. d. Cytokinins are a class of plant hormone produced in the roots. The functions of cytokinins include stimulating cell division and differentiation during plant growth.

49. a. Cytokinins inhibit protein breakdown, stimulate RNA and protein synthesis, and mobilize nutrients. These attributes are thought to be involved in the retardation of aging in some plant organs.

50. c. Although green stems do perform photosynthesis, the leaves are the most important photosynthetic organs in most plants.

51. d. Parenchyma cells, relatively unspecialized and usually lacking secondary walls, carry on most of the plant's metabolic functions.

52. c. Photoperiodism is the physiological response of any organism to day length.

III. Other Concepts You Should Be Familiar With

The following are not formal divisions of your health occupations entrance exam; however, concepts within them overlap with the subjects previously mentioned and may find their way into some of the questions.

A. *The Scientific Method*
1. General
The scientific method is employed by all sciences to study the natural world, regardless of the particular subject matter. Science studies only those aspects of nature that can be perceived by the senses.

2. Steps
Ideally, the scientific method involves the following steps, though the process is never as smooth as that outlined here, and steps may be taken out of order:

  ▪ Formulate the problem, the solution to which explains an order or process in nature.

- Collect data via observations, measurements, and review of the past—look for regularity and relationships between the data.
- Form a hypothesis, an educated guess as to what is going on, using inductive logic (specific to general) to infer a general or universal premise. The hypothesis must be logical and testable. Then formulate the hypothesis using deductive logic (general to specific—If . . . , then . . .).
- Test the hypothesis by experimentation and gathering of new data. A hypothesis can be disproved, but never absolutely proved—it may change with tomorrow's evidence. Experiments must be free of bias and sampling error, with control and experimental groups. An adequate amount of data and/or adequate numbers of individuals must be tested, and experiments must be reproducible by other scientists.
- Decide whether the hypothesis is to be accepted, modified, or denied.
- Formulate a new hypothesis and start again, if necessary.

3. The Science of Biology

Biology applies the scientific method to living organisms in order to attempt to arrive at an understanding of them. It looks at life using chemical and physical approaches, mainly those processes that involve transformation of matter and energy. There are vast numbers of kinds of living entities and therefore many branches of biology.

B. The Origin of Life

1. The Mechanistic View

Held by most scientists, the mechanistic view of the origin of life holds that Earth is billions of years old and that life occurred at a point in time along a continuum of increasingly complex matter. Biologists postulate a natural origin for life.

2. Distinction between Living and Nonliving Entities

Many biologists regard the distinction between living and nonliving entities as arbitrary, believing instead that there is a continuum, generally involving complexity.

Overall, however, there is a difference, in that living entities ordinarily are capable of self-regulation, metabolism, movement; irritability (response to stimuli in its internal and external environments); growth (increase in mass through use of materials from the environment); adaptation (a tendency to change, resulting in improved capacity to survive); and reproduction (production of new individuals like themselves).

C. Classification of Living Entities

1. Systems of Classification

The classification of living entities is an artificial construct. There are various systems, ranging from 3-domain to 7-kingdom classifications. Following are three examples:

- 3-domain classification: Bacteria, Archaea, Eukarya
- 7-kingdom classification: Bacteria, Archaea, Protozoa, Chromista, Fungi, Plantae, Animalia
- Ecological classification: Autotrophs, including green plants and some bacteria; heterotrophs, including herbivores, carnivores, omnivores, scavengers, decomposers, and parasites

2. Linnaean System

The hierarchical system most widely used is the Linnaean system, devised by Swedish botanist Carolus Linnaeus (Carl von Linné, 1707–1778). This system consists of Kingdom, Phylum, Class, Order, Family, Genus, and Species.

3. Binomial Nomenclature

A system also devised by Linnaeus, binomial nomenclature is still used for naming species of an organism. The first part is the generic name, the second the specific—the creature's genus (capitalized) and species (lowercase) are reflected in the name. For example, the common house cat is called *Felis silvestris*; a bacterium that causes one type of streptococcal pneumonia is called *Streptococcus pneumoniae*.

D. Social Behavior of Animals

1. Humans

A heated debate continues to rage over the distinction termed "nature versus nurture." Some scientists, particularly sociobiologists, believe that aspects of human behavior shared across cultures, such as avoidance of incest, can be viewed as innate, somehow evolutionarily programmed. Others insist that such cultural features as taboos would be unnecessary if behavior were truly innate; therefore, they say, much of what we view as particularly human behavior is learned. Those on the "nurture" side of the debate often point to altruistic behavior, which exists to a much greater extent in humans than in any other species. Those on the "nature" side of the debate insist that most altruistic behavior, if carefully looked at, does in some way enhance the individual, even when it causes that individual's death.

2. Other Species

Although much of the social behavior between members of a species involves cooperation, it is still the case that individuals act in their own best interest, and that a good deal of competitive behavior arises in all animal populations. Important aspects of social interaction include:

- agnostic behavior/competitive behavior—for example, for food or a mate—involving a

contest in which individuals threaten one another until one backs down. Often such behavior is ritualistic, as natural selection would favor individuals able to settle a contest without injury.
- dominance hierarchies
- territoriality
- courtship rituals
- communication among individuals
- altruistic behavior, though to a lesser extent than in humans

Questions

53. In science, which of the following is most nearly synonymous with the word "theory"?
    a. a proven fact
    b. a hypothesis that has withstood repeated testing
    c. an untested supposition
    d. a body of published data

54. Which of the following is a key characteristic of fungi?
    a. single-celled
    b. undergo photosynthesis
    c. reproduce asexually
    d. produce seeds

55. The majority of primary producers in an ecosystem are
    a. autotrophs.
    b. carnivores.
    c. detrivores.
    d. herbivores.

56. Two organisms would be most closely related if they shared the same
    a. phylum.
    b. order.
    c. genus.
    d. species.

57. An alternative view of the mechanistic origin of life holds that at least some organic compounds, including amino acids, originated in the hundreds of thousands of meteorites and comets that hit the earth during its early formation—that is, that life had extraterrestrial origins. This idea is called
   a. abiotic synthesis.
   b. panspermia.
   c. protobiotic aggregation.
   d. the Oparin hypothesis.

58. From the point of view of the scientific method, the most important requirement for a sound hypothesis is that it be
   a. able to be confirmed.
   b. intuitively possible.
   c. useful in a practical sense.
   d. testable through experimentation.

59. Altruistic behavior in humans can be explained as an innate behavior because it
   a. occurs in all cultures.
   b. is culturally encouraged.
   c. also benefits the individual.
   d. leads to the individual's death.

60. The primary feature that distinguishes life from nonlife is that living organisms are capable of
   a. reproduction.
   b. entropy.
   c. chemical evolution.
   d. atomic bonding.

Answers

53. b. A theory has undergone testing. The word is often mistakenly used to mean "just a guess." This misuse is seen in such a statement as, "Evolution is just a theory." In fact, evolution is regarded in the scientific community as a hypothesis that is so well-supported by data as to be fact.

54. c. One of the key characteristics of fungi is that they reproduce asexually. Fungi are also generally multicellular and are usually classified as decomposers.

55. a. The primary producers of an ecosystem are autotrophs, most of them photosynthetic organisms that synthesize organic compounds directly from light energy. All the other choices are consumers, directly or indirectly dependent on photosynthetic products for nutrition.

56. d. The Linnaean classification scheme classifies living things using seven levels: kingdom, phylum, class, order, family, genus, and species. The more levels that are shared by two organisms, the more closely they are related. Organisms of the same species are the most closely related, followed by organisms of the same genus.

57. b. The theory of panspermia gained strength in 1986 when spacecraft flying near Halley's Comet showed that the comet contained far more organic material than had previously been thought.

58. d. A hypothesis that is not testable is useless from a scientific point of view. Hypotheses can never be absolutely confirmed (choice **a**). Hypotheses frequently fly in the face of intuition (choice **b**); for instance, a flat Earth probably seems more intuitively right than a spherical one. Many scientific hypotheses have no immediately recognizable practical applications (choice **c**); an example might be David Reznik's hypotheses concerning guppy populations in Trinidad.

59. c. Innate behaviors, those that are considered to be due to "nature," have a genetic component and therefore must allow an individual to pass on all or part of its genetic material, even if that behavior leads to the individual's death. So the individual must also benefit on some level when it behaves altruistically.

60. a. All the other choices are properties of both living and nonliving entities.

8 ▶ CHEMISTRY REVIEW

CHAPTER SUMMARY

This chapter is a general outline and review of the important chemistry concepts that are tested by many health occupations entrance exams. It begins with a topic outline of the chemistry subjects covered, then reviews these important chemistry concepts in the same outline format.

Chemistry Review: Important Concepts

I. General Introduction

A. Description of How Health Occupations Entrance Exams Test Chemistry

This chapter reviews essential concepts in chemistry that are covered in many health occupations entrance exams. Some tests contain specific chemistry or science sections; others ask you to be able to recognize important ideas and terms.

Some of these key concepts are atomic structure, periodic table, chemical bonds, chemical equations, stoichiometry, energy and states of matter, reaction rates, equilibrium, acids, bases, oxidation-reduction, nuclear chemistry, and organic compounds.

B. How to Use This Chapter

This chapter is presented in outline form as a systematic presentation of important chemistry topics to help you review for your exam. This chapter does not constitute a comprehensive chemistry review—use it as an aid to help you recall concepts you have studied and to identify areas in which you need more study.

Read each topic in this chapter and answer the questions that follow. After answering the sample test questions, you can pinpoint where you want to concentrate your efforts. If a question poses particular difficulty for you, study more problems of this type. The more you hone your problem-solving skills, understand basic principles, and recognize core terms, the more relaxed and confident you will feel on test day.

STUDY TIPS FOR CHEMISTRY

- Review the topics covered in this chapter carefully. Keep a copy of one or more of the suggested resource books handy for more extensive review.
- Don't try to review all topics in one or two study sessions. Tackle a couple of topics at a time. Focus more in-depth study on the items within a topic that you feel least confident about first.
- Complete each group of practice questions after you study each topic, and check your answers.
- Review all the answer choices carefully before making your selection. The wrong answers often give you hints at the correct one, and also help you confirm that you really do know the correct answer. Remember that recognition is not necessarily understanding.
- When checking your answers to practice questions with the answer key, be sure you understand why the identified choice is the correct one. Practice writing out your reasoning for choosing a particular answer and checking it against the reasoning given in the answer key.
- Practice pronouncing chemical terminology aloud. If you can pronounce a term with ease, you are more likely to remember the term and its meaning when reading it.
- Review carefully the visual aspects of chemistry, such as the use of symbols, arrows, and sub- and superscripts. If you know the circumstances under which particular symbols are used, you will have immediate clues to right and wrong answers.
- Focus on developing problem-solving skills. Almost all chemical problems require the analysis, sorting, and understanding of details.

II. Main Topics

A. Atoms

1. Atomic Structure

An **atom** is the basic unit of an element that retains all the element's chemical properties. An atom is composed of a nucleus (which contains one or more protons and neutrons) and one or more electrons in motion around it.

An **electron** is of negligible mass compared to the mass of the nucleus and has a negative charge of −1.

A **proton** has a mass of 1 amu (atomic mass unit) and a positive charge +1.

A **neutron** has a mass of 1 amu also but no charge.

Atoms are electrically neutral because they are made of equal numbers of protons and electrons.

2. Dalton's Atomic Theory

In 1808, John Dalton proposed his hypotheses about the nature of matter that became the basis of Dalton's atomic theory:

- All elements are made of tiny, indivisible particles called atoms (from the Greek *atomos*, meaning indivisible).
- Atoms of one element are identical in size, mass, and chemical properties.
- Atoms of different elements have different masses and chemical properties.
- Compounds are made up of atoms of different elements in a ratio that is an integer (a whole number) or a simple fraction.
- Atoms cannot be created or destroyed. They can be combined or rearranged in a **chemical reaction**.

Later experiments completed the understanding of atoms:

- **J. J. Thomson** discovered the electron.
- **Ernest Rutherford** established that the atom is composed of negatively charged electrons moving in the empty space surrounding a dense, positively charged nucleus.
- **Henri Becquerel** and **Marie Curie** discovered that the decay of radioactive (unstable) nuclei resulted in the release of particles and energy.

3. Mass Number

Mass number is the sum of protons and neutrons in the nucleus of the atom. It varies with the isotopes of each element. The mass number is indicated by the number to the upper left of the element symbol: ^{23}Na.

4. Atomic Number

Atomic number is the number of protons in the atom, specific for each element. The atomic number is indicated by the number to the lower left of the element symbol: $_{11}Na$.

5. Isotopes

Isotopes are atoms of the same element that have the same number of protons (same atomic number) but different number of neutrons (different mass number). Isotopes have identical chemical properties (same reactivity) but different physical properties (for example, some decay while others are stable).

ISOTOPES OF HYDROGEN	
^1H	protium
^2H (or D)	deuterium
^3H (or T)	tritium

The **atomic weight** (or mass) of an element is given by the weighted average of the isotopes' masses.

6. Classification of Matter
a. Elements

Elements are substances that are composed of only one type of atom. Elements have chemical symbols (letters of their names) that are used for their representation in the periodic table. The heaviest named element is oganesson, or Og, element 118.

In nature, atoms of one element may be chemically bonded to other atoms of the same element. For example, hydrogen and oxygen are always diatomic; that is, they exist as H_2 and O_2, respectively. Elemental sulfur exists as S_8. Many atoms—for example, sodium—exist as single atoms in their elemental form.

b. Compounds

A **compound** is a combination of two or more atoms of different elements in a precise proportion by mass. In a compound, atoms are held together by attractive forces called *chemical bonds*.

c. Mixtures

A **mixture** is a combination of two or more compounds (or substances) interacting but not bonded chemically with one another. Substances that make up a mixture can be separated by physical means.

7. Properties of Atoms

Law of conservation of mass: In a chemical reaction, matter cannot be created or destroyed; that is, the mass of the reagents equals the mass of the products. Likewise, the number of each type of atom will be equal on each side of the reaction.

Law of constant (definite) proportion: A chemical compound will always have the same proportion of elements by mass—for example, water (H_2O) will always be $\frac{8}{9}$ oxygen and $\frac{1}{9}$ hydrogen by mass.

Law of multiple proportions: If two elements form more than one compound between them, then the ratios of the masses of the second element that combine with a fixed mass of the first element will be ratios of small whole numbers. For

example, 16 grams of oxygen will react with 14 grams of nitrogen to form NO and with 28 grams of nitrogen to form N_2O (1:2 ratio).

Questions

1. Which of the following statements about atoms is true?
   a. They have more protons than electrons.
   b. They have more electrons than protons.
   c. They are electrically neutral.
   d. They have as many neutrons as they have electrons.

2. What is the mass number of an atom with 60 protons, 60 electrons, and 75 neutrons?
   a. 120
   b. 135
   c. 75
   d. 195

3. What is the atomic number of an atom with 17 protons, 17 electrons, and 20 neutrons?
   a. 37
   b. 34
   c. 54
   d. 17

4. Two atoms, L and M, are isotopes. Which of the following properties would they NOT have in common?
   a. atomic number
   b. atomic weight
   c. chemical reactivity
   d. the number of protons in the nucleus

5. An atom with an atomic number of 58 and an atomic mass of 118 has
   a. 58 neutrons.
   b. 176 neutrons.
   c. 60 neutrons.
   d. 116 neutrons.

6. Dalton's theory included the concept that
   a. atoms are mostly made up of empty space.
   b. electrons balance the charge of the nucleus.
   c. atoms can neither be created nor destroyed.
   d. unstable nuclei can undergo radioactive decay.

7. An atom has 12 protons and 10 electrons. What is the charge of the atom?
   a. +1
   b. +2
   c. −1
   d. −2

8. The majority of the space of an atom is made up of its
   a. electrons.
   b. protons.
   c. nucleus.
   d. neutrons.

9. Which of the following is an element?
   a. hydrochloric acid
   b. carbon dioxide
   c. methanol
   d. oxygen gas

10. Which of the following is true of an atom?
   a. It consists of protons, neutrons, and electrons.
   b. It has a nucleus consisting of protons, neutrons, and electrons.
   c. The protons are equal in number to the electrons, so the nucleus is electrically neutral.
   d. All of the above are true.

Answers

1. c. Atoms are electrically neutral; the number of electrons is equal to the number of protons.

2. b. Mass number is the number of protons plus the number of neutrons: $60 + 75 = 135$.

3. d. The atomic number is the number of protons—in this case, 17.

4. b. By definition, isotopes have different numbers of neutrons. Therefore, they differ in atomic weight.

5. c. The number of neutrons is equal to the atomic mass minus the atomic number (the number of protons): $118 − 58 = 60$.

6. c. Dalton proposed that atoms cannot be created or destroyed, only recombined or rearranged in chemical reactions. The other concepts were all discovered later by other scientists.

7. b. Protons have a charge of +1 and electrons have a charge of −1. If there are two more protons than electrons, the charge would be +2.

8. a. The nucleus of an atom contains the protons and neutrons and is responsible almost entirely for the mass of the atom. The electrons orbiting the nucleus take up most of the space of an atom.

9. d. An element is a substance composed of only one atom. Oxygen gas is an example of an element. Hydrochloric acid, carbon dioxide, and methanol are all compounds.

10. a. An atom consists of protons, neutrons, and electrons; the nucleus contains protons and neutrons. The protons are equal in number to the electrons, but the nucleus itself is not electrically neutral.

B. Periodic Table (page 192)
1. Periodic Law
Periodic law is when the properties of the elements are a periodic function of their atomic number.

Periodic table is an arrangement of the elements according to similarity in their chemical properties and in order of increasing atomic number.

2. Properties of the Periodic Table
a. Periods
Periods are the horizontal rows of the periodic table. Elements in the same period have the same number of electron shells (or levels).

1 IA	2 IIA	3 IIIB	4 IVB	5 VB	6 VIB	7 VIIB	8	9 VIIIB	10	11 IB	12 IIB	13 IIIA	14 IVA	15 VA	16 VIA	17 VIIA	18 VIIIA
1 H 1.00794																	2 He 4.002602
3 Li 6.941	4 Be 9.012182											5 B 10.811	6 C 12.0107	7 N 14.00674	8 O 15.9994	9 F 8.9984032	10 Ne 20.1797
11 Na 22.989770	12 Mg 24.3050											13 Al 26.981538	14 Si 28.0855	15 P 30.973761	16 S 32.066	17 Cl 35.4527	18 Ar 39.948
19 K 39.0983	20 Ca 40.078	21 Sc 44.955910	22 Ti 47.867	23 V 50.9415	24 Cr 51.9961	25 Mn 54.938049	26 Fe 55.845	27 Co 58.933200	28 Ni 58.6934	29 Cu 63.546	30 Zn 65.39	31 Ga 69.723	32 Ge 72.61	33 As 74.92160	34 Se 78.96	35 Br 79.904	36 Kr 83.80
37 Rb 85.4678	38 Sr 87.62	39 Y 88.90585	40 Zr 91.224	41 Nb 92.90638	42 Mo 95.94	43 Tc (98)	44 Ru 101.07	45 Rh 102.90550	46 Pd 106.42	47 Ag 107.8682	48 Cd 112.411	49 In 114.818	50 Sn 118.710	51 Sb 121.760	52 Te 127.60	53 I 126.90447	54 Xe 131.29
55 Cs 132.90545	56 Ba 137.327	57 La* 138.9055	72 Hf 178.49	73 Ta 180.9479	74 W 183.84	75 Re 186.207	76 Os 190.23	77 Ir 192.217	78 Pt 195.078	79 Au 196.96655	80 Hg 200.59	81 Tl 204.3833	82 Pb 207.2	83 Bi 208.98038	84 Po (209)	85 At (210)	86 Rn (222)
87 Fr (223)	88 Ra (226)	89 Ac** (227)	104 Rf (265)	105 Db (268)	106 Sg (271)	107 Bh (270)	108 Hs (277)	109 Mt (276)	110 Ds (281)	111 Rg (280)	112 Cn (285)	113 Nh (286)	114 Fl (289)	115 Mc (289)	116 Lv (293)	117 Ts (294)	118 Og (294)

* Lanthanide series	58 Ce 140.116	59 Pr 140.90765	60 Nd 144.24	61 Pm (145)	62 Sm 150.36	63 Eu 151.964	64 Gd 157.25	65 Tb 158.92534	66 Dy 162.50	67 Ho 164.93032	68 Er 167.26	69 Tm 168.93421	70 Yb 173.04	71 Lu 174.967
** Actinide series	90 Th 232.0381	91 Pa 231.03588	92 U 238.0289	93 Np (237)	94 Pu (244)	95 Am (243)	96 Cm (247)	97 Bk (247)	98 Cf (251)	99 Es (252)	100 Fm (257)	101 Md (258)	102 No (259)	103 Lr (262)

b. Groups

Groups are the vertical column of elements with the same number of electron(s) in their outermost shell. The groups are numbered 1–18 from left to right. An older system that uses Roman numerals to indicate the number of valence (or outermost) electrons is also sometimes used. Both numbering systems are shown in the periodic table above. Elements in the same group share similar chemical properties.

c. Metals

A **metal** is an element that is a good conductor of heat and electricity in addition to being shiny (reflecting light), malleable (easily bent), and ductile (made into wire). Metals are electropositive, having a greater tendency to lose their valence electrons. They are grouped in the left of the periodic table (groups 1-13 or IA-IIIA, IB-VIIIB).

d. Nonmetals

A **nonmetal** is an element with poor conducting properties. They are electronegative and accept electrons in their valence shell. They are found in the upper right-hand corner of the periodic table.

e. Metalloids

A **metalloid** is an element with properties that are intermediate between those of metals and nonmetals, such as semiconductivity. They are also found between metals and nonmetals in the periodic table.

3. Electronic Structure of Atoms
a. Bohr Atom

Niels Bohr's planetary model of the hydrogen atom, in which a nucleus was surrounded by orbits of electrons, resembles the solar system. Electrons could be excited by **quanta** of energy and move to an outer orbit (excited level). They could also emit radiation when falling to their original orbit (ground state).

b. Orbitals

An **orbital** is the space where one or two paired electrons can be located. These are mathematical functions (or figures) with restricted zones, called **nodes**, and specific shapes—for example, *s* orbitals are spherical; *p* orbitals are dumbbell-shaped.

c. Quantum Numbers

There are four quantum numbers that describe an electron in an atom. They are the principal quantum number (n), the orbital quantum number (l), the magnetic quantum number (m_l), and the spin quantum number (m_s).

- **Principal quantum number (n)** determines the overall energy level of the electron; n is a positive integer ($n = 1, 2, 3, \ldots$). For a given principal quantum number (n), there are n possible orbital quantum numbers ($0, 1, 2, \ldots, n - 1$). There is a maximum of n^2 orbitals in an energy level (and $2n^2$ electrons).
- **Orbital quantum number (l)** determines the shape of the orbital in which the electron resides ($0 = s, 1 = p, 2 = d, 3 = f$, etc.). For a given orbital quantum number, l, there are $2l + 1$ orbitals.
- **Magnetic quantum number (m_l)** corresponds to a specific orbital in which the electron resides. For a given orbital quantum number, there are $2l + 1$ magnetic quantum numbers ($-l, -l + 1, -l + 2, \ldots, 0, \ldots, l - 2, l - 1, l$).
- **Spin quantum number (m_s)** describes the direction of the electron's spin, which may be either up ($+\frac{1}{2}$) or down ($-\frac{1}{2}$). Therefore, for two electrons to occupy the same orbital, they must be of opposite spins.

d. Pauli Exclusion Principle

The **Pauli exclusion principle** states that no two electrons can possess the same four quantum numbers. As a consequence, each orbital holds a maximum of two electrons and only if they are of opposite spin.

e. Electron Configuration

Electron configuration describes the exact arrangement of electrons (given in a superscript number) in successive shells (indicated by numbers 1, 2, 3, and so on) and orbitals (s, p, d, f) of an atom, starting with the innermost orbital.

For example, $1s^2 2s^2 2p^6$.

f. Hund's Rule

Hund's rule states that the most stable arrangement of electrons in the same energy level is the one in which electrons have parallel spins (same orientation).

g. Outer Shell (or valence shell)

The **outer shell** is the last energy level in which loosely held electrons are contained. These are the electrons that engage in bonding and are therefore characteristic of the element.

You Should Review

- periodic table: structure; specific names of the different groups (group 1 or IA: alkali metal, group 2 or IIA: alkaline earth, group 17 or VIIA: halogens, etc); the location of metals, nonmetals, and metalloids
- Bohr atom
- ground state
- quantization of energy
- quantum number
- Heisenberg uncertainty principle
- the maximum number of electrons that can be held in each energy level

Questions

11. Which element has the electron configuration $1s^2 2s^2 2p^6$?

   a. neon
   b. calcium
   c. helium
   d. lithium

12. Choose the proper group of symbols for the following elements: potassium, silver, mercury, lead, sodium, iron.
a. Po, Ar, Hr, Pm, So, Fm
b. Pb, Sl, Me, Le, Su, Io
c. Pt, Sr, My, Pd, Sd, In
d. K, Ag, Hg, Pb, Na, Fe

13. What is the maximum number of electrons that each *p* orbital can hold?
a. 8
b. 2
c. 6
d. 4

14. What is the maximum number of electrons that the second energy level can hold?
a. 8
b. 6
c. 2
d. 16

15. What is the name of the individual who proposed that the atom was similar to a solar system, with a dense nucleus and concentric circles around it?
a. Hund
b. Dalton
c. Pauli
d. Bohr

16. The horizontal rows of the periodic table are called
a. families.
b. groups.
c. representative elements.
d. periods.

17. Which of the following is an alkali metal (group 1 or IA)?
a. calcium
b. sodium
c. aluminum
d. alkanium

18. Who stated that an orbital can hold as many as two electrons if they have opposite spins, one clockwise and one counterclockwise?
a. Hund
b. Dalton
c. Pauli
d. Bohr

19. Based on its position in the periodic table, which element would be expected to be the best conductor of electricity?
a. nickel
b. argon
c. bromine
d. boron

20. If the electron configuration of an element is written $1s^2 2s^2 2p^6 3s^2 3p^3$, the element's atomic
a. number is 15.
b. number is 5.
c. weight is 15.
d. weight is 5.

Answers

11. a. Neon has 10 electrons. The electron configuration for neon is $1s^2 2s^2 2p^6$, meaning that there are two electrons in the 1*s* orbital, two electrons in the 2*s* orbital, and six electrons in the 2*p* orbital.

12. d. See the periodic table.

13. b. Each *p* orbital holds two electrons. There are three *p* orbitals, holding a total of six electrons.

14. a. The second energy level has one s orbital and three *p* orbitals, holding a total of eight electrons.

15. d. Bohr proposed the model defined in the question.

16. d. By definition, the periods are the horizontal rows on the periodic table.

17. b. Sodium is an alkali metal.

18. c. The question defines the Pauli exclusion principle.

19. a. The position of nickel shows that it is a transition metal. Transition metals are generally good conductors of electricity. Argon and bromine are nonmetals and boron is a metalloid, and all are poor conductors of electricity.

20. a. Since the element has 15 electrons, it also has 15 protons and an atomic number of 15.

C. Chemical Bonds

1. Octet Rule

Octet rule is when atoms bond by surrounding themselves with eight (octet) outer electrons (two electrons for H). They tend to acquire the stability of their closest noble gases in the periodic table, either by losing (metals), gaining (nonmetals), or sharing electrons in their valence shell.

2. Ions

a. Anions

When an atom gains one or more electrons, it becomes a negatively charged entity called an **anion**. Most anions are nonmetallic. Their names are derived from the elemental name with the suffix, -*ide*. For example, a chlor*ide* ion (Cl^-) occurs when a chlorine atom (Cl) has gained one electron to achieve the octet structure of Argon, or Ar. An ox*ide* ion (O^{2-}) occurs when an oxygen atom (O) has acquired two electrons in its valence shell and has the same, stable electron configuration as Neon, or Ne.

b. Cations

A **cation** results when an atom loses one or more electrons, becoming positively charged. Most cations are metallic and have the same name as the metallic element. For example, lithium ion (Li^+) has one electron fewer than lithium atom (Li), having acquired the noble gas electron structure of Helium, or He.

3. Ionic Compounds

Ionic compounds are compounds formed by combining cations and anions. The attractive electrostatic forces between a cation and an anion is called an **ionic bond**.

4. Molecular Compounds

a. Covalent Bonds

A **covalent bond** is a type of bond formed when two atoms share one or more pairs of electrons to achieve an octet of electrons.

b. Lewis Structures

Lewis structures are formulas for compounds in which each atom exhibits an octet of valence electrons. These are represented as dots (or a line for a shared pair of electrons, leaving unshared pairs of electrons as dots).

unshared pairs of electrons

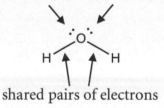

shared pairs of electrons

c. Valence Shell Electron Pair Repulsion (VSEPR) Theory

The **VSEPR model** is based on electrostatic repulsion between electron pair orbitals. By pushing each other away as far as possible, electron pairs dictate which geometry or shape a molecule will adopt. Molecules should be written as Lewis structures (see the electron-dot notation above).

d. Electronegativity and Dipoles

Electronegativity is the ability of an atom in a bond to attract the electron density more than the other atom(s) in the bond. Electronegativity increases from left to right and from bottom to top in the periodic table. Thus, fluorine (F) is the most electronegative element of the periodic table, with the maximum value of 4.0 in the Pauling scale of electronegativity. The Pauling scale is a range of electronegativity values based on fluorine having the highest value at 4.0. These values have no units. Metals are electropositive (with a minimum electronegativity value of 0.8 on the Pauling scale for most alkali metals).

A **dipole** results in a covalent bond between two atoms of different electronegativity. Partial positive ($\delta+$) and negative charges ($\delta-$) develop at both ends of the bond, creating a dipole (i.e., two poles) oriented from the positive end to the negative end.

For example: $H^{+\delta}-Cl^{-\delta}$

5. Hydrogen Bonds

Hydrogen bonds are weak bonds that form between dipoles of consecutive polar molecules (intermolecular) or polar groups of macromolecules (intramolecular), such as proteins and DNA, in which they play an important structural role.

Electronegative atoms (such as F, N, or O) covalently bonded to H atoms are considered hydrogen bond donors. Electronegative atoms with free lone pairs in their Lewis structures act as hydrogen bond acceptors.

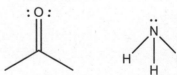

The oxygen atom in acetone [$(CH_3)_2CO$] is a hydrogen bond acceptor. The nitrogen atom in ammonia (NH_3) can act as either a hydrogen bond donor or acceptor. Similarly, the oxygen atom in water can act as either a hydrogen bond donor or acceptor.

6. Polyatomic Ions

Polyatomic ions are groups of two or more covalently bonded atoms that possess a positive or negative charge. They form ionic compounds in the same way as single-atom ions. Polyatomic ions can be as simple as hydroxide (OH^-). Other common examples are ammonium (NH_4^+), phosphate (PO_4^{3-}), carbonate (CO_3^{2-}), nitrate (NO_3^-), and sulfate (SO_4^{2-}).

You Should Review

- polyatomic ions
- molecular structures
- structures of water molecules and of biological compounds

Questions

21. The bond between oxygen and hydrogen atoms in a single water molecule is
    a. a hydrogen bond.
    b. a polar covalent bond.
    c. a nonpolar covalent bond.
    d. an ionic bond.

22. Which of the following is a nonpolar covalent bond?
    a. the bond between two carbons
    b. the bond between sodium and chloride
    c. the bond between two water molecules
    d. the bond between nitrogen and hydrogen

23. The type of bond formed between two molecules of water is a
    a. polar covalent bond.
    b. hydrogen bond.
    c. nonpolar covalent bond.
    d. peptide bond.

24. Which of the following elements has the highest electronegativity?

　　a. lithium

　　b. radon

　　c. silicon

　　d. chlorine

25. If X (atomic number 4) and Y (atomic number 17) react, the formula of the compound formed will be

　　a. XY_2.

　　b. YX_2.

　　c. X_2Y_2.

　　d. XY_4.

26. To acquire an outer octet, an atom of element 19 has to

　　a. lose one electron (and acquire a charge of +1).

　　b. lose two electrons (and acquire a charge of +2).

　　c. gain one electron (and acquire a charge of −1).

　　d. gain two electrons (and acquire a charge of −2).

27. The most common ions of the elements of group 17 (VIIA) have electrical charges of

　　a. +7.

　　b. −7.

　　c. +1.

　　d. −1.

28. Which of the following is true according to the octet rule?

　　a. Ions of all group 2 (IIA) elements have electron configurations that conform to those of the noble gases and have charges of +1.

　　b. Ions of all group 17 (VIIA) elements have electron configurations that conform to those of the noble gases and have charges of −2.

　　c. An ion of a metallic element that has lost electrons to achieve noble gas configuration is less stable than an atom of the same element.

　　d. The most reactive elements are generally those whose atoms are nearest, but not equal, to noble gas configurations.

29. Which of the following is true about the polyatomic ion NH_4^+?

　　a. Its N and H atoms are ionically bonded.

　　b. It can form an ionic compound with Cl^-.

　　c. Each atom in the ion has a charge of +1.

　　d. The +1 charge is located on the N atom.

30. How many electrons does the ion O^{2-} have in its outer shell?

　　a. four

　　b. six

　　c. eight

　　d. ten

Answers

21. b. A covalent bond exists between H and O in an H_2O molecule. Since the bond is formed between two different elements, it is polar.

22. a. The bond formed is covalent. Since it is between two identical elements, it is nonpolar.

23. b. Hydrogen bonds from the H of one water molecule to the O of another hold water molecules together weakly.

24. d. Electronegativity increases as you move left to right across the periodic table and as you move from bottom to top of the periodic table. Chlorine is toward the top and right of the periodic table and is the most electronegative of the elements listed.

25. a. The electron configuration of X is $1s^2 2s^2$, and the electron configuration of Y is $1s^2 2s^2 2p^6 3s^2 3p^5$. X needs to give away two electrons to achieve the stable noble gas configuration of He, which is $1s^2$. Y needs to accept one electron to achieve the outer octet. Therefore, two Y are needed to accept two electrons.

26. a. The electron configuration of element 19 is $1s^2 2s^2 2p^6 3s^2 3p^6 4s^1$. To achieve the outer octet, it must give away one electron.

27. d. Group 17 (VIIA) elements need to accept one electron to achieve the outer octet.

28. d. The alkali metals (group 1 or IA) and the halogens (group 17 or VIIA) have atoms that are near but not equal to noble gas configurations.

29. b. Polyatomic ions can form ionic compounds with oppositely charged ions just like single atom ions. The atoms within a polyatomic ion are covalently bonded and the charge is distributed among all the atoms in the ion, giving the ion the overall charge that it is labeled with.

30. c. The neutral oxygen atom has two electrons in its inner shell and six electrons in its outer shell. The O^{2-} ion has two additional electrons in its outer shell and a stable outer shell of eight electrons.

D. Chemical Equations and Stoichiometry

1. Molecular Weight

Molecular weight is the sum of the atomic weights of all the atoms in a molecular formula. It is the same as the molar mass (in grams) without the unit.

2. Moles

A **mole** of a particular substance is defined as the number of atoms in exactly 12 g of carbon-12. Experiments established that number to be $6.02214199 \times 10^{23}$ particles (Avogadro's number).

3. Chemical Equations
a. Balancing Equations

Chemical reactions can be balanced by a "trial-and-error" method.

- Write the correct formulas for all reactants and products.
- Compare the number of atoms on the reactant and product(s) sides.
- Rebalance and recheck if necessary.
- Always balance the heavier atoms before trying to balance lighter ones, such as H.
- Use fractions if necessary to reduce coefficients or use the smallest possible whole number.
- Verify (again!) that the number of atoms of each element is balanced.

b. Use of Moles in Chemical Equations

Stoichiometry establishes the quantities of reactants used and products obtained based on a balanced chemical equation.

$$\text{\# moles} = \frac{\text{mass (in g)}}{\text{molar mass (in } \frac{\text{g}}{\text{mol}})}$$

4. Theoretical Yield

Theoretical yield is the amount of product expected in a chemical reaction based on the mass of the starting materials and the stoichiometry of the balanced chemical equation.

5. Percentage Yield

When a chemical reaction is run, often the amount of product recovered is less than what is predicted by stoichiometry. The **percentage yield** is the ratio of the experimental (actual) yield of the product divided by the theoretical yield.

$$\% \text{ yield} = \left(\frac{\text{actual yield}}{\text{theoretical yield}}\right) \times 100\%$$

6. Basic Types of Chemical Reactions

- Combination reactions:

  $A + B \rightarrow C$

  $H_2 + \frac{1}{2}O_2 \rightarrow H_2O$

- Decomposition reactions:

  $C \rightarrow A + B$

  $CaCO_3 \rightarrow CaO + CO_2$

- Single displacement reactions:

  $A + BC \rightarrow B + AC$

  $Zn + 2HCl \rightarrow H_2 + ZnCl_2$

- Double displacement reactions:

  $AB + CD \rightarrow AC + BD$

  $HCl + NaOH \rightarrow H_2O + NaCl$

You Should Review

- balancing equations and using polyatomic ions in balancing equations

Questions

31. Which of the following is the percentage yield for a reaction that is expected to yield 2.5 grams of a product, but actually yields 2.4 grams of the product?
a. 0.96%
b. 1.04%
c. 96%
d. 104%

32. The formula of carbon dioxide is CO_2. Its molecular weight is 44 amu. A sample of 11 grams of CO_2 contains
a. 1.0 mole of carbon dioxide.
b. 1.5 grams of carbon.
c. 3.0 grams of carbon.
d. 6.0 grams of oxygen.

33. How many grams are contained in 0.200 mol of calcium phosphate, $Ca_3(PO_4)_2$?
a. 6.20
b. 62.0
c. 124
d. 31.0

34. A chemical reaction produced 0.1 grams of hydrogen gas (H_2). How many moles of hydrogen gas did the reaction produce?
a. 0.05 moles
b. 0.2 moles
c. 5 moles
d. 20 moles

35. In the reaction $CaCl_2 + Na_2CO_3 \rightarrow CaCO_3 + 2NaCl$, if 0.5 mole of NaCl is to be formed,
a. 1 mole of Na_2CO_3 is needed.
b. 0.5 mole of $CaCO_3$ is also formed.
c. 0.5 mole of Na_2CO_3 is needed.
d. 0.25 mole of $CaCl_2$ is needed.

36. In the reaction $2Cu_2S + 3O_2 \rightarrow 2Cu_2O + 2SO_2$, if 24 moles of Cu_2O are to be prepared, then how many moles of O_2 are needed?
a. 24
b. 36
c. 16
d. 27

37. Which of the following equations is balanced?
a. $2H_2O_2 \rightarrow 2H_2O + O_2$
b. $Ag + Cl_2 \rightarrow 2AgCl$
c. $KClO_3 \rightarrow KCl + O_2$
d. $Na + H_2O \rightarrow NaOH + H_2$

38. Butane (C_4H_{10}) burns with oxygen in the air according to the following equation:

$2C_4H_{10} + 13O_2 \rightarrow 8CO_2 + 10H_2O$.

In one experiment, the supply of oxygen was limited to 98.0 g. How much butane can be burned by this much oxygen?
a. 15.1 g C_4H_{10}
b. 27.3 g C_4H_{10}
c. 54.6 g C_4H_{10}
d. 30.2 g C_4H_{10}

39. What type of chemical equation is
$2NH_3 \rightarrow N_2 + 3H_2$?
a. combination reaction
b. decomposition reaction
c. single displacement reaction
d. double displacement reaction

40. Which of the following equations is balanced?
a. $Mg + N_2 \rightarrow Mg_3N_2$
b. $Fe + O_2 \rightarrow Fe_2O_3$
c. $C_{12}H_{22}O_{11} \rightarrow 12C + 11H_2O$
d. $Ca + H_2O \rightarrow Ca(OH)_2 + H_2$

Answers

31. c. The percentage yield is found by dividing the actual yield, 2.4 grams, by the expected yield, 2.5 grams, and multiplying the result by 100.

32. c. $11 \text{ g CO}_2 \times \frac{\text{mol C}}{44 \text{ g CO}_2} \times \frac{12 \text{ g}}{\text{mol C}} = 3.0 \text{ g}$

33. b. 1 mole of $Ca_23(PO_4)_2 = 310$ g;
$0.200 \text{ mol} \times \frac{310 \text{ g}}{\text{mol}} = 62.0 \text{ g}$

34. a. The molar mass of hydrogen gas, H_2, is 2.01588 grams/mole, which means that one mole of hydrogen gas has a mass of 2.01588 grams. The number of moles of gas produced is found by dividing the mass of the hydrogen gas, 0.1 grams, by the molar mass, 2.01588 grams/mole.

35. d. One mole of $CaCl_2$ would be needed to get 2 mol NaCl. Since 0.5 mol of NaCl, or 25% of 2 moles, is to be formed, 0.25 mol $CaCl_2$ (25% of 1 mole) is needed.

36. b. $24 \text{ mol Cu}_2O \times \frac{3 \text{ mol O}_2}{2 \text{ mol Cu}_2O} = 36 \text{ mol O}_2$

37. a. There are 4 H in the reactants and 4 H in the products, and 4 O in the reactants and 4 O in the products.

38. b. Normally 2 moles of C_4H_{10} react with 13 moles of O_2. The supply of oxygen is limited to 98 g, or 3.06 moles; $98.0 \text{ g O}_2 \times \frac{\text{mol O}_2}{32.0 \text{ g O}_2} \times \frac{2 \text{ mol C}_4H_{10}}{13 \text{ mol O}_2} \times \frac{58.0 \text{ g}}{\text{mol C}_4H_{10}} = 27.3 \text{ g}$.

39. b. A decomposition reaction takes the form $C \rightarrow A + B$.

40. c. There are 12 C on both sides, 22 H on both sides, and 11 O on both sides.

E. Energy and the States of Matter
1. Solids
A **solid** is the state of matter characterized by a definite volume and shape. Solids are not compressible.

2. Liquids
A **liquid** is a fluid state of matter characterized by a definite volume but no definite shape. Liquids are also slightly compressible.

3. Gases
All gases behave according to the following characteristics:

- Gases expand to assume the volume and shape of their container.
- Many gases mix evenly and completely when confined in the same container.
- Gas molecules collide with each other; they do not attract or repel each other.
- Gas molecules have higher kinetic energy at higher temperatures.

4. Pressure
Pressure is force exerted over an unit area. The atmospheric pressure exerted by Earth's atmosphere is a function of the altitude and the weather conditions. It decreases with higher altitude. Some useful units of pressure and how they relate are: 1 atm (atmosphere) = 760 mm Hg = 760 torr = 101,325 Pa (pascals).

5. Gas Laws
a. Boyle's Law (at constant temperature)
The volume of a sample of gas decreases as its pressure increases ($P \propto \frac{1}{V}$): $P_1V_1 = P_2V_2$.

b. Charles's Law (at constant pressure)

The volume of a sample of gas maintained at constant pressure increases with its temperature ($V \propto T$): $\frac{V_1}{T_1} = \frac{V_2}{T_2}$.

c. Gay-Lussac's Law (at constant volume)

The pressure of any sample of gas increases (maintained at constant volume) with the temperature ($P \propto T$): $\frac{P_1}{T_1} = \frac{P_2}{T_2}$.

d. Avogadro's Law (at constant T and P)

The volume of gas increases with the number of moles of gas present at constant temperature and pressure ($V \propto n$): $\frac{V_1}{n_1} = \frac{V_2}{n_2}$.

Standard temperature and pressure (STP) condition is achieved at 273 K and 1 atm (760 torr) when one mole (or 6.02×10^{23} particles) of any gas occupies a volume of 22.4 liters (molar volume at STP).

e. Dalton's Law of Partial Pressure

In a mixture of gases, individual gases behave independently so that the total pressure is the sum of partial pressures; $P_T = P_1 + P_2 + P_3 + \ldots$

f. Graham's Law of Effusion

Graham's law of effusion is that:
$$\frac{\text{Effusion rate of A}}{\text{Effusion rate of B}} = \frac{k_A}{k_B} = \sqrt{\frac{\text{MW of B}}{\text{MW of A}}}.$$

Graham's law states that the rate of effusion of two gases is inversely proportional to the square root of their molecular weights. For example, if hydrogen (H_2, MW = 2 g/mol) and oxygen (O_2, MW = 32 g/mol) are used to fill a balloon and a small pinhole is introduced, hydrogen will escape four times faster than oxygen.

$$\frac{k_{H^2}}{k_{O^2}} = \sqrt{\frac{32 \text{ g/mol}}{2 \text{ g/mol}}} = 4$$

g. Ideal Gas Law

An ideal gas is a gas whose pressure, volume, and temperature obey the relation, $PV = nRT$ (a com-bination of Boyle's, Charles's, and Avogadro's laws), R being the gas constant. The same relation can also be expressed by: $\frac{P_1 V_1}{T_1} = \frac{P_2 V_2}{T_2}$.

You Should Review

- properties of gases, liquids, and solids
- kinetic theory of gases
- kinetic theory and chemical reactions

Questions

41. A pressure of 740 mm Hg is the same as
- **a.** 1 atm.
- **b.** 0.974 atm.
- **c.** 1.03 atm.
- **d.** 0.740 atm.

42. According to Graham's law, which of the following gases will effuse fastest?
- **a.** NO_2
- **b.** CO_2
- **c.** SO_2
- **d.** N_2O

43. Charles's Law describes the relationship between
- **a.** temperature and pressure.
- **b.** pressure and volume.
- **c.** volume and temperature.
- **d.** pressure, volume, and temperature.

44. Which of the following laws is related to this expression: $P_T = P_1 + P_2 + P_3$?
- **a.** Boyle's law
- **b.** Charles's law
- **c.** Gay-Lussac's law
- **d.** Dalton's law

45. A substance has a definite volume. Which of the following could the substance be?
- **a.** only a liquid
- **b.** only a solid
- **c.** a liquid or a solid
- **d.** a gas, a liquid, or a solid

46. Gases that conform to the assumptions of kinetic theory are referred to as
  a. kinetic gases.
  b. natural gases.
  c. ideal gases.
  d. real gases.

47. What does the term *pressure* mean when applied to a gas?
  a. weight
  b. how heavy the gas is
  c. mass divided by volume
  d. force exerted per unit area

48. A sample of helium at 25°C occupies a volume of 725 ml at 730 mm Hg. What volume will it occupy at 25°C and 760 mm Hg?
  a. 755 ml
  b. 760 ml
  c. 696 ml
  d. 730 ml

49. A sample of nitrogen at 20°C in a volume of 875 ml has a pressure of 730 mm Hg. What will be its pressure at 20°C if the volume is changed to 955 ml?
  a. 750 mm Hg
  b. 658 mm Hg
  c. 797 mm Hg
  d. 669 mm Hg

50. A mixture consisting of 8.0 g of oxygen and 14 g of nitrogen is prepared in a container such that the total pressure is 750 mm Hg. The partial pressure of oxygen in the mixture is
  a. 125 mm Hg.
  b. 500 mm Hg.
  c. 135 mm Hg.
  d. 250 mm Hg.

Answers

41. b. 760 mm Hg is equal to 1 atmosphere; $\frac{740 \text{ mm}}{760 \text{ mm}} = 0.974$.

42. c. Graham's law states that the rate of effusion of a gas is proportional to the inverse square root of its molar mass. Thus, gases with higher molar masses have faster rates of effusion. Sulfur dioxide (SO_2) has the highest molar mass of the gases listed, 64 g/mol.

43. a. Charles's Law describes the relationship between temperature and pressure. It states that the volume of a gas increases with temperature.

44. d. Dalton's law states that $P_T = P_1 + P_2 + P_3$.

45. c. Gases, liquids, and solids can be classified based on whether they have definite volume and definite shape. Gases do not have a definite volume or a definite shape. Liquids and solids both have a definite volume, but only solids also have a definite shape. A substance with a definite volume could be a liquid or a solid, but not a gas.

46. c. The assumptions are applied to ideal gases.

47. d. Pressure refers to the force exerted per unit area.

48. c. Use Boyle's law: $P_1 V_1 = P_2 V_2$.
  $730 \times 725 = 760 V_2$
  $529,250 = 760 V_2$
  $\frac{529,250}{760} = V_2$
  $696 \text{ ml} = V_2$

49. d. Again, use Boyle's law: $P_1 V_1 = P_2 V_2$.
  $730 \times 875 = P_1 \times 955$
  $638,750 = 955 P_1$
  $\frac{638,750}{955} = P_1$
  $669 \text{ mm} = P_1$

50. d. $8.0 \text{ g O}_2 \times \frac{\text{mol O}_2}{32.0 \text{ g O}_2} = 0.25 \text{ mol O}_2$; $14 \text{ g N}_2 \times \frac{\text{mol N}_2}{28.0 \text{ g N}_2} = 0.50 \text{ mol N}_2$; $PO_2 = \frac{0.25}{0.25 + 0.50} \times 750 \text{ mm Hg} = 250 \text{ mm Hg}$

F. Solutions

1. Properties

Solution is a homogeneous mixture.

Solute is a substance dissolved in a solvent.

Solvent is a medium in which a solute is dissolved.

Solvation is the process of dissolving solute molecules in a solvent.

2. Solubility

Solubility is the maximum amount of solute (in grams) that can be dissolved in a certain amount of solvent (in ml) at a particular temperature.

a. Pressure

Solubility increases with pressure for a gas immersed in a liquid. Solubility of solids and liquids does not vary significantly with pressure.

b. Temperature

Solubility of most solids and liquids increases with increasing temperature while decreasing for gases dissolved in liquids (gas molecules tend to escape).

3. Concentration of Solutions

Percent concentration expresses the concentration as a ratio of the weight (or the volume) of the solute over the weight (or the volume) of the solution. This ratio is then multiplied by 100.

$$\frac{\text{Weight}}{\text{volume}}\% = \frac{\text{grams of solute}}{100 \text{ ml of solvent}}$$

$$\frac{\text{Volume}}{\text{volume}}\% = \frac{\text{volume of solute}}{100 \text{ ml volume of final solution}}$$

$$\frac{\text{Weight}}{\text{weight}}\% = \frac{\text{grams of solute}}{100 \text{ g of solution}}$$

4. Molarity

Molarity (M) expresses the number of moles of solute per liter of solution. A 0.1 M NaOH aqueous (water) solution has 0.1 mol of solute (NaOH) in 1 liter of solution.

5. Dilution

$M_i V_i = M_f V_f$ (i = initial; f = final) establishes the equivalence between the initial and final concen-trations. In dilution, equivalence must be achieved between the initial and final number of moles.

Since M (mol/L) $\times V$ (L) gives units of moles, this equation states that the amount of a substance must be constant before and after a dilution occurs (i.e., if 1 L of an aqueous solution containing 0.1 mol [5.8 g] NaCl is diluted by adding an additional liter of water, there will still be 0.1 mol [5.8 g] NaCl in the solution).

6. Colloids

Colloids are stable mixtures in which particles of rather large sizes (ranging from 1 nm [nanometer] to 1 μm [micrometer]) are dispersed throughout another substance. Aerosols (liquid droplets or solid particles dispersed in a gas) such as fog can scatter a beam of light. This is called the **Tyndall effect**.

7. Water

a. Properties

Water is the most abundant (and important, besides oxygen) substance on Earth. Its O-H bonds are highly polar, and water molecules form networks of hydrogen bonds. It is found in large amounts in cells and blood. Water is an excellent solvent and has a high boiling point, high surface tension, high heat of vaporization, and low vapor pressure.

b. High Heat Capacity and High Heat of Vaporization

Heat capacity is the amount of energy required to raise the temperature of a substance by one degree Celsius. The specific heat capacity is the energy required to raise 1 g of a substance by 1°C. Water has high heat capacity, absorbing and releasing large amounts of heat before changing its own temperature. It thus allows the body to maintain a steady temperature even when internal and/or external conditions would increase body temperature.

Specific heat of vaporization is the heat required to evaporate 1 gram of a liquid. Water's large heat of vaporization (540 calories/gram) requires large amounts of heat in order to vaporize it into gas. During perspiration, water evaporates from the skin and large amounts of heat are lost.

c. Reactivity

Water is not reactive with most biological substances, so it can serve to transport substances in the body. It takes part in most metabolic transformations (hydrolysis and dehydration reactions).

You Should Review

- the characteristics of solutions and the properties of true solutions
- the types of solutions and how they compare
- saturated solutions
- supersaturated solutions
- dilute solutions
- concentrated solutions
- how water dissolves ionic compounds
- how water dissolves covalent compounds
- hydrates

Questions

51. In a dilute solution of sodium chloride in water, the sodium chloride is the
a. solvent.
b. solute.
c. precipitate.
d. reactant.

52. To prepare 100 ml of 0.20 M NaCl solution from stock solution of 1.00 M NaCl, you should mix
a. 20 ml of stock solution with 80 ml of water.
b. 40 ml of stock solution with 60 ml of water.
c. 20 ml of stock solution with 100 ml of water.
d. 25 ml of stock solution with 75 ml of water.

53. How many grams of NaOH would be needed to make 250 ml of 0.200 M solution? (molecular weight of NaOH = 40.0)
a. 8.00 g
b. 4.00 g
c. 2.00 g
d. 2.50 g

54. The number of moles of NaCl in 250 ml of a 0.300 M solution of NaCl is
a. 0.0750.
b. 0.150.
c. 0.250.
d. 1.15.

55. Which of the following properties of water is not dependent on the polar nature of water?
a. color
b. high boiling point
c. solvent power
d. high heat of vaporization

56. Which change would increase the solubility of a salt in water?
a. decreasing the surface area of the salt
b. increasing the temperature of the water
c. decreasing the pressure on the water
d. increasing the pressure on the salt

57. How many grams of sugar are needed to make 500 ml of a 5% (weight/volume) solution of sugar?
a. 20
b. 25
c. 50
d. 10

58. Which of the following types of bonds forms when a hydrogen atom binds to a highly electronegative atom and also partially binds to another atom?
  a. coordinate covalent bond
  b. hydrogen bond
  c. ionic bond
  d. covalent bond

59. The heat of vaporization of methanol is 43.5 kilojoules/mole. This indicates that 43.5 kilojoules of heat
  a. is required to raise the temperature methanol by 1° Celsius.
  b. is released when one mole of methanol evaporates.
  c. is required to evaporate one mole of methanol.
  d. is released as each molecule of methanol evaporates.

60. Which of the following is NOT a factor that affects solubility?
  a. temperature
  b. pressure
  c. particle size
  d. properties of the solvent

Answers

51. b. The substance being dissolved is the solute, by definition.

52. a. You need 20 ml of stock solution; you would fill the container with water to the 100 ml mark (80 ml H_2O).
$$M_i \times V_i = M_f \times V_f$$
$$1.0\ M \times V_i = 0.2\ M \times 100\ ml$$
$$1.0\ V_i = 20$$
$$V_i = \frac{20}{1} = 20\ ml$$

53. c. $250\ ml \times \frac{0.2\ M\ NaOH}{1,000\ ml} = 0.05\ mol$; 0.05 moles $\times 40\ g = 2.00\ g$

54. a. $250\ ml \times \frac{0.3\ M\ NaCl}{1,000\ ml} = 0.0750\ mol$

55. a. The other properties listed are due to the polar nature of water.

56. b. One way to increase the solubility of liquids and solids is to increase the temperature of either the liquid or solid. In this case, increasing the temperature of the liquid solvent would increase the solubility of the salt.

57. b. $5\%\ \frac{w}{v} = \frac{5\ g\ solute}{100\ ml\ solution}$
$$\frac{5\ g}{100\ ml} = \frac{x\ (solute\ needed)}{500\ ml\ (final\ volume)}$$
$$\frac{5 \times 500}{100} = x$$
$$25\ g = x$$

58. b. Hydrogen atoms are capable of forming a partial bond between a highly electronegative atom and another atom.

59. c. Heat of vaporization is a measure of the amount of heat or energy needed to evaporate a substance. It is commonly measured as kilojoules/mole or calories/gram.

60. c. Temperature, pressure, and the properties of the solvent all affect solubility.

G. Reaction Rates and Equilibrium

1. Equilibrium

Equilibrium is reached when two opposing reactions occur at the same rate. No change is observed in the system; for example, for the reaction A ⇆ B, the rate at which A is converted to B is the same rate at which B is converted to A.

2. Equilibrium Constant

The **equilibrium constant**, *K*, for a reaction describes the concentrations of reactants and products for a chemical reaction at equilibrium. *K* is often dependent on temperature. For a balanced chemical equation the equilibrium constant is written as:

$$wA + xB \leftrightarrows yC + zD \qquad K = \frac{[C]^y[D]^z}{[A]^w[B]^x}$$

where [*A*], [*B*], [*C*], and [*D*] are concentrations of reactants and products and *w*, *x*, *y*, and *z* are the coefficients used to balance the chemical equation.

If one of the reactants or products is a solid, it is not included in the equilibrium expression.

3. Activation Energy

Activation energy is the minimum amount of energy required for reactants to be transformed into products (i.e., to overcome the energy barrier between reactants and products). The higher the activation energy, the slower the reaction.

4. Endothermic vs. Exothermic Reactions

Endothermic reactions are reactions that consume energy in order to take place. Anabolic reactions are examples.

Exothermic reactions are energy-releasing reactions. Most catabolic and oxidative reactions are examples.

5. Factors Affecting the Rate of Reaction

a. Temperature

Rates of reactions increase with temperature, as more collisions between particles occur at higher temperatures.

b. Particle Size

Smaller particles react faster, as they collide often at any given temperature and concentration.

c. Concentration

A high concentration of reacting particles increases the rate of chemical reactions between them.

d. Catalysis

Catalysts speed the reaction rate by lowering the activation energy of the reaction. They are not consumed in the reaction.

6. Reversible Reactions

A double arrow ($\leftrightarrows$) designates reversible (two-way) chemical reactions. If arrows differ in length, the longer arrow indicates the major (faster) direction in which the reaction proceeds.

7. Le Chatelier's Principle

Le Chatelier's principle states that when a system at equilibrium experiences a change (e.g., in concentration, temperature, or partial pressure), it will respond to counteract this change and establish a new equilibrium. For example, increasing the concentration of compounds on the right side of a chemical equation will shift the equilibrium to the left.

You Should Review

- Le Chatelier's principle and the different stresses that can be placed on chemical processes
- equilibrium constants
- energy diagrams

Questions

61. Which of the following is NOT true of reversible chemical reactions?
- **a.** A chemical reaction is never complete.
- **b.** The products of the reaction also react to reform the original reactants.
- **c.** When the reaction is finished, both reactants and products are present in equal amounts.
- **d.** The reaction can result in an equilibrium.

62. Which is an example of an exothermic change?
- **a.** sublimation
- **b.** condensation
- **c.** melting
- **d.** evaporation

63. Which of the following would decrease the rate of a reaction?
- **a.** decreasing the particle size
- **b.** using a more dilute reactant
- **c.** increasing the temperature
- **d.** adding a catalyst

64. The following reaction is exothermic: $AgNO_3 + NaCl \leftrightarrows AgCl + NaNO_3$. How will the equilibrium be changed if the temperature is increased?

   a. Equilibrium will shift to the right.

   b. Equilibrium will shift to the left.

   c. The reaction will not proceed.

   d. Equilibrium will not change.

Answers

61. c. The fact that a reaction is complete does not mean that both reactants and products are present in equal amounts.

62. b. Condensation is an example of a reaction in which energy is given off.

63. b. Using a more dilute reactant would decrease the rate of a reaction. Decreasing the particle size, increasing the temperature, and adding a catalyst would all increase the rate of a reaction.

64. b. When the temperature is increased, the equilibrium shifts to the left.

H. Acids and Bases
1. Definitions

Acids are proton donors (according to Bronsted theory) or electron acceptors (according to Lewis theory). Acids release protons (H^+) and form anionic conjugate bases (negatively charged ions). Strong acids completely dissociate in water. Acids have a sour taste.

COMMON STRONG ACIDS
Hydrochloric (HCl)
Hydrobromic (HBr)
Hydroiodic (HI)
Perchloric (HClO$_4$)
Sulfuric (H$_2$SO$_4$)

Bases are proton acceptors (Bronsted) or electron donors (Lewis). When dissolved in water, strong bases such as NaOH dissociate to release hydroxide ions and cationic conjugate acids (positively charged ions). Bases have a bitter taste and feel slippery like soap.

2. Reactions of Acids

Common reactions include:

- metal + acid → salt + hydrogen gas
  $Zn + 2HCl \rightarrow ZnCl_2 + H_2$
- base + acid → salt + water
  $NaOH + HNO_3 \rightarrow NaNO_3 + H_2O$
- metal oxide + acid → salt + water
  $CaO + 2HNO_3 \rightarrow Ca(NO_3)_2 + H_2O$
- metal carbonate + acid → salt + carbonic acid (unstable)
  $NaHCO_3 + HCl \rightarrow NaCl + H_2CO_3$
  $(H_2CO_3 \rightarrow H_2O + CO_2)$

3. Autoionization of Water

In pure water, $2H_2O \leftrightarrows H_3O^+ + OH^-$.

The molar concentration of H_3O^+ is equal to molar concentration of OH^- (i.e., $[H_3O]^+ = [OH^-]$).

The ion product of water is K_w; $K_w = [H_3O^+] \times [OH^-] = 1 \times 10^{-14}$. Thus, in pure water: $[H_3O^+] = [OH^-] = 1 \times 10^{-7}$ moles/liter.

4. pH

$pH = - \log [H^+]$ The **pH** measures the negative logarithm (for presentation of very small numbers in a large scale) of the hydrogen ion concentration (in moles/liter). The pH scale runs from 0 to 14 with acids in the lower end of the scale (smaller than pH 7) and bases at the higher end (greater than pH 7).

5. Buffers

Buffer is a solution of a weak base and its conjugate acid (weak also) that prevents drastic changes in pH. The weak base reacts with any H^+ ions that could increase acidity, and the weak conjugate acid reacts with OH^- ions that may increase the basicity of the solution.

a. Carbonic Acid/Bicarbonate Buffer

The pH of blood plasma must be maintained at pH 7.40 by a buffer system consisting of H_2CO_3 and HCO_3^-.

Neutralization of acid:

$$HCO_3^- + H^+ \rightarrow H_2CO_3$$

Neutralization of base:

$$H_2CO_3 + NaOH \rightarrow NaHCO_3 + H_2O$$

b. Phosphate Buffer

The principal buffer system inside cells consists of $H_2PO_4^-$ and HPO_4^{-2}.

Neutralization of acid:

$$HPO_4^{-2} + H^+ \rightarrow H_2PO_4^-$$

Neutralization of base:

$$H_2PO_4^- + OH^- \rightarrow HPO_4^{-2} + H_2O$$

6. Titration

Titration is a technique used to determine the unknown concentration of substance of interest by reacting it with a known quantity of a reagent. In an acid–base titration, an acid or base of unknown concentration is reacted with a known amount of base or acid.

a. Equivalence Point

In an acid–base titration, the **equivalence point** is reached when the amount of titrant (acid or base of known concentration) is equal to the amount of analyte (base or acid of unknown concentration), and the solution is of neutral pH.

b. Normality (N)

Normality is the number of equivalents of the solute per liter of solution. 1 N solution of acid (or base) contains 1 equivalent, that is, 1 mole of H^+ ions (or OH^- ions), of an acid (or base) per liter of solution.

You Should Review

- monoprotic, diprotic, and triprotic acids
- organic and inorganic acids
- Arrhenius acids and bases
- Bronsted-Lowry acids and bases
- reactions of acids
- activity series of metals
- solubilities of salts
- ionic equations
- buffer systems in the body
- metabolic acidosis and alkalosis
- respiratory acidosis and alkalosis

Questions

65. What is the hydrogen ion concentration of a solution with a pH of 2.6?
   a. $0.6 \times 10^{-2.0}$
   b. $1.0 \times 10^{-2.6}$
   c. $1.0 \times 10^{-11.4}$
   d. $2.0 \times 10^{-0.6}$

66. What is the formula of the hydronium ion?
   a. H^+
   b. NH_4^+
   c. H_3O^+
   d. H_2O^+

67. The pH of a blood sample is 7.40 at room temperature. The pOH is therefore
   a. 6.60.
   b. 7.40.
   c. 6×10^{-6}.
   d. 4×10^{-7}.

68. As the concentration of hydrogen ions in a solution decreases,
   a. the pH numerically decreases.
   b. the pH numerically increases.
   c. the product of the concentrations $[H^+] \times [OH^-]$ comes closer to 1×10^{-14}.
   d. the solution becomes more acidic.

69. Which of the following best explains why hydrofluoric acid (HF) is considered a weak acid?

   a. It only partially dissociates in water.
   b. It contains only one hydrogen atom.
   c. It is neutralized by water molecules.
   d. It is a highly corrosive substance.

70. Which of the following acids is a weak acid?

   a. H_2SO_4
   b. HCl
   c. HNO_3
   d. H_3PO_4

71. An acid is a substance that dissociates in water into one or more _____ ions and one or more _____.

   a. hydrogen . . . anions
   b. hydrogen . . . cations
   c. hydroxide . . . anions
   d. hydroxide . . . cations

72. A pH of 4 denotes _____ times fewer _____ than a pH of 3.

   a. 10 . . . hydrogen ions
   b. 4 . . . hydrogen ions
   c. 10 . . . water molecules
   d. 20 . . . hydroxide ions

73. Which of the following is considered to be neutral on the pH scale?

   a. pure water
   b. pure saliva
   c. pure blood
   d. pure urine

74. A substance that functions to prevent rapid, drastic changes in the pH of a fluid by changing strong acids and bases into weak acids and bases is called a(n)

   a. salt.
   b. buffer.
   c. enzyme.
   d. coenzyme.

75. Complete the following equation:
$NaHCO_3 + HCl \rightarrow NaCl +$

   a. HCO_3.
   b. H_2CO_3.
   c. HCl.
   d. H_2PO_4.

Answers

65. **b.** $pH = -\log [H^+]$, so $[H^+] = 1.0 \times 10^{-pH}$
   $= 1.0 \times 10^{-2.6}$.

66. **c.** The formula is H_3O^+.

67. **a.** $[H^+][OH^-] = 1 \times 10^{-14}$

   $[OH^-] = \dfrac{1 \times 10^{-14}}{[H^+]} = \dfrac{1 \times 10^{-14}}{1 \times 10^{-7.40}} = 1 \times 10^{-6.60}$

   $pOH = 6.60$
   or
   $pH + pOH = 14.00$
   $pOH = 14.00 - 7.40 = 6.60$

68. **b.** As the concentration of hydrogen ions decreases, the pH increases.

69. **a.** A strong acid fully dissociates in water, whereas a weak acid only partially dissociates in water. Hydrofluoric acid only partially dissociates in water and so is a weak acid.

70. **d.** Sulfuric acid (H_2SO_4), hydrochloric acid (HCl), and nitric acid (HNO_3) are all strong acids. Phosphoric acid (H_3PO_4) is a weak acid.

71. **a.** By definition, when an acid dissociates in water, it produces one or more H^+ and one or more anions.

72. **a.** An increase of one pH unit is a tenfold decrease in hydrogen ions.

73. a. The pH of pure H_2O is 7. $[H^+] = [OH^-]$
74. b. This is the definition of a buffer.
75. b. Metal bicarbonate + an acid → salt + carbonic acid.

I. Oxidation-Reduction
1. Oxidation State

Oxidation state (or **oxidation number**) is the number of charges carried by an ion in an atom, or the number of charges that an atom would have in a [neutral] molecule if electrons were transferred completely. Oxidation numbers enable the identification of oxidized (increase in oxidation number) and reduced (reduction in oxidation number) elements.

The sum of the oxidation numbers of all atoms in the formula of a neutral compound is zero (or equal to the charge on the ion for a polyatomic ion).

2. Oxidation-Reduction (Redox) Reactions

Oxidation corresponds to a loss of electrons.
Reduction corresponds to a gain of electrons.

Redox (reduction-oxidation) reaction involves an electron transfer between the oxidizing (oxidizes another by accepting its electrons) and the reducing (reduces another by donating electrons) agents.

Example:

$$Na \rightarrow Na^+ + e^-$$

Oxidation Number: 0   +1   −1
(Na is oxidized to Na^+)

Example:

$$Cl + e^- \rightarrow Cl^-$$

Oxidation Number: 0   −1   −1
(Cl is reduced to Cl^-)
Sum: $Na + Cl \rightarrow Na^+ + Cl^-$

You Should Review

- redox reactions: cellular respiration, combustion, rusting
- oxidizing agents
- reducing agents

Questions

76. The number of electrons lost during oxidation must always equal the
  a. charge of the ion.
  b. total change in oxidation number.
  c. number of electrons gained in the reduction.
  d. number of electrons gained by the reducing agent.

77. In a redox reaction, the oxidation number of solid cadmium increases from 0 to +2. Which of the following correctly describes the reaction?
  a. Cadmium is oxidized and is the oxidizing agent.
  b. Cadmium is oxidized and is the reducing agent.
  c. Cadmium is reduced and is the reducing agent.
  d. Cadmium is reduced and is the oxidizing agent.

Answers

76. c. The number of electrons lost during oxidation must always equal the number of electrons gained in the reduction.
77. b. The oxidation number of the cadmium atom has increased, which means the atom has lost electrons and cadmium has been oxidized. In a redox reaction, the substance that is oxidized is the reducing agent.

J. Nuclear Chemistry
1. Characteristics of Radioactivity

Radioactivity is the process by which unstable nuclei break down spontaneously, emitting particles and/or electromagnetic radiation (i.e., energy) also called **nuclear radiation.**

Heavy elements (from atomic numbers 83 to 92) are naturally radioactive and many more (the transuranium elements: atomic number 93 to 118) have been generated in laboratories.

2. Alpha Emission

An **alpha particle** (symbol: ^4_2He or α) corresponds to the nucleus of a helium atom (having two protons and two neutrons) that is spontaneously emitted by a nuclear breakdown or decay.

α-particles are of low energy and therefore low penetrating (a lab coat is sufficient to block their penetration), but dangerous if inhaled or ingested.

3. Beta Emission

A **beta particle** (symbol: $^0_{-1}\text{e}$ or β^-) is an electron released with high speed by a radioactive nucleus in which neutrons are converted into protons and electrons (β-particles). β-particles are medium-penetrating radiation requiring dense material and several layers of clothing to block their penetration. They are dangerous if inhaled or ingested.

4. Gamma Emission

Gamma rays (symbol: γ) are a massless and chargeless form of radiation (pure energy). They are the most-penetrating form of radiation, similar to X-rays, and can only be stopped by barriers of heavy materials such as concrete or lead. They are extremely dangerous and can cause damage to the human body.

5. Transmutation

Nuclear **transmutation** is the conversion of one element or isotope into another. This process may be spontaneous (through α or β decay) resulting in lighter elements, or it may occur when nuclei are bombarded by other particles (protons or neutrons) or nuclei, resulting in heavier elements. During a nuclear reaction, there is:

1. Conservation of mass number
2. Conservation of atomic number

For example, ^{238}U undergoes a decay to form ^{234}Th:

$$^{238}_{92}\text{U} \rightarrow\, ^{234}_{90}\text{Th} +\, ^4_2\text{He}$$

6. Half-Life

Half-life (symbol: $t_{\frac{1}{2}}$) is the time required for the concentration of the nuclei in a given sample to decrease to half of its initial concentration. Half life is specific to a radioactive element and varies widely (from a fraction of a second for ^{43}Tc to millions of years for ^{238}U).

7. Nuclear Fusion

Nuclear fusion is the process in which small nuclei are combined (fused) into larger, more stable ones with the release of a large amount of energy. Fusion reactions take place at very high temperatures. They are also known as thermonuclear reactions. Examples are the reactions that happen in our Sun and H-bombs.

8. Nuclear Fission

Nuclear fission is the process in which a heavier, usually less stable, nucleus splits into smaller nuclei and neutrons. The process releases a large amount of energy and neutrons that can set up a **chain reaction** (or self-sustaining nuclear fission reaction) with a more and more uncontrollable release of energy (a highly exothermic reaction) and neutrons.

9. Radioactive Isotopes

Radioactive isotope (radioisotope) is an unstable isotope of an element that decays into a more stable isotope of the same or a different element. They are of great use in medicine as tracers in the body to help monitor particular atoms in chemical and biological reactions. In this way, they aid with diagnosis and treatment. Doctors use Iodine (-131 and -123) and Technetium-99 because of their short half-lives. A short half-life means a radioisotope decays into a stable (nonradioactive) substance in a relatively short time.

You Should Review

- nuclear reactions
- writing balanced nuclear equations
- radiocarbon dating

- the principles of nuclear power
- the use of radioisotopes and their detection in nuclear medicine
- the dangers of ionizing radiation
- radiation sickness/biological effects of radiation
- units of radiation measurement

Questions

78. The time required for $\frac{1}{2}$ of the atoms in a sample of a radioactive element to disintegrate is known as the element's
   a. decay period.
   b. life time.
   c. radioactive period.
   d. half-life.

79. The least penetrating radiation given off by a radioactive substance consists of
   a. alpha particles.
   b. beta particles.
   c. gamma rays.
   d. X-rays.

80. The half-life of a given element is 70 years. How long will it take 5.0 g of this element to be reduced to 1.25 g?
   a. 70 years
   b. 140 years
   c. 210 years
   d. 35 years

81. If element $^{210}_{83}A$ gives off an alpha particle, what is the atomic number and mass of the resulting element B?
   a. $^{210}_{81}B$
   b. $^{206}_{81}B$
   c. $^{206}_{83}B$
   d. $^{204}_{81}B$

82. If element $^{238}_{92}U$ gives off a beta particle and gamma rays, what is the resulting element?
   a. $^{238}_{93}Np$
   b. $^{234}_{90}Th$
   c. $^{239}_{92}U$
   d. $^{239}_{91}Pa$

83. Iodine-123 has a half-life of 13 hours. How many grams of a 10-gram sample of iodine-123 will remain after 39 hours?
   a. 8.75 grams
   b. 5 grams
   c. 2.5 grams
   d. 1.25 grams

84. What is the missing product?
   $$^{60}_{24}A \rightarrow ^{60}_{24}B + ?$$
   a. $^{4}_{2}He$
   b. γ
   c. $^{0}_{-1}e$
   d. $^{0}_{1}\beta$

Answers

78. d. The question gives the definition of half-life.

79. a. Alpha particles give off the least penetrating radiation.

80. b. In 70 years, there will be $\frac{1}{2} \times 5.0 = 2.5$ g. In 70 more years (140 total), there will be $\frac{1}{2} \times 2.5 = 1.25$ g.

81. b. Giving off an alpha particle is equivalent to giving off a helium nucleus.
   $$^{210}_{83}A - ^{4}_{2}He = ^{206}_{81}B$$

82. a. When a beta particle is given off, the nucleus has the same mass number, but the atomic number is greater by one since a neutron is converted to a proton and an electron.

83. d. The half-life is the time it takes for half of the atoms in a sample to degrade. After 39 hours, iodine-123 has gone through three half-lives. The mass of the element remaining is found by dividing the initial mass in half three times.

84. b. Gamma rays are not particles and therefore do not change the atomic number or atomic mass.

K. Organic Compounds

1. Definition

Organic compounds are compounds made of carbon and hydrogen (hydrocarbon) and heteroatoms such as oxygen, nitrogen, the halogens, phosphorus, sulfur, and others.

2. Stereoisomers

Stereoisomers are two molecules having the same molecular formula and structure but different spatial orientation with respect to the median axis or plane of the molecule. Their three-dimensional shapes are, therefore, very different.

3. Carbohydrates

a. Function

Carbohydrates (or sugars) serve as the main source of energy for living organisms. They are made of one, two, or more rings of carbon, hydrogen, and oxygen. The names of carbohydrates end with the suffix *-ose* (for example, *glucose* and *fructose*).

b. Monosaccharides

Monosaccharides are the simplest carbohydrate structures made of one ring that can contain five C atoms, called a **pentose**, or six C atoms, called a **hexose**. An example of a pentose is ribose, which is a constituent of RNA. One example of a hexose is galactose, that is derived from milk-sugar lactose.

c. Disaccharides

Disaccharides are dimeric sugars made of two monosaccharides joined together in a reaction that releases a molecule of water (dehydration). The bond between the two sugar molecules is called glycosidic linkage and can have either an axial (β-glycoside) or an equatorial (α-glycoside) orientation with respect to the ring conformation.

Examples:

Maltose is two glucose molecules joined together, found in starch.

Lactose is one galactose joined to one glucose, found in milk.

Sucrose is one fructose joined to one glucose, found in table sugar.

d. Polysaccharides

Polysaccharides are polymers, or a long chain of repeating monosaccharide units.

- **Starch** is a mixture of two kinds of polymers of α glucose (linear amylose and amylopectin). Amylose contains glucose molecules joined together by α-glycosidic linkages while amylopectin has an addition of branching at C-6. They are used to store energy in plants.
- **Glycogen** consists of glucose molecules linked by α-glycosidic linkage (C-1 and C-4) and branched (C-6) by α-glycosidic linkage. Glycogen is the storage form of glucose in animals (in liver and skeletal muscle).
- **Cellulose** consists of glucose molecules joined together by β-glycosidic linkage. Cellulose is found in plants and is not digested by humans (they lack the necessary enzyme).

e. Condensation and Hydrolysis

Condensation is the process of bonding together separate monosaccharide subunits into a disaccharide and/or a polysaccharide. It is also called **dehy-**

dration synthesis, as one molecule of water is lost in the process. It is carried out by specific enzymes.

Hydrolysis is the reverse process of condensation as a water molecule and specific enzymes break the glycosidic linkages in disaccharides and polysaccharides into their constituting monosaccharides.

4. Lipids

a. Function

Lipids are a diverse group of compounds that are insoluble in water and polar solvents but soluble in nonpolar solvents. Lipids are stored in the body as a source of energy (twice the energy provided by equal amounts of carbohydrates).

b. Triglycerides

Triglycerides are lipids formed by condensation of glycerol (one molecule) with fatty acids (three molecules). They can be saturated (with fatty acids containing only C-C single bonds) or unsaturated (presence of one or more C=C double bonds). Triglycerides are found in the adipose cells of the body (neutral fat) and are metabolized by the enzyme lipase (an esterase) during hydrolysis, producing fatty acids and glycerol.

c. Ketone Bodies

Three ketone bodies are formed during the breakdown (metabolism) of fats: acetoacetate, β-hydroxybutyrate, and acetone. They are produced to meet the energy requirements of other tissues. Fatty acids—produced by hydrolysis of triglycerides—are converted to ketone bodies in the liver. They are removed by the kidneys (ketonuria), but if they are found in excess in the blood (ketonemia), ketone bodies can cause a decrease of the blood pH and ketoacidosis may result. In ketoacidosis, acetone is exhaled via the lungs. The whole process is called ketosis. Ketonuria and ketonemia are common in patients with diabetes mellitus and cases of prolonged starvation.

d. Phospholipids

Phospholipids are lipids containing a phosphate group. They are the main constituents of cellular membranes.

e. Steroids

Steroids are organic compounds characterized by a core structure known as gonane (three cyclohexane—six carbon rings and one cyclopentane— or five C rings fused together). Steroids differ by the functional groups attached to the gonane core. Cholesterol is an example of a steroid and is a precursor for the steroid hormones such as the sex hormones (androgens and estrogens) and the corticosteroids (hormones of the adrenal cortex).

5. Proteins

a. Functions

Every organism contains thousands of different proteins with a variety of functions: structure (collagen, histones), transport (hemoglobin, serum albumin), defense (antibodies, fibrinogen for blood coagulation), control and regulation (insulin), catalysis (enzymes), and storage.

b. Structure

Proteins (also called polypeptides) are long chains of amino acids joined together by covalent bonds of the same type (peptide or amide bonds). There are 20 naturally occurring amino acids, each characterized by an amino group at one end and a carboxylic acid group at the other end. Different proteins have different numbers and kinds of additional functional groups.

The sequence of amino acids in the long chain defines the primary structure of a protein.

A secondary structure is determined when several residues, linked by hydrogen bonds, conform to a given combination (for example, the α-helix or β-turns).

Tertiary structure refers to the three-dimensionally folded conformation of a protein. This is the biologically active conformation (crystal structure).

A **quaternary structure** can result when two or more individual proteins assemble into a multi-subunit complex.

Conjugated proteins are complexes of proteins with other biomolecules (for example, glycoproteins, also called sugar proteins).

c. Enzymes

Enzymes are biological catalysts whose role is to increase the rate of chemical (metabolic) reactions without being consumed in the reaction. They do so by lowering the activation energy of a reaction by binding specifically (in the active site) to their substrates in a "lock and key" or "induced-fit" mechanism (enzyme-substrate complex). They do not change the nature of the reaction (in fact, any change is associated with a malfunctioning enzyme, the onset of a disease) or its outcome. (See diagram at bottom.)

Enzyme activity is influenced by:

- temperature; proteins can be destroyed at high temperatures and their action is slowed at low temperature.
- pH; enzymes are active in a certain range of the pH.
- concentration of cofactors and coenzymes (vitamins).
- concentration of enzymes and substrates.
- feedback reactions.

Enzyme names are derived from their substrate names with the addition of the suffix, -ase. An example is *sucrase* (substrate is sucrose). There are categories of enzymes according to the reactions they catalyze (for example, the kinases, or phosphorylation).

Enzymes are often found in multienzyme systems that operate by simple negative feedback.

d. Protein Denaturation

Protein denaturation occurs when the protein configuration is changed by the destruction of the secondary and tertiary structures (reduced to the primary structure). Common denaturing agents are alcohol, heat, and heavy metal salts.

You Should Review

- stereoisomers
- the structure of monosaccharides and hemiacetals
- the structure of disaccharides and acetals, glycosides
- reducing sugars
- stereoisomers and enzymes in carbohydrate metabolism
- digestion and synthesis of carbohydrates
- ketoacidosis, ketonemia, acetone breath, chemical structures of ketone bodies, gluconeogenesis
- functions of proteins
- protein synthesis and amino acid structures
- organic functional groups in proteins
- enzyme-catalyzed reactions
- vitamins, metal ion activators
- enzyme nomenclature
- multienzyme systems, simple negative feedback

Questions

85. The elements found in carbohydrates are
   a. oxygen, carbon, and hydrogen.
   b. zinc, hydrogen, and iron.
   c. carbon, iron, and oxygen.
   d. hydrogen, iron, and carbon.

$$E \quad + \quad S \quad \rightarrow \quad ES \quad \rightarrow \quad E \quad + \quad P$$

enzyme　　　substrate　　enzyme-substrate　　enzyme　　　product
　　　　　　　　　　　　　　complex

86. Hemoglobin is a specialized protein that functions in the transport of
   a. enzymes.
   b. oxygen and carbon dioxide.
   c. glucose.
   d. androgens and estrogens.

87. The primary function of food carbohydrates in the body is to
   a. provide for the storage of glycogen in cells.
   b. maintain the constancy of the blood sugar.
   c. maintain energy production within the cells.
   d. contribute to the structure of the cells.

88. A high level of ketone bodies in urine indicates marked increase in the metabolism of
   a. carbohydrates.
   b. fats.
   c. proteins.
   d. nucleic acids.

89. Which polysaccharide is a branched polymer of α-glucose found in the liver and muscle cells?
   a. amylase
   b. cellulose
   c. glycogen
   d. amylopectin

90. The sequence of amino acids that make up a protein is referred to as the protein's
   a. primary structure.
   b. secondary structure.
   c. tertiary structure.
   d. quaternary structure.

91. The site on an enzyme molecule that does the catalytic work is called the
   a. binding site.
   b. allosteric site.
   c. lock.
   d. active site.

92. In the multienzyme sequence shown here, molecules of E are able to fit to the enzyme E_1 and prevent the conversion of A to B. What is this action of E called?

$$A \xrightarrow{E_1} B \xrightarrow{E_2} C \xrightarrow{E_3} D \xrightarrow{E_4} E$$

   a. effector inhibition
   b. allosteric inhibition
   c. feedback inhibition
   d. competitive inhibition by nonproduct

93. Which type of lipid contains a gonane core?
   a. fatty acid
   b. phospholipid
   c. steroid
   d. triglyceride

94. The bonds between amino acids in a polypeptide are
   a. glycosidic bonds.
   b. ester bonds.
   c. peptide bonds.
   d. hydrogen bonds.

Answers

85. a. By definition, carbohydrates are made of oxygen, carbon, and hydrogen.

86. b. Hemoglobin is a protein present in the blood. Its function is to transport carbon dioxide and oxygen through the body.

87. c. Glucose, the monosaccharide, is the primary energy source in the body.

88. b. Ketone bodies are formed from free fatty acids.

89. c. Glycogen is a branched polymer of α-glucose, which is found stored in limited amounts in the liver and muscle cells.

90. a. Proteins can be described by their primary, secondary, tertiary, and quaternary structure. The primary structure is the most basic structure and refers to the sequence of amino acids that make up the protein.

91. d. The active site is where the substrate is acted on.

92. c. E stops E_1 from converting A to B.

93. c. Steroids are characterized by a gonane core, which is three six-carbon rings (cyclohexanes) and one five-carbon ring (cyclopentane) fused together.

94. c. Peptide bonds are formed between adjacent amino acids in a polypeptide chain.

III. Other Concepts You Should Be Familiar With

A. The Scientific Method

1. General

The scientific method is based upon **observations** that lead to the formulation of a **hypothesis** in an attempt to make a comprehensive guess. Only **experiments** (reproducible ones) will confirm the hypothesis and develop into a **theory** supported by all the facts.

2. The Science of Chemistry

Chemistry is the study of the structures, properties, and transformation of atoms and molecules.

B. Metric System

Metric system is the standard system for recording measurements. It is a decimal system (the basic unit and its subunits are separated by increasing and decreasing powers of ten). Some of the basic units of measurement are:

- Length: meter (m)
- Volume: liter (l)
- Mass: kilogram (kg)
- Time: the second (s)
- Temperature: Kelvin (K)
- Amount of substance: mole (mol)

C. Unit Conversion: The Factor Label Method

Conversion factor establishes a relationship of equivalence in measurement between two different units. It is expressed as a fraction. For instance, for 1 kg = 2.2 lbs., the conversion factor is: $\frac{1 \text{ kg}}{2.2 \text{ lbs.}}$ or $\frac{2.2 \text{ lbs.}}{1 \text{ kg}}$.

Example:

Convert 50 cm to m:

Since 100 cm = 1 m, the conversion factor is

$\frac{1 \text{ m}}{100 \text{ cm}}$ or $\frac{100 \text{ cm}}{1 \text{ m}}$

So, 50 cm $\times (\frac{1 \text{ m}}{100 \text{ cm}}) = 0.50$ m

Example:

How many grams are in 0.45 lbs.? (1 lb. = 453.6 g)

Conversion factor: $\frac{1 \text{ lb.}}{453.6 \text{ g}}$ or $\frac{453.6 \text{ g}}{1 \text{ lb.}}$

Since we need an answer in grams, we will use the conversion factor that has the grams in the numerator.

So, 0.45 lb. $\times (\frac{453.6 \text{ g}}{1 \text{ lb.}}) = 204.1$ g.

D. Significant Figures

The number of significant figures in any physical quantity or measurement is the number of digits known precisely to be accurate. The last digit to the right is inaccurate. The rules for counting significant figures are the following:

- Zeros sandwiched between nonzero digits are significant. For example, both 400.005 and 400,005 have six significant figures.
- Zeros that locate the decimal place (place holder) on the left are not significant. For example, 0.045 ml, 0.0045 ml, and 0.00045 ml each have two significant figures.
- Trailing zeros to the right of the decimal point are significant if the number is greater than 1. For example, 4.56000 has six significant figures.
- For numbers smaller than 1, only zeros to the right of the first significant digit are significant. For example, 0.020 has two significant figures.
- Trailing zeros are not significant in a non-decimal number. For example, 5,500 has two significant figures.

E. Error, Accuracy, Precision, and Uncertainty

Error is the difference between a value obtained experimentally and the standard value accepted by the scientific community.

Accuracy establishes how close in agreement a measurement is with the accepted value.

Precision of a measurement is the degree to which successive measurements agree with each other (average deviation is minimized).

Uncertainty expresses the doubt associated with the accuracy of any single measurement.

F. Functional Groups in Organic Chemistry

1. Alkene

2. Alcohol

3. Aldehyde

4. Ketone

5. Carboxylic Acid

6. Amine

7. Amide

8. Ester

9. Aromatic

10. Alkyne

11. Ether

12. Disulfide

9 ▶ GENERAL SCIENCE REVIEW

CHAPTER SUMMARY

This chapter highlights the core concepts that you need to know for the general science section of most health occupations entrance exams—essential topics such as the scientific method, formation of the universe, evolution, and biodiversity. Use this chapter as a study aid to review important concepts and test yourself with sample questions.

General Science Review: Important Concepts

I. General Introduction

A. *Description of How Health Occupations Entrance Exams Test General Science*

Not all health occupations entrance exams measure scientific knowledge in the same way. The natural sciences section of the Health Occupations Aptitude Exam (HOAE), made up of approximately 65 multiple-choice questions, tests your knowledge of general science. Other entrance exams, like the Health Occupations Basic Entrance Test (HOBET), require only that you can read and understand college-level scientific material, and do not have a separate science test section.

The following subject areas are important for you to know for your exam: history and methods of science, the cosmos, basics of matter, evolution and life, earth works, biodiversity, ecology, and global environmental challenges.

B. How to Use This Chapter

Use the information about core topics and the practice questions in this chapter to guide you as you prepare for your exam, but remember that this chapter should not be your only resource. Review scientific concepts more comprehensively in your own textbooks.

After you read each subject heading in this chapter, answer the practice questions that follow. These questions are designed to reflect the type of questions you will find on your health occupations entrance exam. Once you have answered the sample questions, you can target the content areas where you need the most review.

Plan your study time effectively so that you have enough preparation for the test. Familiarizing yourself with real test questions and brushing up on important natural science topics in a good college-level textbook will build your confidence and lessen your test anxiety.

II. Main Topics

A. History and Methods of Science

Everywhere you look, science is evident from the technology of medicine to our understanding of how stars are made. Here you have an overview of what science is and how it works.

1. Giants of Science

How did science begin? Who were the early discoverers of this way of exploring nature? It is important to look back and review some of the influential figures in this field.

a. Ancient Greeks

(Some dates are approximate.)

Thales (624–546 B.C.E.), called the "father of philosophy," said the universe was ultimately made of water (one of the four ancient Greek elements of water, fire, earth, and air).

Pythagorus (560–480 B.C.E.) discovered the mathematics of musical harmony and the properties of right triangles (triangles with one 90° angle in them).

Hippocrates (460–370 B.C.E.) was called the "father of medicine."

Plato (427–347 B.C.E.) was a major philosopher who wrote the dialogues of Socrates, championing logical thinking.

Aristotle (384–322 B.C.E.) was a student of Plato and tutor of Alexander the Great. He wrote volumes on the knowledge of everything, from plants to the heavens and politics.

Euclid (325–270 B.C.E.) conducted significant work in geometry.

Archimedes (287–212 B.C.E.), according to legend, ran down the street naked after discovering the law of buoyancy and density during a bath, which allowed a king to verify the amount of gold in a crown. He accomplished major work in geometry and was first to calculate the surface area and volume of a sphere.

b. Originators of Modern Science

Nicholas Copernicus (1473–1543), Polish. His book showed that the motions of the Sun, Moon, and planets in the sky could be explained by assuming that the planets go around the Sun and that Earth is a planet as well. The book had so much influence that we still talk about the "Copernican Revolution."

Tycho Brahe (1546–1601), Danish. His observations and notes of planetary motion were the foundation of his student Johannes Kepler's later work.

Francis Bacon (1561–1626), English. He wrote early books on how to do science, emphasizing experimentation and inductive reasoning (to make generalizations).

Galileo Galilei (1564–1642), Italian. Galileo studied the swing of a pendulum, found that bodies of different masses fall at the same rate, and distinguished acceleration from velocity. He first saw the moons of Jupiter and craters on Earth's Moon. He was branded a heretic and condemned to house arrest for his assertions of his findings.

Johannes Kepler (1571–1630), German. Kepler described the laws of planetary motion and declared that the paths of planets around the Sun are ellipses, not circles.

René Descartes (1596–1650), French. This father of modern philosophy invented coordinate geometry (the *x–y* axis) and said, "I think, therefore I am."

Robert Hooke (1635–1703), English. Hooke published the book *Micrographia*, with detailed drawings of life under a microscope. He named the little units he saw in cork "cells," which became the general word used in biology.

Antonie van Leeuwenhoek (1632–1723), Dutch. He perfected the microscope and made many discoveries, such as human sperm cells.

Sir Isaac Newton (1643–1727), English. Newton discovered the law of gravity, discovered how a prism splits light into colors, invented calculus, and set forth the laws of motion (such as "every action has an equal and opposite reaction").

Pierre Simon Laplace (1749–1827), French. Laplace applied math to the solar system in a new level of detail and correctly surmised that the solar system was formed by condensation from a gas nebula.

c. Science Goes Full Tilt

James Hutton (1726–1797), Scottish. This "father of geology" realized the antiquity of Earth.

John Dalton (1766–1844), English. Dalton was a chemist whose theory of atoms explained why elements combined into molecules in constant proportions.

Sir Charles Lyell (1797–1875), Scottish. This geologist championed "uniformitarianism," the idea that small constant changes over time created today's Earth.

Baron von Humboldt (1769–1850), German. Baron von Humboldt was a geologist and world traveler. The "Humboldt Current" off South America is named after him.

Matthias Jacob Schleiden (1804–1881), German. Schleiden contributed the cell theory for plants that says that all plants are made of cells.

Charles Darwin (1809–1882), English. Darwin's book *The Origin of Species by Means of Natural Selection* started a new field of science, evolutionary biology. He traveled extensively in South America and discovered many new species both modern and extinct.

Theodor Schwann (1810–1882), German. Schwann contributed the cell theory for animals that says that all animals are made of cells and coined the term "metabolism."

Gregor Mendel (1822–1884), Austrian. Mendel studied the heredity of pea plants, which led to genetics.

Louis Pasteur (1822–1895), French. Pasteur invented biochemistry, discovered right-handed and left-handed crystals, worked with yeast and proved that life only came from other life, and developed the germ theory of disease.

Thomas Huxley (1825–1895), English. Huxley championed the theory of evolution for technical and popular audiences, and became known as Darwin's "bulldog."

Lord Kelvin (1824–1907), Scottish. Kelvin made new calculations on heat and analyzed the history of Earth.

James Clerk Maxwell (1831–1870), Scottish. Maxwell developed mathematical laws of electromagnetism, now known as "Maxwell's equations."

Dmitri Mendeleyev (1834–1907), Russian. Mendeleyev arranged elements in repeating sequences of properties, and thereby created the first periodical table of chemistry. He predicted new elements, which were, in fact, found.

Ernst Mach (1838–1916), Austrian. Mach was a physicist honored by our use of the name "Mach 1" for the speed of sound, "Mach 2" for twice the speed of sound, and so forth.

Sigmund Freud (1856–1939), Austrian. Freud developed a theory of dreams and the unconscious.

d. The Last 100 Years

Albert Einstein (1879–1955), German-Swiss. Einstein computed the size of atoms. He developed the special and general theories of relativity, for light and gravity, respectively. He also described the concept of four-dimensional space-time and made famous the equation $E = mc^2$.

Marie Curie (1867–1934), Polish. Curie was the first person to win two Nobel prizes, for her pioneering studies of radioactivity.

Ernest Rutherford (1871–1937), New Zealand. Rutherford's work with nuclear physics led the way for modern understanding of atomic structure. His "gold-foil" experiment revealed that atoms were mainly empty space with most of their mass located in a central nucleus.

Alfred Wegener (1880–1930), German. Wegener proposed that all continents were once a single large one and had drifted apart in a "continental drift."

Niels Bohr (1885–1962), Danish. He described the "Bohr" model of the atom, in which electrons rotate around a nucleus like planets around the Sun.

Werner Heisenberg (1901–1976), German. Heisenberg developed the uncertainty principle of quantum physics.

Linus Pauling (1901–1994), American. Pauling studied electronegativity and chemical bonds and is considered one of the most influential chemists of the twentieth century.

Francis Crick (1916–2004), English. Crick was codiscoverer of the double helix structure of DNA.

Erwin Schrödinger (1887–1961), Austrian. Schrödinger developed wave mechanics to explain the structure of atoms.

James Watson (1928–), American. Watson was also codiscoverer of the double helix structure of DNA and a leader in the recent Human Genome Project.

2. Methods

What makes science special are its specific methods that uncover the truths of nature, in ways that can be repeated by anyone. For example, after Galileo saw the moons of Jupiter, anyone could look at Jupiter through a telescope and see them. Science does not accept any revelations said to be available only to visionary individuals.

a. Scientific Method

The scientific method is used in all branches of science to study the natural world. The method outlines a series of five principal steps that scientists must undertake in order to test and verify their ideas. Let's review it again.

1. **Formulate the problem:** Develop a question, the solution to which explains an order or process in nature.
2. **Collect data:** Research background information and make observations that are related to the problem.
3. **Form a hypothesis:** Develop an educated guess based on your observations and background research that will answer the question. The hypothesis must be logical and testable—experiments must be possible that can disprove the hypothesis.

4. **Do experiments:** Conduct experiments to test the hypothesis. A hypothesis can be disproved, but never absolutely proved—it may change with new evidence! Experiments must be repeatable, free of bias, and adequately controlled.

5. **Analyze the data:** Look at the results of your experiments. Determine if they are consistent with your hypothesis. If not, develop a new hypothesis that is consistent with all available data. Begin the scientific method again with this new hypothesis!

Successful hypotheses lead scientists to make predictions about the natural world that allow the hypothesis to be tested further.

b. Conducting Good Experiments

Experiments are tests designed to evaluate a hypothesis. In a good experiment, only one variable is changed at a time and all other variables are kept constant; this is to ensure that any change is a result of only that variable. Often in an experiment, two systems are compared; in one system nothing is changed (the **control**), and in the other system the aspect to be tested is altered (the formal **experiment**). The results of the two systems are compared.

Example: Louis Pasteur took two flasks of sterilized meat broth and configured their long necks so air could go into both. But for one (the experiment), dust normally in the air was blocked. In the other (the control), the dust along with the air could get in (as would usually be the situation, note the baseline is the control).

In Pasteur's experiment, he observed that the meat broth spoiled in the control flask open to both air and dust but not in the other experiment flask where dust was excluded. Experiments consist of independent variables, which are usually consciously varied by the experimenter (in Pasteur's case, the presence or absence of dust). Experiments also have dependent variables, which, in our example, is state of the broth, which is affected by (and therefore is dependent upon) the independent variables. Often, experiments are not a simple two-part system, but include some variable that is shifted across a range of values, to be compared to the control. If you were Pasteur, you might predict that using a different kind of meat broth would give the same results, thus confirming the original experiment. More remarkably, you might predict the existence of small, invisible organisms in the dust of air as the cause of the spoiling of the meat broth (microbes in air were in fact discovered).

Hypothesis and theory: The process of experiment is cyclic. That is, the experiment leads to new ideas for further experiments. The cycle of the scientific method is repeated.

c. How Truth Is Forged

The ancient Greeks never formalized the process of experimentation in the way that Europeans did after Galileo's time.

Laws versus rules. When phenomena eventually become explained, they become laws of science. This term is most appropriate in physics and chemistry. Biology, in contrast, includes so many creatures and types of ecosystems, that there are often exceptions to the norm. Biologists refer to rules instead of laws.

What determines scientific truth? The famous philosopher of science, Karl Popper, said experiments never prove, they only fail to disprove. He therefore said one should design experiments with the aim to falsify. Popper's concept has been influential. So how is truth known? As more and more experiments fail to falsify a specific hypothesis, the hypothesis comes to be known as true.

Paradigm shift is a term coined by the philosopher of the process of science, Thomas Kuhn, that refers to what happens when new scientific discoveries overturn an entire body of knowledge.

Einstein's theories of relativity were a paradigm shift.

Reductionism occurs when smaller entities interacting as a system explain a phenomenon. **Holism** is sometimes contrasted to reductionism—it looks to the context, the larger system surrounding the phenomenon being studied, as key to the explanation.

Truth changes as science progresses. Does that mean that anything goes, that anything is possible? All scientific truth is tentative but not arbitrary. Truth is won by many practitioners, checking each other's results and trying new ideas for experiments, over and over.

d. Graphs, Calculations, and Models

Detailed data from experiments are often plotted as points or lines on **graphs** with x- and y-axes.

> **x-axis:** the horizontal axis, that by convention, varies along the numerical range of the independent variable (either time or some other property being changed by the experimenter, such as temperature).
> **y-axis:** the vertical axis that contains the result being measured, which is called the dependent variable.

Three-dimensional graphs are graphs that use two horizontal axes for two independent variables (x,y) and a vertical axis called the z-axis for the dependent variable.

Calculations are crucial to science. Important tools are measurements, which then might be analyzed by algebra (to relate variables), calculus (to look at changes in time, and changes in rates of processes in time), and statistics (to look at large amounts of data that have inherent variability).

Models are conceptual or mathematical systems that serve as explanations for phenomena. Models can be simple, such as Copernicus's model of the solar system. But usually the term *model* refers to conceptual systems that are more complex, such as

today's computer models of the weather that include hundreds of equations.

3. Measurements

Measurements are so important to science that a practitioner once said that "the only things that count are things that can be counted." This goes too far, but it captures the importance of measurement. For example, the Egyptians knew how to lay out right triangles to measure areas of land and to site the pyramids. The word *geometry* comes from ancient Greek, meaning "Earth-measurement."

a. Units Are Crucial

Two types of units are used in the world: the metric system and the English system (used only in the United States). The units in the English system include pounds, quarts, feet, inches, miles, and degrees Fahrenheit. The modern metric system (also known as the International System of Measurements or SI), used by most of the world and by scientists, is the universal language of science. Here are some units in the metric system, which uses factors of ten smaller or larger to develop the names.

> *Length:* meter (m)
> micrometer (μm), also called a micron (0.000001 m)
> millimeter (mm) (0.001 m)
> centimeter (cm) (0.01 m)
> kilometer (km) (1,000 m)
> *Time:* second (s). Time in the metric system does not use factors (or powers) of ten, except for units under a second (hundredths of a second, milliseconds, microseconds, and so forth).
> minute (min.)
> hour (h. or hr.)
> day (d.)
> year (y. or yr.)

Note that there is another "second" in use as well. Consider: For degrees latitude and longitude, the 360 degrees of the circle is divided into smaller units called "minutes" (60 to each degree, note this is not a minute of time) and "seconds" (60 seconds to a minute of degree).

Mass: gram (g)
   micrograms (μg) (0.000001 g)
   milligrams (mg) (0.001 g)
   gram (g)
   kilograms (kg) (1,000 g)
   metric tons (t) (1,000 kilograms)

Volume: liter (L)
   milliliters (mL) (0.001 L)
   the cubic meter (1,000 L = 1 m³)

Temperature: The degree Centigrade (°C, sometimes also called degree Celsius). An interval of one degree C is $\frac{9}{5}$ times larger than the interval of one °F. To convert the numerical scale of °F into the numerical scale of °C, use the equation $x°C = \frac{5}{9}(y°F - 32)$. The freezing point of water is 0°C or 32°F.

Energy: The joule (J), or calorie (cal); 1 cal = 4.184 J. Note that 1 calorie of energy in food (Cal) is actually a kilocalorie of energy in the metric system. Therefore, 1 Cal = 1,000 cal = 1 kcal. Also, power is energy summed up over time. Therefore, another term for energy is the kilowatt-hour (kW-h) [or joule second (J-s)].

Power: watt (W)
   milliwatts (mW)
   kilowatts (kW)

b. Powers of Ten and Constants

Powers of ten with prefix names in the metric system:

10^{-12} pico (p), one-trillionth
10^{-9} nano (n), one-billionth
10^{-6} micro (μ), one-millionth
10^{-3} milli (m), one-thousandth
10^{-2} centi (c), one-hundredth
10^{3} kilo (k), thousand
10^{6} mega (M), million
10^{9} giga (G), billion

10^{12} tera (T), trillion
10^{15} peta (P), quadrillion

Constants: Relating properties in the calculations of science has resulted in universal constants for major laws. These constants have units that make the total units equal on both sides of scientific equations. You do not have to memorize the numbers, but you should be familiar with the existence and use of these constants.

Avogadro's number N_A or (*n*): In a "mole" of atoms of any element, for example, there is an Avogadro's number of atoms. This number can also be used for the number of molecules of a substance in a mole of a pure compound.

$N_A = 6.022 \times 10^{23}$ mole^{-1}

Speed of light in a vacuum (*c*): $3.0 \times 10^8 \frac{m}{s}$.

Universal gas constant (*R*): used to relate pressure, temperature, and volume of a gas in the gas law.

$$R = 8.314 \ \frac{J}{mol \times K} \ \text{or} \ 0.08206 \ \frac{L \times atm}{mol \times K}$$

Stefan-Boltzmann constant (σ). It is used to relate the energy of radiation of a material body (such as the Sun) to its surface temperature.

$$\sigma = 5.67 \times 10^{-8} \ \frac{J}{s \times m^2 \times K^4}$$

You Should Review

- major scientists
- major experiments and findings
- units of metric system
- powers of ten

Questions

1. This man wrote *The Origin of Species by Means of Natural Selection,* which established the theory of evolution.
   a. Charles Darwin
   b. Gregor Mendel
   c. Aristotle
   d. René Descartes

2. If you are measuring how water chemistry changes in a river in the days after a flood, the time measurement is the
　a. independent variable.
　b. independent constant.
　c. dependent variable.
　d. dependent constant.

3. In the metric system, the prefix *tera-* refers to which number?
　a. thousand
　b. trillion
　c. ten thousand
　d. three

4. This codiscoverer published one of the giant papers in the history of science in 1953, on the double helix of DNA.
　a. Albert Einstein
　b. Francis Crick
　c. Ernst Mach
　d. Niels Bohr

5. Mathematics provides science with analytical tools. The branch of mathematics that deals with the rates of changes of variables over time is
　a. algebra.
　b. calculus.
　c. statistics.
　d. tensor analysis.

6. To compute the number of molecules in 2 moles of oxygen gas, you would use
　a. Avogadro's number.
　b. Einstein's speed of light.
　c. the Stefan-Boltzman constant.
　d. Planck's constant.

7. Who was the first to win two Nobel Prizes, for groundbreaking work on radioactivity?
　a. Niels Bohr
　b. Marie Curie
　c. Ernest Rutherford
　d. Erwin Schrödinger

8. You predict that salt will increase the boiling point of water. Which answer best defines the nature of your "prediction"?
　a. It is an experiment.
　b. It is scientific theory.
　c. It is an observation.
　d. It is a hypothesis.

9. How many milliwatts are in 10 watts?
　a. 10,000
　b. 1,000
　c. 100
　d. 10

10. Which of the following is the metric (SI) unit for energy?
　a. watt (W)
　b. Centigrade (°C)
　c. joule (J)
　d. ampere (A)

Answers

1. a. Darwin's world-shaking book on evolution was published in 1859, in England. See pages 220–222 for the others.

2. a. The independent variable in this case is time, because that is what is changing by itself. On the other hand, the river chemistry is the dependent variable, changing as a function of time. Choices **b** and **d** are made up.

3. b. The prefix *tera-* refers to trillion. For example, a teragram is a trillion grams.

4. b. Francis Crick not only described the double helix of DNA, but went on to figure out the genetic code that coded for amino acids that are assembled into proteins. See pages 220–222 for the others.

5. b. Calculus can take derivatives of variables, which gives rates of changes in the variables.

6. a. Avogadro's number is a specific number of atoms or molecules (a very large number!). Planck's constant is a constant of quantum physics. See pages 220–222 for the others.

7. b. Marie Curie was the first person to win two Nobel Prizes, one in physics in 1903 and one in chemistry in 1911.

8. d. A hypothesis or educated guess is a formulated idea or prediction that can then be tested with experiments.

9. a. Because there are 1,000 milliwatts in one watt, in 10 watts there are 10,000 milliwatts.

10. c. The joule (J) is the metric (SI) unit used for measuring energy. Watts measure power, Centigrade (°C) measures temperature, and ampere (A) measures electric current.

B. The Cosmos

1. First Billion Years of the Universe

Nearly 14 billion years ago, our universe began with an event called the Big Bang and by a billion years or so later, galaxies had formed.

a. Evidence for the Expanding Universe

In the 1920s, American astronomer Edwin Hubble measured the distances to a number of galaxies and their spectra of light, which provided crucial evidence that the universe is expanding.

Spectra: All elements, if above 0 K (absolute zero, the K or Kelvin scale of temperature, which is referenced to absolute zero, approximately −273° C), glow at particular wavelengths. These are along different parts of the electromagnetic (EM) spectrum, which spans the very long wavelengths of radio waves to the ultra short wavelengths of X-rays. The wavelengths that our eyes see are called visible light. Visible red is a longer wavelength than blue. The particular wavelengths for each element form patterns, which are characteristic of that element, and which might be called *photon-prints*, after the patterns of the EM photons. As the numerous EM emissions from a star pass through gases that contain particular elements, elements also absorb wavelengths in their characteristic patterns. Thus both emission spectra and absorption spectra can provide astronomers with information about the elements out in space.

Hubble's Observations: By examining spectra, Hubble found that compared to the photon-prints of elements on Earth, those elements found in the galaxies of deep space are shifted toward the red; in other words, the wavelengths are longer. This could only occur if the galaxies were moving away from Earth. (If the galaxies were moving toward us, the shift in the wavelengths of the patterns would have been toward the blue, which was not observed.)

Hubble had discovered the expanding universe. By extrapolating the expansion back in time, astronomers concluded that the expansion started with a single explosive event known as the Big Bang.

If all galaxies are moving away from us, does that imply that we are at the center? No, because inhabitants of any galaxy would also observe that they appear to be at the center. To illustrate this phenomenon, think of raisins in an expanding raisin bread. To each raisin, all the others are moving away.

We can look back in time, as we look out into space, because the light reaching us was emitted long ago. Because the speed of light is finite (fast but finite), the light emitted from stars in our own galaxy hundred of thousands of years ago or from stars in other galaxies billions of years ago is just now reaching us.

b. The Big Bang

The Big Bang occurred about 13.7 billion years ago (with an uncertainty of a few hundred million years).

At one microsecond (following the Big Bang): The universe as a whole had a temperature of about one trillion K. Matter as we know it, as stable atoms, does not exist at this temperature.

Between the first microsecond and one second: Matter and antimatter nearly annihilated each other.

Antimatter is a form of matter that is the mirror opposite of matter in all aspects. For a positively charged particle, for example, the antiparticle is negatively charged. Particles and their antiparticles have the same masses. The key point is that when particles and antiparticles meet, they explode into pure energy, in an amount according to Einstein's famous equation $E = mc^2$. We know that antiparticles exist because they can be made in high-energy physics experiments.

In the early universe, there was an imbalance between matter and antimatter, to the extent of about one part in 200 million. Therefore, in the matter-antimatter annihilation, only one part in 200 million remained as matter, and the rest became energy.

At one second: The universe was about one billion K. This was "cool" enough for protons, neutrons, and electrons to exist as stable particles, what physicists call "subatomic" particles, because they are basic constituents of atoms.

Note that the proton by itself is the nucleus of a hydrogen atom.

c. Formation of First Atoms

At around 300,000 years after the Big Bang, the temperature of the universe had dropped to about 3,000 K (close to the temperature of our Sun's surface). This was cool enough for electrons to remain bound to nuclei of protons and neutrons, creating atoms. (In contrast, at hotter temperatures, electrons are stripped off nuclei and atoms cannot exist.)

Astronomers talk about this event by saying that the "universe became transparent." Before this point, freely moving electrons (in the state of matter known as **plasma**, a kind of matter-energy "fog") blocked the propagation of electromagnetic

radiation. This crucial event separated matter and energy. Except for small amounts absorbed over time by interactions with matter, this energy has been traveling throughout the universe ever since, as the universe stretches and cools with the ongoing expansion.

In 1965, this radiation was detected. It is called the **cosmic background radiation**. Its temperature, which represents the average temperature of the current state of the universe, is 2.7 K, very close to absolute zero. (Locally, places like Earth and the Sun, of course, are much hotter.)

At this point of formation of atoms, both theoretical calculations and actual measurements have shown that matter consisted of 76% hydrogen and 24% helium (with a trace of lithium). No other elements existed.

d. Formation of Stars and Galaxies

Stars and galaxies formed between one million and one billion years after the Big Bang. Stars are created when gas clouds in space condense, pulled together by gravity. During the condensation, the gas becomes hotter and hotter. If the density and temperature are high enough, the protostar ignites and is sustained as a glowing star by nuclear fusion.

Stars are within large gravitationally bound groupings called **galaxies**. Our Milky Way galaxy has about 100 billion stars, which go through birth, life, and death. In special cases, extremely large masses can contract so much that light itself cannot escape; they are called **black holes**. Many galaxies are believed to have black holes in their centers. Our galaxy has a central black hole.

The contraction of the matter of the universe into galaxies could only have occurred from some initial lumpiness in the universe, which was predicted to be present in the cosmic background radiation. Satellites such as the Cosmic Background Explorer did indeed find such **inhomogeneities**, which indicate differences in the distribution of energy in space from the time the universe became transparent. These differences are small, only + or

−27 microdegrees warmer and cooler than the average 2.7 K, but they are a crucial confirmation for the Big Bang theory. Our universe now contains about 100 billion galaxies.

2. Birth of Chemical Elements in Stars

All elements heavier than the primordial triplet of elements, primarily hydrogen and helium with a trace of lithium, are created in stars.

a. Nuclear Fusion

Stars are hot and are able to throw radiation into space because of fusion reactions deep within their cores. For atoms from hydrogen up to the atomic weight of iron, energy is released when atoms are fused to make larger atoms. This is because the protons and neutrons inside the nuclei of the larger atoms (again, up to iron) contain less mass per subatomic particle and therefore less energy according to Einstein's equation. The excess energy of fusion is released as heat and radiation.

b. Sequence of Births of Elements

Inside stars, the first element to be fused is hydrogen, the most abundant primordial element. Under intense temperature and pressure, two hydrogen atoms are fused into one atom of helium, releasing energy and making stars hot, thus sustaining further fusion reactions. When the hydrogen is used up, helium is fused into carbon, and then the carbon and some helium are fused into oxygen. All the elements up to iron can be made in this way. Note the sequence of how elements are made: Hydrogen (H) → Helium (He) → Carbon (C) → Oxygen (O). All these fusion reactions release energy.

c. Supernovas and the Dispersal of Elements

Stars can run out of matter to fuel fusion; they can "die." Some stars die by throwing off gases, then withering into small, smoldering white dwarfs.

Very massive stars, on the order of ten times the mass of our Sun, can create supernova explosions at their deaths. One supernova, for example, which occurred in our galaxy in A.D. 1066, is now the Crab Nebula. Ancient people observed this bright new star in the sky before it faded.

Supernovas are important parts of how our universe works. They do two special things. First, all elements heavier than iron (such as gold and uranium) are made in the intense heat and pressure of the supernova. Second, the supernovas disperse all the elements inside the former star out into space. We can see these elements in the emission and absorption spectra in the regions surrounding former sites of supernovas. In the dispersal of elements by supernovas, there are elements made earlier in fusion reactions during the long, ordinary lifetime of the star, as well as the new elements made only in the supernova itself.

The elements dispersed into space can eventually gather into gas clouds and might contract, after mixing with remnants of other supernovas, into totally new stars and their planets.

3. Formation of Earth
a. Ages of Sun and Earth

About five billion years ago, a gas cloud condensed into the star that is now our Sun, which has been burning since that birth.

Around the Sun, the gas cloud condensed into smaller bodies (picture small whirlpools of contraction around a large, central one). What started as dust grains coalesced into rocks, then boulders, then objects the size of mountains. By collisions and gravitational attraction, which held the bodies together, the objects grew. Sometimes, the collisions created smaller bodies but, on the whole, growth in size ruled. Earth formed about 4.5 billion years ago.

b. Methods of Dating

To date the formation of stars and planets, scientists use radioactive clocks. Very large atoms, such as those of uranium, can have unstable nuclei. These unstable nuclei restructure into nuclei that are slightly smaller by giving off radioactive particles (there is also a kind of radioactive decay that only gives off energy). The new atom might also be radioactive, and thus, the process continues until it reaches an atom that is perfectly stable. Lead-206, for example, is the stable daughter-product of what started as Uranium-238 (the numbers refer to the atomic weights). When molten or gaseous, the lead-206 is driven off; the radioactive clock is thereby "reset." We can use the clock to date when rocks formed. The oldest Earth rocks are 3.9 billion years old, the oldest Moon rocks 4.1 billion years old, and most meteorites about 4.6 billion years old. Because the Moon and Earth would have been molten even after they formed (see below), the date of the meteorites is taken to be that time that Earth condensed (4.6 billion years ago, or, rounded to the nearest half billion, about four and a half billion years ago).

c. Formation of the Moon

Though it was once thought that the Moon might have condensed separately around Earth, scientists believe the following scenario to be true (from multiple lines of evidence). A few hundred million years after the formation of Earth, a rogue body about the size of Mars, which had an odd orbit around the Sun, smashed into Earth. Material from both the colliding body and Earth flew off and condensed around Earth to form the Moon. The Moon was much closer and has been slowly moving away from Earth ever since.

4. Exploration of the Solar System

From the dawn of time, humans have looked up at the stars. Only in the past half century have we been able to look back on Earth itself with satellite cameras and even human eyes.

a. From Satellites to Humans in Space

Sputnik, which means "fellow traveler" in Russian, was launched by the U.S.S.R. in 1957. It was the first artificial satellite in orbit.

Vanguard was the first U.S. satellite, in 1958.

In the manned U.S. space program, the *Mercury* program put solo humans in orbit, the *Gemini* program put teams of two into orbit, and the *Apollo* program, with teams of three, aimed for the Moon. The first manned Moon landing came in 1969. The Russians had the first space station, called *Mir* (for "peace"), but eventually it could not be maintained and fell to Earth. The International Space Station, led by the efforts of the United States, is currently in orbit, and every half year or so, there are changes of crew. Russia has supplied the rockets for these changes in recent years, following the grounding of the U.S. space shuttles, after the second total loss of a space shuttle crew in 2003, during a disastrous reentry into Earth's atmosphere. The space shuttle program was reinstated in 2005 was retired July 21, 2011.

b. Discoveries from Venus

Astronomers cannot see surface features of the planet Venus because of its thick clouds. Several U.S. and Russian probes have measured properties of the Venusian atmosphere and even mapped the surface from orbit, using various wavelengths that can penetrate the clouds. Despite its similar size to Earth, Venus is very different from Earth. It is extremely hot, partly because it is closer to the Sun, but mostly because the atmosphere is about 600 times more massive than that of Earth, and is mostly carbon dioxide. This amount of CO_2 produces an intense greenhouse effect, keeping the planet hot. There is no water vapor or oxygen in the atmosphere.

c. Discoveries from Mars

In the mid-1970s, the Viking probe successfully landed on Mars and measured properties of the soil, seeking signs of life. None was found, but scientists now believe there is a possibility for life in cracks in rocks, well beneath the surface. Unusual bacteria are found in similar sites deep under the surface of Earth.

In 2004, the United States successfully deployed two more rovers on the surface of Mars, and in 2012 landed yet another. They have analyzed minerals and have concluded, through multiple lines of evidence, that Mars was once wet. Rivers flowed; there was possibly a shallow ocean. Again, compared to Earth, the atmosphere of Mars is very foreign. The thin atmosphere (about 2% the thickness of that of Earth) is, like that of Venus, mostly carbon dioxide. There is only a faint trace of oxygen and little nitrogen (the two most abundant gases in Earth's atmosphere).

5. Mysteries of the Cosmos
a. Dark Matter

When astronomers use the law of gravity to compute what the spin of galaxies (such as ours) should be, given the presence of a known amount of matter, they find that there must be a significant amount of matter that is "dark," unseen, and unknown.

The dark matter is about six times the mass of the known, ordinary matter of stars and gas clouds.

b. Dark Energy

Certain kinds of supernovas explode with a fixed real brilliance. Astronomers have mapped these "standard candles," and, knowing their real brilliance, their apparent brilliance to us on Earth, and their red shifts, can calculate their distances and ages. A startling fact has emerged, which has been borne out by other lines of evidence as well: The expansion of the universe has been accelerating since the Big Bang.

What is causing the expansion? It is some kind of energy that we cannot currently see. It is therefore known as **dark energy**.

Using Einstein's equation $E = mc^2$, any amount of energy can be computed as an equivalent mass. Therefore, scientists can ask about the amounts of dark energy, dark matter, and the universe's third constituent of known, ordinary matter and energy. Here are the results:

Dark energy: 73% (the most of the substance of the universe)
Dark matter: 23%
Ordinary matter and energy: 4%

c. Life and Intelligence Elsewhere

Are we alone? The research program called SETI (the Search for Extraterrestrial Intelligence) seeks answers to this question. It assumes that other intelligent civilizations might send out signals to space. So far, no definite signals have been found.

By measuring wobbles in stars, which are caused by planets circling the stars and perturbing the stars with their gravity, astronomers were able to locate very large planets, assumed to be similar to Jupiter and Saturn, the gas giants of our solar system. In 2009, the U.S. launched the *Kepler* space telescope, which was able to detect much smaller planets. Thanks to *Kepler*, more than 3,500 planets around other stars are currently known, some of which are Earth-sized and capable of supporting life. The first stars of the universe could not have had planets of heavy elements, such as iron. Early planets could not have had carbon, a crucial element for life as we know it. This is because iron and carbon are made in the fusion reactions inside stars. Therefore, the density of carbon increases over time, as stars go through lifetimes and more stars form. Is there a critical density of carbon needed for life? Perhaps we are alone (or nearly so), because just around the time of formation of Earth the density of carbon reached a value high enough to form life. This is a possible explanation for our apparent aloneness, but more work on the history and composition of the cosmos needs to be done.

You Should Review

- Big Bang theory
- formation of stars and galaxies
- dating methods
- supernovas
- formation of Earth and Moon
- characteristics of planets in the solar system
- discoveries from space exploration
- dark matter and dark energy

Questions

11. What feature of our universe is demonstrated by the "red shift"?
   a. an increase in supernovas
   b. the contraction of black holes
   c. the expansion of the universe
   d. the decrease in gravity

12. The universe formed approximately how long ago?
   a. 13.7 thousand years ago
   b. 13.7 million years ago
   c. 13.7 billion years ago
   d. 13.7 trillion years ago

13. What is the current temperature of the universe, as indicated by the cosmic background radiation?
   a. 2.7°C
   b. −2.7 K
   c. −2.7°C
   d. 2.7 K

14. In the stages of nuclear fusion inside stars, which element in the list, compared to the others, is the ultimate building block for all the others?
   a. hydrogen
   b. helium
   c. carbon
   d. oxygen

15. A supernova is observed in a star that is a distance of 500 light-years from Earth. That means we now see the star
   a. as it was 500 years in the past.
   b. as it was 500 years after the Big Bang.
   c. as it will be 500 years in the future.
   d. as it is, basically, today.

16. We can date very old rocks because of what fact?
   a. Uranium turns into platinum.
   b. Uranium turns into lead.
   c. Lead turns into uranium.
   d. Gold turns into uranium.

17. How did the Moon form?
   a. A large body crashed into Earth soon after its own formation.
   b. A gas cloud condensed around Earth at the same time Earth itself condensed.
   c. The early Earth was unstable and split into the Moon and what became Earth.
   d. The Moon was captured by Earth early on.

18. Which planet is about the same size as Earth, has a blanket of thick clouds, and has a surface temperature that could melt lead?
   a. Mercury
   b. Jupiter
   c. Titan
   d. Venus

19. What was *Sputnik*?
   a. the first satellite launched into Earth's orbit
   b. the first spacecraft to reach the moon
   c. the first manned spacecraft to orbit Earth
   d. the first manned space station

20. What is the main piece of evidence for dark energy?
   a. black holes found in the centers of most galaxies
   b. discovery of cosmic background radiation
   c. rotations of galaxies not explained by our known, ordinary matter and energy
   d. acceleration of the expansion of the universe

Answers

11. c. All galaxies have red shifts in the signatures of elements in their spectra of light, which shows us that the galaxies are all moving away from each other and therefore that the universe is expanding.

12. c. Based upon observations by Edwin Hubble, the universe is expanding. Scientists believe our expanding universe originated in an event known as the Big Bang, approximately 13.7 billion years ago.

13. d. 2.7 K. K for Kelvin refers to the temperature scale that uses absolute zero as the "zero" point. Note that it is written as just "K" rather than "° K." You can figure this out if you know that 0 K refers to absolute zero and that the average temperature of the universe is very close to absolute zero. Negative K makes no sense. Choices **a** and **c** are too warm, given that 0°C is about 273 K.

14. a. Hydrogen is the building block for other elements inside stars. It is the simplest element, with one proton and one electron.

15. a. We see the star as it was 500 years in the past, because light can only travel at a finite speed (fast but finite, the *c* in Einstein's famous equation). A light-year is the distance that light travels in a year. When we look out into space, we also are looking back in time.

16. b. Uranium, a radioactive element, turns into lead, which is stable. The amount of a particular isotope of lead gives the amount of time that has passed since the rock formed and any lead previously present would have been purged during a gaseous or molten state.

17. a. A large body crashed into Earth soon after its own formation. From this collision, material went into space and recondensed to form the Moon as well as restructuring the surface of Earth. This was after Earth had already condensed.

18. d. Venus has a super-thick atmosphere of carbon dioxide that creates high surface temperatures. Choice **c** is not a planet, but a moon of Saturn.

19. a. *Sputnik* was the first artificial satellite launched into Earth's orbit. The satellite was launched by the Soviet Union on October 4, 1957, and spurred the U.S.–Soviet "space race" and exploration of space as we know it today.

20. d. The existence of dark energy is evidenced by the accelerating expansion of the universe. We know this by measuring the distances to certain types of supernovas in distant galaxies, which serve as standard candles of known brightness.

C. Basics of Matter
1. Physics
Physics is the study of the constituents and forces that govern matter at its most elementary level.

a. Atoms
The word **atom** comes from the ancient Greek, meaning "indivisible." Atoms are the most finely divided parts of matter that possess the characteristics of a particular element, such as copper, gold, carbon, or hydrogen.

Atoms are not actually indivisible. Atoms not in molecules or ions are electrically neutral and contain equal amounts of positive and negative electrical charges. The positive charge is concentrated in a tiny central massive region called the **nucleus**. The negative charge is in one or more tiny electrons, which "whir" around the nucleus, bound to it by electrical attraction.

The nucleus, too, has parts: **protons** and **neutrons**. Protons are positively charged, neutrons are neutral. Their masses are nearly (but not exactly) the same. The mass of a proton or neutron is about 2,000 times the mass of an electron.

Quantum theory made the picture of the atom more complete though more difficult to visualize. According to quantum mechanics, the electrons do not orbit the nucleus like planets around a star, but are more like clouds of probability, in which an electron can exist anywhere in its cloud (its range of possible places), popping in and out of existence in different sites within its cloud, which fades out with distance from the nucleus.

The atoms of a particular element all have the same number of protons in their nuclei (which determines the charge of the nucleus, thus the number of electrons around the nucleus, and thus the chemistry of the element). But atoms of elements can vary in the number of neutrons in their nuclei. Therefore atoms of an element can vary in their masses. Atoms with the same number of protons (same element), but a different number of neutrons (different atomic mass), are referred to as **isotopes**.

Example:

Most atoms of the element carbon contain 6 protons and 6 neutrons in their nuclei. This is carbon-12 (atomic number 6, atomic weight 12). About 1 in 100 atoms of carbon have 6 protons and 7 neutrons in their nuclei. This is carbon-13 (atomic number 6, atomic weight 13). An even smaller fraction of carbon is carbon-14. It has 6 protons and 8 neutrons in the nucleus. Also, it is radioactive, which means it is inherently unstable and will decay in the following manner. One neutron converts to a proton plus an electron that is shot out at great energy from the nucleus (note that the electron was created by the conversion; it was not "in" the nucleus). This is beta decay, governed by the weak nuclear force. After beta decay, the atom is no longer carbon, it is nitrogen, with 7 protons and 7 neutrons, and now is perfectly stable. Other radioactive isotopes, such as those of uranium, can decay in another manner called alpha decay, when a bound particle of 2 protons and 2 neutrons (an He nucleus) is ejected.

b. Quarks and Charges

From the discoveries of quantum mechanics, protons and neutrons were found to be made of **quarks**. There are six flavors (types) of quarks according to the Standard Model (the current framework used to describe elementary particles): up, down, top, bottom, charm, and strange. Combinations of quarks make up some subatomic particles. For example, the proton is made of two "up" quarks and the neutron is one "up" quark and two "down" quarks. Other combinations of quarks create other kinds of particles in a quantum mechanical "zoo," such as **mesons**. This zoo also contains chargeless particles called **neutrinos** with a mass much less than that of electrons.

c. Essential Concepts

Velocity (*v*) is distance (*d*) covered per unit time (*t*): $v = \frac{d}{t}$.

Acceleration (*a*) is the change in velocity over an interval of time. It can be written as $a = \frac{\Delta v}{\Delta t}$ (Δd = difference, or, in the terms of calculus, **derivative**). If velocity is a change in position, acceleration is the change in velocity.

Newtonian concept of force (*F*): $F = m \times a$. It takes force to accelerate a mass (*m*) (stepping on the gas pedal of a car, which causes more gasoline to be burned and converted into the car's forward motion). Honoring Newton, the metric unit of force is called a Newton (*N*). Its units are $\frac{kg \times m}{s^2}$ (the force it takes to accelerate one kilogram by one meter by second over the course of one second).

Momentum is mass times velocity. A car traveling at 60 mph has twice the momentum of a car of the same mass traveling at 30 mph.

Objects traveling not in straight lines but in curved paths have angular properties—**angular velocity**, **angular acceleration**, and **angular momentum**. In the governing equations one must also account for the change in the angle. Earth has a huge angular momentum because of its huge mass.

Forces can be **static** as well as **dynamic**. **Pressure** (for example the pressure that exists inside a balloon blown up with air) is expressed as $\frac{N}{m^2}$, a force per area on the inner surface of the balloon. But once it is blown up, the balloon does not keep expanding. This is because there is an equal and opposite force exerted by the stretched skin of the balloon as well as by the outside air pressure. The balloon remains at the same size (except for slowly leaking) because the two forces, from air and skin, balance each other exactly.

Electricity is an entire special topic in physics.

Voltage is the difference in electrical force that can drive electrons from one place to another; the unit is the volt.

Amperage is the actual amount of flow of electricity, or electrons; the unit is the ampere or amp.

Resistance is the resistance to the flow of electricity, which varies among materials; the unit is the ohm. The watt (*W*) is the amount of power that flows when 1 amp flows through an electrical force of 1 volt.

Another important topic in physics is waves. **Waves** are characterized by frequency (cycles per time) and by wavelength (distance traveled by one cycle). Amplitude (strength) is another characteristic. For example, sound consists of traveling waves of compression and expansion in air (or water). Light waves (standing waves) are electromagnetic, which can travel in a vacuum.

d. Basic Forces

Physicists recognize four forces that are ultimately fundamental.

1. **Gravity** attracts two masses toward each other. Mass accelerates due to the gravity at Earth's surface, which is approximately 9.8 m/s^2. Newton wrote the main equation of gravity, and Einstein's general theory of relativity more completely explained gravity as a warping by matter of space-time. The force of gravity obeys an inverse-square law: The force falls off as the square of the distance from the source.

2. **Electromagnetism** (*EM*) is the force that exists between charged particles. It is attractive when the charges are opposite (positive and negative) and repulsive when the charges are the same (both positive or both negative). Electromagnetism holds atoms together—the EM force in various forms is the secret to the chemical bond. The EM force, like gravity, obeys an inverse square law. Its main theoretical formulation is in Maxwell's equations.

3. **Weak nuclear force**, which has a very short range and is responsible for certain kinds of interactions within the atom, governs a particular kind of radioactive decay called **beta decay**, in which a neutron converts to a proton plus an electron and antineutrino.

4. **Strong nuclear force** is the major stabilizer of the atomic nucleus, governing interactions among the quarks that make up the protons and neutrons. Unlike forces such as gravity and EM that diminish with distance, strong nuclear force strengthens with distance. The more quarks are separated, the more strongly they are bound to each other. This is why free quarks have never been observed.

2. Chemistry

Chemistry studies the interactions of atoms, how they form molecules, and the interactions of those molecules, which range from simple ions to complex organic molecules.

a. Atoms and the Periodic Table

The naturally occurring elements contain from 1 proton (hydrogen) to 92 protons (uranium) in the nuclei of their atoms. Elements with more protons have been made artificially in experiments of high-energy physics.

The electrons around each nucleus fill, in sequence, what are called **shells**. These shells, and the number of electrons in them, determine the chemical properties of the elements, such as crystal geometry, electrical conductivity, and, most importantly, their bonding properties with other atoms into molecules.

The first shell, K, can hold 2 electrons. The second shell, L, can hold 8 electrons (in two subshells of s with 2 and p with 6). The third shell, M, can also hold 18 electrons (in three subshells of s with 2, p with 6, and d with 10), and so on. Things become more complicated as the elements move into higher **atomic numbers** (the number of protons in their nuclei), with, for example, phenomena such as a lower subshell filling after a more outer shell contains electrons. But basically, for most chemistry we need to consider, the outermost shell will have 8 electrons when it is "full." (Note that the first shell only holds 2 electrons.)

These shells of electrons, and the fact that shells can be full or less than full, creates **cycles** in the properties of elements. For example, elements with full shells include helium, neon, and argon. These elements are in the family of elements called **noble gases**, which tend not to combine with other elements (they don't need the other elements to create a full shell of electrons, because they already are full).

There is a tendency, driven by energy considerations, for atoms to achieve complete shells of electrons. They may do this by either losing or gaining electrons, depending on which direction makes creating the full shell "easier."

For example, elements with one electron in an outer shell will tend to give up that electron in a chemical bond with a different atom. Elements with 7 electrons in the outer shell will tend to grab an electron in a chemical bond with another atom. An example is table salt, NaCl. By themselves, atoms of sodium (Na) have one outer electron, whereas those of chlorine (Cl) have seven outer electrons. In chemical contact, sodium gives up an electron to chlorine, thereby both achieving full shells. They bond into a solid crystal (salt) of an alternating, three-dimensional lattice of Na ions and Cl ions.

The outer shell that is chemically active by virtue of this tendency to give up or gain electrons is called the **valence shell** of atoms.

Depending on the strength of the tendency to gain or lose electrons, and on the "needs" of chemical partners, **chemical bonds** exist in different types. **Ionic bonds** occur when one element completely gives up electrons and the other element gains. An example is table salt, where the sodium atoms, having lost electrons, become ions with a positive charge (of +1), and the chlorine atoms, having gained electrons, become ions with a negative charge (of −1). In another kind of bond, called a **covalent bond**, electrons are shared in pairs. In a covalent bond, the resulting atoms in the bond do not become ions, but still can have a slight charge polarization. The complexities of forces between atoms in chemical bonds and between molecules with charged surfaces create other types of bonds (for example, hydrogen bonds and the bonds from van der Waal forces).

b. Chemical Reactions

Chemical reactions occur when chemical reactants change into products. Reactions can be as simple as iron rusting, or as complex as two organic molecules brought together into a larger one in the presence of an enzyme. Parts on the left-hand side of a reaction equation are called the **reactants**. Parts on the right-hand side are called the **products**. By convention, reactions are written with an arrow taking reactants into the state of products.

Chemical reactions must be balanced according to the **law of conservation of matter**: Matter can be neither created nor destroyed. (Changes in the nucleus, for example, from nuclear fusion, nuclear fission, or radioactive decay are not considered chemical reactions, which involve only the electrons of atoms, not their nuclei.) For instance, the number of atoms of oxygen in the reactants has to equal the number of atoms of oxygen in the products.

Reactions can give off energy (**exothermic**). These tend to occur spontaneously (but not instantaneously). Some reactions can require energy supplied from the environment—these are called **endothermic**.

Many important chemical reactions are known as **oxidation-reduction reactions**. One element gains electrons (is reduced). A different element loses electrons (is oxidized). The word **reduced** refers to the fact that the gain in electrons reduces the charge of the element to a more negative value.

Acids are substances whose dissolution creates hydrogen ions (H^+) in water. **Bases** are substances whose dissolution accepts hydrogen ions (H^+) in water. The **pH scale** is the measure of acidity.

c. States of Matter

Solid: the state of matter in which the atoms or molecules are bound tightly and move together as a unit. Some solids are mathematically regular in their atomic structure (such as crystals). Other solids can be more amorphous (such as coal).

Liquid: the state of matter in which the atoms or molecules can glide past each other, loosely bound but not attached to specific neighbors. However, in liquids, the molecules still have some degree of coherence to each other.

Gas: the state of matter in which atoms or molecules are totally free of each other. In air, for example, the molecules of nitrogen and oxygen travel as independent units, only bumping into other molecules (this bumping creates the gas pressure).

The different states of matter contain different amounts of energy. The energy required to change a substance from solid to liquid is called the **heat of fusion** (fusion here means melting). The energy required to change a substance from liquid to gas is called the **heat of vaporization**. The heats of fusion and vaporization occur at constant temperatures. It requires energy to heat water to the boiling point, but then more energy is needed—at that constant boiling point temperature—to turn the water into steam. Only after the water has become steam can more energy raise the temperature of the steam itself. These heats of fusion and vaporization are unique for all substances, as are the freezing and boiling temperatures.

Water, for example, has a heat of vaporization of 549 calories per gram.

When temperatures are extreme (as in the center of the Sun), electrons are stripped from their nuclei. The resulting state of matter is called a **plasma** (often plasma is called a fourth state of matter).

d. Organic and Inorganic Molecules

Basically, organic molecules contain a reduced form of carbon, in other words, carbon with a slightly negative charge from the stronger attraction for electrons (electron affinity) that it shares with other atoms, notably hydrogen. Carbon has four electrons in an outer energy level, thus requiring four more to complete the shell of eight. It is special. Carbon can bond with itself in chains, a virtually unique feature of its atomic structure (silicon also has this special characteristic). Pure forms of carbon include diamonds, graphite, and the recently discovered form of carbon in hollow spheres of 60 atoms called "buckyballs."

Organic molecules are the stuff of life. Therefore, organic chemistry is the chemistry of life itself. There are important classes of organic molecules in living things.

Proteins are organic molecules made from smaller organic components called **amino acids**. Amino acids contain the element nitrogen. **Enzymes** and many structural parts of cells are all types of proteins. **Hemoglobin** in our blood is a protein.

Carbohydrates are organic molecules of carbon in chains that are fairly short, with side groups that branch off the chains and consist of hydrogen and hydrogen-oxygen pairs (hydroxyl groups). The chemical formulae for carbohydrates often look like they consist of carbon plus multiples of water (for example, $C_6H_{12}O_6$)—thus, the name **carbohydrates**. Examples are sugars such as sucrose and lactose, and starch. The important structural molecule of plants—cellulose—is also a carbohydrate.

Lipids are very long chains of carbon atoms, with side groups that are primarily single hydrogen atoms. Other side groups also occur. Examples of lipids are the molecules in various kinds of oils (saturated versus unsaturated). Lipids are crucial in the membranes of cells, which all consist of complex lipids called **phospholipids**, because they have a phosphate group at one end. Most lipids are insoluble in water.

Nucleic acids, such as DNA and RNA, are important coding molecules for the genetics of living things and are located inside cells.

Inorganic chemistry deals with the chemistry of everything that is not organic. This includes, for example, the chemical reactions between simple charged ions dissolved in water, and the structures of crystals, with their different planes of cleavage. Inorganic chemistry includes many kinds of reactions among molecules in Earth's atmosphere.

3. Energy
a. First Law of Thermodynamics

Work is force times distance, which has the same units as energy. The metric unit of energy is the joule (J, therefore $1 J = 1 N \cdot m$). The unit is named after James Prescott Joule (1818–1889), one of the founders of the concept of the conservation of energy.

In the first law of thermodynamics, energy is neither created nor destroyed, but only transformed.

One of the amazing discoveries in the history of science was the gradual realization that types of energy can be equivalent in value (the manifestation of the first law). How can the warmth of our body or the strength of our arms come from the food we eat? Joule discovered that, indeed, mechanical motion and heat could be put into equivalent terms as forms of energy. In heat, the unit is the calorie. In the mechanical equivalent of heat, 4.18 J = 1 calorie. One feature shared by all forms of energy is that they can be converted into heat, or work.

b. Second Law of Thermodynamics

All forms of energy can be converted to heat; however, heat cannot be converted to all other forms of energy with equal efficiency. In a sense, heat is the most degraded form of energy, because it is least convertible into the other forms. This fact—that not all forms of energy are equal in "quality"—led to what is known today as the second law of thermodynamics.

The second law states that **entropy** always increases. Entropy is often taken to mean "disorder." Indeed, there is a relationship between the order of matter and its entropy content. Thus, a gas has a higher entropy than a solid, because compared to the molecular chaos of a gas, the solid has atoms and molecules in relatively neat arrangements.

Physicist Ludwig Boltzman (1844–1906) worked out the relationship between entropy and the number of states possibly occupied by a state of matter. He had the equation for entropy put on his gravestone.

In general, entropy will increase over time. Disorder increases. A hot cup of tea placed in an ordinary room will cool off. Its energy goes into the room's air. Thus, the tea cooled off by many degrees as the room warmed up a tiny amount of temperature (because it has a bigger mass). Because the heat, as energy, went from a more concentrated state (in the tea) to a more diffuse state (in the room's air), there was an increase in entropy of the tea-and-room considered as a system. A concentrated amount of heat at a high temperature is not as degraded as a diffuse amount of heat at a lower temperature. In fact, the unit of entropy is the heat per unit degree Centigrade, in other words, the $\frac{calorie}{°C}$. (Note from this definition that one calorie of heat at a lower temperature has a higher entropy than one calorie at a higher temperature.) A state of higher entropy is a more disorderly and a more degraded state of energy. These considerations are essential for the industrial world—for example, in the design and operation of the electrical power plants.

Entropy can sometimes decrease. Energy can become more useful (less degraded). For example, in plant photosynthesis, carbon dioxide and water are transformed into carbohydrates, which are food energy that we can eat. The carbon dioxide and water have a higher entropy than the same atoms arranged into the carbohydrate molecules. In this case, entropy decreased, an apparent violation of the law. But photosynthesis takes sunlight—solar energy—which itself is a very high quality (low entropy) form of energy. One can compute the efficiency of photosynthesis, which is the efficiency of the conversion of solar energy into chemical energy of food. The wasted light (this waste is an unavoidable part of the process) goes off as heat from the plant. This heat is an increase in entropy. When we combine the entropies for the two processes (1. some part of the sunlight, along with carbon dioxide and water, goes into carbohydrates in an entropy decrease; 2. the other part of sunlight goes into heat in an entropy increase), it turns out that the increase dominates.

Local decreases in entropy have always been found to co-occur with increases in entropy at a larger scale, when more factors are included. Therefore, some prefer to state the second law as the fact that in any process that transforms energy, the entropy of the universe always increases.

c. Types of Energy

Heat (also called **thermal energy**), on a molecular scale, whether for a solid, liquid, or gas, is the motion of molecules. In a solid, the atoms or molecules do not go anywhere, they vibrate in place. In a gas, higher temperatures mean faster velocities for the molecules. As a cup of hot tea cools, the fast molecules of the tea hit the molecules of the tea cup, which causes them to vibrate faster; these, in turn, come in contact with the molecules of air around the cup, causing the air molecules to move faster. The air molecules that are faster collide into the slower ones, causing them to move. Thus, the heat moves outward as the cup cools. In addition to this conduction of heat, heat can also move by **convection**, as when waves of air waft upward from a hot highway during midday in summer. Heat can also move by **radiation**, which is why your hands held near a campfire are warmed.

Mechanical energy is the sum of a system's potential energy (stored energy) and its kinetic energy (energy of motion). Mechanical energy can be represented by the example of water in a waterfall turning a turbine. As a very high quality (low entropy) form of energy, mechanical motion can be easily converted into other high-quality forms, such as electricity.

Light is an electromagnetic wave or particle (referred to as wave-particle duality) that travels in a vacuum at the universal constant velocity, the speed of light. The energy of an individual quantum packet of light in this wave (the photon) is higher for shorter wavelengths. Thus, a blue photon has higher energy than a red photon, and an ultraviolet photon has even higher energy. A very high energy photon would be the X-ray. A low energy photon is the microwave.

Electricity is moving electrons. In direct current (DC, as from a battery), electrons actually move from the negative pole to the positive pole. Eventually, the battery becomes dead when the electrons that can move have all done so. In alternating current (AC, 60 cycles per second in the United States), electrons are vibrated back and forth, first toward one direction in the wire, then toward the other direction. So they do not actually travel any real distance because they end up where they started. We use AC for most power needs, because it is safer at the high voltages needed for long-distance transmission from the power plants to individual homes.

Nuclear energy is the energy inherent in the nuclei of certain atoms. For example, nuclear power plants use the nuclear energy of a uranium isotope (U-235), which can be split in a controlled chain reaction of nuclear fission. This source of energy turns water to steam to spin a turbine and thereby generate electricity. In the Sun, the form of nuclear energy is nuclear fusion, in which hydrogen is fused to helium, with the release of energy.

Work is formally defined as force times distance ($w = F \times d$). For example, to lift a heavy box from the ground is work. You exert a force, counter to that of gravity, to lift the mass through a distance. Work has the same units as energy. Work requires the expenditure of energy. Where has the energy gone? Some went into body heat as your muscles were used. Some went into lifting the box, now above the ground, and now a form of potential energy.

Gravitational and mechanical potential energy: There are many forms of potential energy, which usually means that energy is held in a static arrangement of matter in some form, with the potential to be released and turned into some other form of energy, such as kinetic or electrical or heat (thermal). An object lifted above the ground has potential energy (thus, every leaf on a tree has potential energy). Potential energy also resides in the mechanical tension of a pressed or stretched spring.

Chemical potential energy exists when any two or more substances are capable of undergoing a chemical reaction that could potentially release energy in an exothermic reaction. One example is food and the oxygen in the air. That pair has the chemical potential to "burn" together and release energy. We do this when consuming the food. Our cells convert the energy into other molecules that can store energy. This stored energy can then be used to construct the other molecules we need to live.

Kinetic energy is a type of mechanical energy and is called the energy of motion. It is proportional to the square of the velocity of an object. $E_k = \frac{1}{2}mv^2$ (m is the mass of the object, and v is the velocity).

You Should Review

- laws of motion, gravitation, momentum
- light and magnetism
- electricity
- structure of the atom
- periodic table
- chemical bonds
- forms of energy
- first and second laws of energy thermodynamics

Questions

21. The atomic number of carbon is 6. Which of the following determines carbon's atomic number?
    a. The six neutrons located in carbon's nucleus.
    b. The six protons located in carbon's nucleus.
    c. The six electrons surrounding carbon's nucleus.
    d. The average masses of all of carbon's isotopes.

22. Which of the following is a true statement?
    a. Velocity is the rate of change of time.
    b. Acceleration is the rate of change of velocity.
    c. Velocity is the rate of change of acceleration.
    d. Acceleration is the rate of change of time.

23. What type of reaction occurs when a substance changes from solid to liquid?
    a. fusion
    b. exothermic
    c. sublimation
    d. vaporization

24. Which force gets stronger as the distance increases?
    a. strong nuclear force
    b. gravity
    c. weak nuclear force
    d. electromagnetism

25. When a sodium atom gives up an electron to enter into an ionic bond with chorine in table salt, it does so because
    a. it requires an electrical charge of +1.
    b. it requires an electrical charge of –1.
    c. it creates a negative potential energy.
    d. it achieves a full outer electron shell.

26. Dissolving H_2SO_4 in water creates an acid by increasing the concentration of
    a. sulfate ions.
    b. water ions.
    c. hydrogen ions.
    d. oxygen ions.

27. Which organic molecule contains nitrogen?
    a. carbohydrate
    b. lipid
    c. cellulose
    d. protein

28. What is the first law of thermodynamics?
    a. Matter can be neither created nor destroyed, but only transformed.
    b. Energy moves from higher forms to lower forms.
    c. Energy can be neither created nor destroyed, but only transformed.
    d. Matter moves from higher forms to lower forms.

29. Which system exhibits the greatest entropy?
    a. a pot of boiling water
    b. a glass of water sitting on the counter
    c. an ice cube in the freezer
    d. a puddle of water in the road

30. Moving electrons are best described as
    a. electricity.
    b. heat.
    c. kinetic energy.
    d. light.

Answers

21. b. The atomic number of any element is determined by the number of protons located in the atom's nucleus.

22. b. Velocity is a change in distance; acceleration is a change in velocity.

23. a. When a substance changes from solid to liquid, it undergoes melting, or fusion. This is an endothermic reaction that requires the input of energy, not an exothermic one.

24. a. The strong nuclear force exhibits this counterintuitive behavior.

25. d. The sodium atom has 1 electron in its outermost shell; by losing 1 electron, it achieves a full outermost (valence) shell (the next innermost one was already full). The sodium atom achieves an electrical charge of +1, which is the result of, not the reason for, giving up an electron.

26. c. Hydrogen ions come directly from putting H_2SO_4 into solution.

27. d. The amino acids that make up proteins all have nitrogen atoms in them. Cellulose is a carbohydrate.

28. c. Thermodynamics covers the properties of energy, and the first law is about the conservation of energy.

29. a. Entropy is the measure of a system's "disorder." The more disordered a system, the greater its entropy. In a pot of boiling water, the water is changing from its liquid form to its gaseous form, steam, which is a more disordered system than solid ice or liquid water alone.

30. a. Electricity is electrons in motion.

D. Evolution and Life

1. Origin of Life

Life on Earth has persisted for nearly four billion years. How did it begin?

a. Formation of Organic Molecules

In 1953, a Nobel Prize–winning experiment by Harold Urey and Stanley Miller created organic molecules by passing a spark through a mixture of gases, such as methane and ammonia, presumed constituents of an early Earth atmosphere. Zapping inorganic molecules with energy—a possible analogy to lightning in ancient Earth's atmosphere—could create certain constituents for life.

Other possible sources of organic molecules are (1) space, because organic molecules do occur in certain types of meteorites, and (2) deep sea vents, where raw chemicals from the inner Earth provide a source of materials and chemical energy.

b. Concentration of Organic Molecules

To form life, organic molecules need to be concentrated. Darwin had the concept of a warm little pond as a site for the origin of life. Lagoons that periodically flooded and then dried up might have concentrated organic molecules during the dry stages.

Scientists are not sure of the temperature of early Earth at the time of the formation of life. Some say that if early Earth was cold enough for ice to at least occasionally form, the freezing of water, which excludes any organic molecules present, could have concentrated organic molecules at the surfaces of ice.

Clay minerals are complex, and some scientists have suggested clay as a material for the concentration and even organization of organic molecules into more complex networks, on the way to life.

As a possible source of organic molecules, deep sea vents are also candidates for their necessary concentration. In fact, in recent years, various lab experiments have increased the odds that the vents—with hot water rich with minerals and abundant complex minerals—were sites for key steps in the origin of life.

c. Membranes

All cells have membranes that separate their insides from the outside environment and regulate the exchange of matter and energy.

Organic molecules (lipids) from certain kinds of meteorites, when added in water, spontaneously form spherical vesicles (liposomes). According to some, these gifts from space could have created the molecular vesicles that became protocells, within which ran self-perpetuating chemical reactions, a step on the way to real life.

The details of how the origin of life went from simple organic molecules, perhaps enclosed in membranes, to real cells with the genetic machinery of proteins and DNA, are still unknown. Many scientists claim that RNA served as the first genetic material, only later supplanted by DNA, at which time RNA then took on the role of helper molecules in that machinery.

d. Evidence in the Rocks

Two types of evidence for early life have been discovered.

An isotope of carbon, carbon-13, is set in a special ratio to ordinary carbon-12 when carbon passes through living metabolisms. Some evidence of this isotopic signature of early life has been found in rocks as old as 3.9 billion years old.

Scientists (micropaleontologists) find ancient rocks, slice them, and look at them through a microscope to seek direct visual evidence of cells. There are indications of cells in rocks from 3.5 billion years ago.

To gain clues to the origin of life, scientists seek organisms generally known as **extremophiles** across Earth. These are bacteria or archaea adapted to (and requiring) extreme conditions of acid or temperature to live (acidophiles, thermophiles, and others).

2. Recipe for Evolution
a. Inheritance, Variation, and Selection

Inheritance is when organisms in each generation share many of the same features of their predecessors, because the DNA is copied from parent to offspring.

Variation: Often, offspring are not exactly like the parents. Variation is key because this serves as the raw material that can be molded by evolution into new types of creatures.

Selection (natural selection) is defined as survival of the fittest. Not all offspring live long enough to put forth the next generation. Those with variations that can withstand drought, or seek out food most efficiently, or run the swiftest, survive. The environment selects certain types of creatures (and their variation) to carry on.

In summary, evolution is modification by natural selection. The process repeats: inheritance, variation, selection. It operates over and over, as generations roll along, and it has been doing so for nearly four billion years.

b. DNA and Mutations

The molecule **DNA (deoxyribonucleic acid)** is key to inheritance and variation. It is the famous double helix, with double strands of alternating sugar and phosphate units, between which are set rungs of the genetic code. The code is made of four bases: adenine (A), cytosine (C), thymine (T), and guanine (G). Base A always pairs with base T, base C always pairs with base G. The double helix allows a way for DNA to make copies. In the copying process, DNA unravels, and because of the rule of pairing (A-T, C-G), the code on both individual strands can be both made double again, as the complementary bases are added, rung by rung. This copying creates faithful inheritance.

Mistakes, or mutations, in the copying sometimes occur randomly. Most mutations have no effect on or are detrimental to the offspring. But some can be beneficial (for example, a mutation might create a more effective pore in the cell membrane for the transport of nutrients into the cell).

The simplest type is **base substitution**, in which, say, a T is removed and an A, C, or G is substituted. In another kind of mutation, entire genes can be duplicated and put somewhere else into the DNA. If the original gene continues with its function, the duplicated gene is free to mutate into possibly a new and beneficial function.

There can be insertions and deletions from sections of the code.

All mutations potentially serve as variation that can be selected for in the process of evolution.

How is the genetic code translated to proteins? Triplets of bases code for single amino acids (there are about 20 of these). Amino acids are assembled in chains that then fold into complex, bulbous shapes of proteins. Many proteins are active enzymes, others are structural. Enzymes facilitate the assembly of other types of molecules through chemical reactions inside cells and perform many other tasks.

c. "Blind Watchmaker" of Natural Selection

Before evolution was accepted, a story about a watch found on a beach was used as a parable to suggest the presence of a creator for all life forms. It was thought that a watch, being so complex, obviously had a watchmaker. The scientist and prominent writer about evolution, Richard Dawkins, coined the phrase the "blind watchmaker" to describe evolution. Evolution creates wondrous organisms, but the process is "blind"—it doesn't know where it is going.

3. Types of Cells
a. Prokaryotes

Prokaryotic cells were the earliest type of cell. They are small and simple. The word *prokaryote* means "before" (*pro*) and "kernel" (*karyote*), signifying that the prokaryotes are single cells with no central nucleus (in other words, no kernel). Prokaryotes have their DNA floating inside, and do not contain membrane-bound organelles. Today, there are two types of prokaryotic organisms: **archaea** and **bacteria**. Prokaryotes reproduce primarily by fission of the cell into two equal daughter cells in a process called **mitosis**. Bacteria also have ways to exchange parts of their genomes with different bacteria of the same species or even other species.

b. Eukaryotes

Eukaryotes are larger cells that make up animal and plant matter and fungi. Some types of single-celled creatures, such as amoebas and paramecia, are also eukaryotes. The word *eukaryote* means "good" (*eu*) and "kernel" (*karyote*), signifying that eukaryotic cells have a central, membrane-bound nucleus, which houses the DNA for these complex cells. Eukaryotic cells also have other membrane-bound organelles inside them, which support special functions for the cells. All eukaryotic cells have **mitochondria**, power-plant organelles that take food nutrients and create high-energy molecules used elsewhere in the cell for various metabolic tasks. Plant cells have another organelle, called the **chloroplast**. It is also membrane bound and contains the photosynthetic machinery for the plant cell. Eukaryotic cells have internal structures, like wires and tent posts, called, respectively, **microfilaments** and **microtubules**. These allow the big cells to take on complex shapes (or even creep along as the amoeba does).

Eukaryotic cells (for example, paramecia or our skin cells) can reproduce by mitosis. In addition, multicellular eukaryotes (animals, plants, fungi) have sexual reproduction of the entire organism, which uses **meiosis** to generate sex cells with half the parent's genetic components (sperm and egg).

c. Cell Evolution by Symbiosis

The eukaryotic cell evolved about two billion years ago, at about the same time that Earth's atmosphere shifted from anaerobic (with virtually no oxygen) to a level of oxygen about ten percent of today's amount. The eukaryotic cell evolved from a symbiotic merger between a large prokaryote and a smaller prokaryote, which eventually became the mitochondrion of the new, eukaryotic type of cell. **Symbiosis** means working together, and the two

cells that merged had specific ways to help the other (probably sharing metabolic products that were needed by the other). Eventually, this merger became permanent. Genes were transferred from the small, embedded cell into the genome of the larger host. One strong piece of evidence of this ancient merger is the fact that today's mitochondria have a remnant of still useful DNA inside them. Also, the mitochondria are about the same size as typical bacteria.

The chloroplast also came about from a symbiotic merger with something like today's **cyanobacteria** (a type of photosynthesizing, chlorophyll-containing bacterium). As in the case of the mitochondrion, most of the DNA from the symbiotic cyanobacteria migrated into the genome of the larger host cell, but there still exists remnant DNA for a few proteins in the modern cell's chloroplast. Again, the chloroplast's size is also about right for the theory.

Because all eukaryotic cells have mitochondria but only some have chloroplasts, the symbiotic event that created the mitochondria came first. Scientists do not know how the nucleus itself evolved.

d. The Universal Tree of Life

All life possesses DNA and much the same genetic machinery. This is strong evidence that all current life shares a universal ancestry. In addition, all organisms manufacture proteins at cell sites called **ribosomes** (where the amino acids are linked into chains, on the way to forming proteins). The ribosome contains some structural RNA as a permanent subunit. All organisms thus contain rRNA (for ribosomal RNA). This rRNA varies from creature to creature, because the rRNA mutated over time. The closer in structure the rRNA is between two creatures, the more closely related they are.

Scientists can construct a tree of all life, using the degree of similarity of rRNA as the metric to distinguish and group organisms. The rRNA tree of life reveals three major lobes: the eukaryotes, the archaea (a type of prokaryote), and the bacteria (another type of prokaryote). Eukaryotes most likely gained some of their genetic material from the archaea and some from the bacteria.

The universal tree of life constructed from the patterns of rRNA shows that most of the organisms near the trunk (prokaryotes living today that presumably are similar to those that lived long ago, when the tree was near its trunk stage in evolutionary time) are **hyperthermophilic** (they require high temperatures). These creatures might indicate a very high temperature origin for life. Such temperatures would have occurred at the deep sea vents, or possibly over the entire Earth.

4. Multicellular Life

The eukaryotic cells gave rise in evolution to true multicellular life forms: fungi, plants, and animals.

a. Earliest Evidence

Evidence of the first multicelled creatures is obscure because their soft bodies meant they were only rarely preserved as fossils. Scientists use fossil and genetic evidence (the universal tree of life) to estimate the date of origin of multicellularity at about one billion years ago. That means that for nearly three-fourths of the history of life, all creatures were single-celled.

Ediacaran fauna was an early type of multicellular life, which lived about 600 million years ago (MYA). Scientists named these strange, flat creatures found in many shapes and sizes after the Ediacara Hills of Australia, where their fossils were first found. Some scientists believe that the Ediacarans went extinct when predators evolved.

b. Cambrian Explosion

The **Cambrian explosion** was the geological time period of ten million years that began around 540 million years ago, in which suddenly all kinds of animals with hard parts (that is why they were preserved) "exploded" into the fossil record. The hard parts—shells of various types—used calcium from ocean water. Except for the absence of vertebrates,

the Cambrian explosion formed most of the basic body plans of animals. The action was all underwater, with **arthropods** (such as **crustaceans** called **trilobites**) and bizarre creatures crawling on the sea floor while others swam and sported formidable jaws. Scientists have not yet determined the trigger for this blossoming of life.

c. Evolution of Trees and Fungi

The **Devonian period** was a period roughly between 300 and 400 million years ago, in which new types of creatures emerged. Important adaptations made this evolution possible. For land plants, these changes included: (1) molecules such as **cellulose** and **lignin** that could give structure to stems and trunks and lift plants up into the air and (2) **vascular tissues** in the stems, trunks, and roots that could transport water and mineral ions up from the roots to the photosynthetic parts (via tubes called the **xylem**) and could transport manufactured food downward from the photosynthetic parts to the roots (via tubes called the **phloem**).

The fossil record shows that plants evolved from tiny, moss-sized beings into tall trees over a period that was only about 20 million years long. No flowering plants (**angiosperms**)—like deciduous trees—existed yet. Fossil evidence shows that fungal cells (visible as microscopic fossils) occurred inside the roots of ancient plants. Apparently, these fungi lived like some kinds of fungus do today, in a symbiotic partnership with plants. Most fungi live as microscopic underground threads, called **hyphae**.

d. Animals

What makes an animal? One defining characteristic is a **blastula stage** (a hollow ball of cells) during early embryonic development.

Vertebrates evolved in the ocean as fish.

Animal life came ashore during the Devonian, as fishlike creatures with four legs (tetrapods). Besides the legs, lungs were another key development for what became **amphibians**.

To become fully terrestrial, vertebrates had to solve the problem of living in the desiccating air. **Reptiles** became terrestrial with adaptations like a water-retaining amnion (sac) in their embryo stages, a waterproof egg, and a watertight skin of scales.

Mammals evolved by around 200 million years ago, from mammal-like reptiles, which had split off from other reptiles about 260 million years ago. Adaptations of mammals include hair and nursing the young with mammary glands.

5. Mass Extinctions

In just the last 20 years, scientists have discovered what they believe to be the cause of the extinction of the dinosaurs. The answer has given new understanding to what factors contributed to the story of life.

a. Origin of the Dinosaurs

Dinosaurs are a group of reptiles that diverged from early reptiles by 220 million years ago. An adaptation of dinosaurs was a new kind of hip joint that allowed many early (and late) dinosaurs to run bipedally. Species of dinosaurs came and went over more than 150 million years of time, until their sudden extinction at 65 million years ago.

b. Evidence for Impacts from Space

Objects from space occasionally strike Earth—evidence includes the meteor crater in northern Arizona and the Sudbury crater in Canada (the result of a much larger impact occurring about two billion years ago). The longer the time period between impacts, the more chance for a devastating impact. (Small objects enter Earth's atmosphere every night, and burn up—shooting stars.) On the Moon and Mars where little or no geological change occurs, scientists see evidence (craters) of large impacts. On Earth, as wind and water shift sediments, as continents rise and fall, most craters are buried or erased.

c. End of Cretaceous and End of Dinosaurs

In the 1980s, an unusually large amount of a rare element called iridium (Ir) was discovered in a centimeter-thick clay layer in rocks in Italy, dating from the time of the dinosaur extinction. This anomaly of iridium was subsequently found all over the world.

Iridium occurs at such concentrations only in meteorites. This discovery pointed to a large impactor (comet or asteroid) as the cause of the iridium and the mass extinction. Such an object would have smashed into Earth at a speed of 20 km/s, and is estimated to have been about the size of Manhattan (10 km or 6 miles in diameter).

A few years later, evidence from gravity patterns (mapped by a Mexican oil company, during prospecting) revealed a crater buried under sediments in the Yucatan Peninsula of Mexico. About 200 km in diameter (about the estimated size of the crater made by a 10-km object), it dates to exactly 65 million years ago, the end of what geologists call the **Cretaceous** (K) and the beginning of the **Paleogene** (Pg), formerly known as the **Tertiary** (T). A wealth of other evidence for the **K-Pg (K-T) impact** has been found, including material ejected close to the impact and shocked minerals, as well as chemical evidence for worldwide fires and other environmental disruptions.

At the K-Pg boundary, 65 million years ago, many other types of life also went extinct, on all scales, all the way down to the plankton. One group of creatures survived that had been alive at the time of the K-Pg extinction and were directly descended from the dinosaurs. These are the birds. And, fortunately for us, mammals survived, too, probably because the mammals back then were only the size of rats, and could weather the catastrophe underground in burrows.

d. End of Permian

Another large extinction occurred 250 million years ago, at the end of the **Permian period**, and beginning of the **Triassic** (the P-Tr boundary). It came just before either dinosaurs or mammals existed, during an age of giant amphibians and early reptiles. Some paleontologists have called this the mother of all mass extinctions. What caused it is not yet known.

e. Other Mass Extinctions

Species are always going extinct. Based on the fossil record, scientists have uncovered a cyclical nature for mass extinctions, with large-scale extinctions occurring approximately every 62 million years for the last 540 million years. The cause of this extinction pattern is still unknown. In some cases, scientists name climate change or large impacts as the cause.

Though the stories of individual mass extinctions are still being assembled from field data, the discovery of the K-Pg impact and the mass extinction of the dinosaurs has given us new insight into how precarious life on Earth has been and how evolution has been subjected to random shocks from space. What if the impact had been larger? And what if it had not taken place? Before the dinosaurs went extinct, mammals had remained small for over a hundred million years. In the millions of years following the demise of the dinosaurs, mammals evolved into a huge variety of species, some of them as big as hippopotamuses and elephants. In terms of evolutionary biology, the mammals radiated. Without the K-Pg extinction, this radiation would not have occurred.

6. Human Evolution
a. Chimps, Gorillas, and the Hominid Tree of Life

The molecular clock, the rate at which certain proteins mutate over time, has been used to date the divergences of evolutionary lineages of humans from the great apes: orangutans, gorillas, and chimpanzees. These are all modern creatures, but we are trying to date their most recent common ancestors.

At about 12–15 MYA, the lineage leading to orangutans diverges.

At about 8–10 MYA, the lineage leading to modern gorillas diverges.

At about 5–7 MYA, humans and chimps branch off from a common ancestor. Many lines of evidence—from morphology to genetics—show that chimpanzees are our closest living animal relative.

b. Many Species of Hominids

Australopithecus is the genus that evolved in Africa after the hominids' divergence from chimps.

Australopithecus africanus is the species thought to be a human ancestor; the fossil called "Lucy" was this species, which lived about 3.5 million years ago. It had a brain size equivalent to the modern chimp's (humans' famed evolutionary brain growth had not yet begun), but the species stood upright and its legs, feet, spine, pelvis, and skull were adapted to upright living. Some paleontologists suggest that living upright freed the hands to carry objects (but no real stone tools yet), and that caused selective pressure for more braininess.

Homo is the genus of modern human, which evolved by 1.5 million years ago. An early important species in genus *Homo* is *Homo erectus*, which evolved in Africa but spread as far as China and other parts of Asia. Some paleontologists think a closely related species, *Homo ergaster*, is more likely our direct ancestor. Compared to *Australopithecus*, the brains and bodies of *Homo erectus* and *Homo ergaster* are larger. Scientists have found evidence of the first stone tools—crudely chipped rocks—which were likely made for cutting meat, scraping, and pounding.

There were other species of genus *Homo* in the time between 500,000 to 200,000 years ago. Paleontologists are still sorting out (and discovering) evidence. Some of these species reached Europe and evolved, by 150,000 years ago, into *Homo neanderthalensis*, the Neanderthals. They were large and powerfully muscular, with brow ridges above their eyes, and slightly bigger brains than humans have today. Though the word Neanderthal is sometimes used to mean "dumb," these creatures are considered intelligent. Why did they go extinct? Was it from competition or interbreeding with our species? Was it climate change? They did survive in Europe and Russia during a deep ice age.

Homo sapiens, the species of modern humans, originated in Africa about 150,000 years ago. *Homo sapiens* migrated from Africa into the Middle East and even shared land with Neanderthals in some cases. Over this span of human evolution, from *Australopithecus africanus* to *Homo sapiens*, brain size increased about threefold. Human brains (relative to body size) are way above the mammalian average and enormous even for the brains of primates.

c. The Creative Explosion

A creative explosion occurred between about 60,000–30,000 years ago and included complex tool making (using animal bones for needles, harpoons, and other craft items), clothing, and elaborate burial practices. An early sculpture from Germany shows what seems to be a standing man with a lion's head. Was this a shaman? Does this signal the birth of myths? (Some scholars claim we will find evidence for art even earlier, when the time period of 100,000 years ago is examined more carefully in Africa.) By 30,000 years ago, we have evidence of paintings deep within caves, elaborate color paintings of animals, usually the animals that were hunted. Were these the sites for rituals? For initiation ceremonies?

A find in the Ukraine, dated at about 15,000 years ago, shows that these people constructed dome homes out of mammoth bones, probably covered with mammoth hides. Thus, they had architecture.

What was their language? Scholars tend to agree that by the time of cave art and elaborate bone tools and carvings, language was used to educate the young and to organize complex social dynamics. But did language come even earlier? And was the creative explosion due to a final genetic advance or was it all cultural? Scientists do not yet have the answers.

d. Evolutionary Psychology

Evolutionary psychology is the study of the evolution of human behavior, considered controversial by some because scientists cannot directly study the minds and emotions of ancestral humans. No other mammal species wages war, although male chimps have been observed in similar behavior, forming a band to kill a solitary individual in a competing band. Humans also cooperate to an unprecedented degree. In a central African jungle lives another kind of chimp called the bonobo. Unlike the male-dominated chimp culture, the bonobo has a female-bonded society and uses sex as a social lubricant. Chimps and bonobos genetically diverged 2–3 million years ago, after their shared lineage diverged from the lineage that led to us. Evolutionary psychologists study chimps and bonobos to investigate how the behavior of humans may have evolved.

The human brain contains an organ that senses danger and creates the emotion of fear (the brain organ is the **amygdala**). Humans share this with other mammals and most vertebrates. But humans can also project into the future more than any other creature. We know we are going to die. Evolutionary psychologists investigate whether this knowledge is lined with the origin of religion.

You Should Review

- cell evolution
- prokaryotic and eukaryotic cells
- major events of evolution
- major adaptations leading to new kinds of organisms
- steps in human evolution
- mass extinctions

Questions

31. The four bases of DNA are
   a. ACEG.
   b. CMEP.
   c. TAGC.
   d. MGPA.

32. Considering the problem of the origin of life on Earth, which is NOT a possible source of organic molecules?
- **a.** dissolution of rocks
- **b.** lightning in the atmosphere
- **c.** deep sea vents
- **d.** meteorites from space

33. Which cell type has a nucleus?
- **a.** bikaryotic
- **b.** prokaryotic
- **c.** eukaryotic
- **d.** postkaryotic

34. For what fraction of the span of life's existence on Earth was life only microbial?
- **a.** $\frac{1}{1}$
- **b.** $\frac{3}{4}$
- **c.** $\frac{1}{2}$
- **d.** $\frac{1}{5}$

35. Based upon the rock record, approximately how long ago did simple cells emerge?
- **a.** 3.5 trillion years
- **b.** 3.5 billion years
- **c.** 3.5 million years
- **d.** 3.5 thousand years

36. What was the mass extinction that ended the reign of the dinosaurs?
- **a.** Cretaceous-Paleogene
- **b.** Permian-Triassic
- **c.** Triassic-Jurassic
- **d.** Carboniferous-Permian

37. The most direct ancestor of the mammals was a
- **a.** mammal-like amphibian.
- **b.** mammal-like reptile.
- **c.** mammal-like fish.
- **d.** mammal-like crocodile.

38. Which animal today is the direct descendant of the dinosaurs?
- **a.** ostrich
- **b.** white shark
- **c.** African lion
- **d.** humpback whale

39. The "Cambrian Explosion" refers to
- **a.** the appearance of the first hominids approximately 3.5 million years ago.
- **b.** the period of widespread volcanic activity on Earth that paved the path for the evolution of life.
- **c.** the collision of a large meteor with Earth, which is believed to have caused the extinction of dinosaurs.
- **d.** the large-scale appearance of animals as indicated by the fossil record.

40. Which is the second oldest, in terms of evolution?
- **a.** *Homo erectus*
- **b.** *Homo sapiens*
- **c.** Neanderthal
- **d.** *Australopithecus*

Answers

31. c. The four DNA bases are tyrosine, adenine, guanine, and cytosine.

32. a. Dissolution of rocks creates ions in water, but this has nothing to do with actually forming organic molecules. All the other choices are definite possibilities.

33. c. Eukaryotic cells have a nucleus in each cell. The word means "good (or true) kernel."

34. b. Life became single celled nearly four billion years ago, but multicellular life did not evolve until about one billion years ago. Therefore, the time period over which life was only microbial was $\frac{3}{4}$ of the total time of life.

35. b. Scientists believe the first cells, the precursors to life, appeared on Earth around 3.5 billion years ago. Evidence of the cells has been found in ancient rocks.

36. a. The Cretaceous-Paleogene event caused the extinction of the dinosaurs, about 65 million years ago. (This is also called the K-Pg boundary—K for Cretaceous, in geologist's terminology.)

37. b. Because fish evolved into amphibians, which evolved into reptiles, the ancestor of mammals was a mammal-like reptile. Crocodiles came much later.

38. a. The ostrich, like all birds, is a descendent of the dinosaurs.

39. d. The Cambrian Explosion refers to the widespread appearance of life approximately 540 million years ago. Prior to this time, most life forms were "soft bodied," not allowing for adequate fossil preservation. The Cambrian period saw the evolution of life with "hard" parts (shells, for example) that were retained in the fossil record.

40. a. *Homo erectus* came after *Australopithecus* but well before the Neanderthal and *Homo sapiens*.

E. Earth Works

1. Continental Drift and Plate Tectonics

a. History

In 1912, German scientist Alfred Wegener proposed that continents could move around, or "drift." One of Wegener's clues to the drift was the fact that the east coast of South America could fit into the lower half of the west coast of Africa, almost like puzzle pieces. Wegener also pointed to evidence in South America, Africa, India, and Australia for ice sheets at about the same time, 300 million years ago, which made no sense with the continents in their present positions, because some of these sites are at today's equator.

Modern geologists have evidence that continents have shifted positions radically throughout Earth's history. For example, when molten rock (**magma**) cools to become solid rock, if the rock is slightly magnetic, it takes on the magnetic field of Earth, which depends on latitude. Rocks near the poles have signatures of ancient latitudes near the equator and vice versa.

b. Seafloor Spreading

In the 1960s, new lines of evidence supported the idea of shifting continents, but the focus changed to the spreading ocean floor. Ships drilled and brought to the surface cores from the ocean's rocky floor, and the cores were analyzed for periodic reversals in Earth's magnetic fields.

On both sides of the Atlantic Ocean's mid-ocean ridge, stripes showed times when Earth's magnetic field was normal and reversed. The ocean's floor had been growing over time, and the Atlantic Ocean was slowly increasing in size. This ocean floor provided a record of the history of seafloor spreading. The Atlantic Ocean spreads at a rate of 1–2 inches per year (consider that rate over tens of millions of years).

Finally, scientists had a mechanism for continental drift. It wasn't that the continents drifted, but that they were moved by changes in the ocean's floor. Seafloor spreading replaced continents drifting.

c. Subduction Zones and Plate Tectonics

If the Atlantic Ocean is growing, what about the other oceans? Because Earth is a constant size, the other oceans cannot be growing, too. However, there is a north-south underwater volcanic ridge in the Eastern Pacific, and that is spreading even several times faster than the Mid-Atlantic Ridge. Eventually, the solution was found in the discovery of what are called **subduction zones**. These are regions ("lines") where ocean crust disappears by diving down into the deep Earth, by subducting. The loss of ocean floor (crust) in subduction zones balances the creation of new ocean floor (crust) in mid-ocean ridges.

The modern theory of **plate tectonics** was thus born. Earth's geological activities have always been called **tectonism**. What about the term **plate**? Think of an egg shell with patterns of cracks in it, creating zones of the shell. That's the crust of Earth. Earth's surface is divided into a number of major plates. Sometimes, continents ride within the areas of the plates; sometimes edges of continents coincide with edges of plates. From some of the edges of the plates emerges new ocean crust from mid-ocean ridges and seafloor spreading. Into other cracks, ocean crust subducts (the western coast of South America and the ocean trench regions of the western Pacific are examples). Plates grow and shrink in size with the geological ages. Thus, continents shift positions.

South America, Africa, and Antarctica were all joined as recently as 200 million years ago.

Plate tectonics is an overarching theory that solves many separate mysteries about geology. What made mountain ranges? Why do earthquakes and volcanoes occur where they do? Why is there a "ring of fire" around the outer edge of the Pacific Ocean, a ring with huge numbers of earthquakes and volcanoes? It turns out that earthquakes and volcanoes tend to occur at the boundaries between two plates, because that is where geological activity happens. The Pacific ring of fire occurs because the Pacific Ocean is ringed by many plate edges. The famous San Andreas fault in California, which is the origin of California's earthquakes, is a plate boundary (here the two plates are sliding past each other, neither subducting nor spreading apart). The towering Andes mountain chain along the western coast of South America has been lifted up by a plate plunging under South America from the west, putting pressure from below to lift the mountains up.

d. Earth Over Time and the Geological Time Scale

Planet Earth coalesced from planetary materials brought together by gravity about 4.6 billion years ago (BYA).

Hadean (4.6–4 billion years ago) was the earliest eon and means "time of hell." Earth still experienced many bombardments from space.

The **Archean** eon (4–2.5 BYA) was when single-celled life originated.

The **Proterozoic** eon (about 2,500–545 millions of years ago) was the time of the first great rise in oxygen and evolution of eukaryotic cell about 2,000 MYA. Near the end of the eon, multicellular life evolved. There is also evidence for massive ice ages, which came close to covering the entire Earth in ice sheets.

The **Paleozoic** eon (545–250 MYA) started with the Cambrian explosion of life and by its end, plants had evolved into tall trees. Giant amphibians and early reptiles were the dominant life on land.

The **Phanerozoic** is the current eon, further divided into eras. The **Mesozoic** era (250–65 MYA) is subdivided into three main periods called the Triassic, Jurassic, and Cretaceous. The Jurassic was the reign of dinosaurs. The mass extinction at 65 MYA ended the dinosaurs' existence and the Mesozoic period.

The **Cenozoic** period (from 65 MYA to today) is the age of mammals. The **Pleistocene** epoch (a subdivision of the Cenozoic period) lasting from 2 MYA to 10,000 years ago, is a time of the growth and then retreat of giant ice sheets, in cycles of about 100,000 years each. During the height of the last ice age, for example, ice sheets a mile thick covered all of Canada and extended as far south as New York City. Sea level was 100 meters lower, and the ocean was therefore far offshore of its present location. At the final deglaciation, about 10,000 years ago, geologists end the Pleistocene and start a new epoch, called the **Holocene** (for "wholly recent"). Because humans are perturbing so much of the planet, there has been the suggestion that we have inaugurated what should be called a new epoch, perhaps the "anthropocene," the "human-made recent."

2. Earth's Layers

a. Core and Mantle

When Earth formed 4.6 billion years ago, the heat generated from all the impacts that formed it, and heat from the high levels of radioactive rock, put Earth into a molten state. Being molten, elements and minerals could separate according to their density. The heavier materials sunk toward Earth's center. The lighter materials floated, so to speak, nearer the surface.

Earth's metallic core is solid near the center and liquid further out. It is about 1,200 kilometers thick and mostly iron, with smaller amounts of nickel and other elements.

Circulation of the liquid iron in the core generates Earth's magnetic field. This field is related to Earth's spin, but the north and south magnetic poles are not in the same locations as the north and south poles of Earth's spin axis.

Outside the core is the layer called the **mantle**. With a thickness of about 2,800 km, the mantle reaches to 10–50 km below the surface. The upper layer of the mantle belongs to the lithosphere (see below). Then, below the lithosphere and about 250 km thick, is a layer of the mantle called the **asthenosphere**. This is crucial because although made of rock, the asthenosphere can move like putty over long time periods. The circulation of the asthenosphere is one main factor in plate tectonics.

When Earth's crust enters subduction zones, the material sinks back down into the asthenosphere (in other words, into the mantle), melting and joining with the deep Earth material.

b. Lithosphere

Lithosphere (literally "rock-sphere"), the uppermost and lightest layer, consists of the outermost crust and a thin upper part of mantle. Below the lithosphere, the rock is malleable (the putty of the asthenosphere). The lithosphere itself, being cooler, is brittle. The border between lithosphere and asthenosphere is defined by this change in behavior of the rock, from brittle to malleable.

The crust under the ocean's water is thin, about 10 km deep.

The crust under the continents is thick, about 50 km deep.

c. Oceans

The average depth of the ocean is about four km. Around the continents, the ocean is shallow, about 100–300 meters deep. This so-called continental shelf is really part of the continental mass. Heading seaward from the continental shelf, the bottom of the ocean drops downward in a steep slope. This region is called the **continental slope**.

Much of the ocean, at its deepest, is in the 3–5 km range of depth. Exceptions are the very deep trenches, formed where slabs of ocean floor are subducting downward into the mantle at plate boundaries. Other exceptions are the mid-ocean ridges, which are mountain ranges underwater where new crust is forming, as described above.

At places on Earth, plumes of magma in semi-permanent columns from the mantle rise into the lithosphere. These are the **hotspots**. For example, the Hawaiian islands have been formed by one of these hotspots. As the Pacific plate moves westward (its motion created by plate tectonics), the plate moves over the hotspot (which remains approximately stationary). The Hawaiian islands have been formed, one by one, sequentially, as the Pacific plate moved over the hotspot over tens of millions of years. Therefore, the oldest Hawaiian island is the one furthest to the west, Kauai. The most recent Hawaiian island, with active volcanoes, is the "big island," called Hawaii itself. Because new ocean floor (crust) is continually being formed and then subducted, the average age of the oldest ocean floor is about 100 million years.

d. Continents

The continents are also part of the crust, much thicker than the ocean-floor crust. Continents that are elevated because of mountain ranges also have deep roots below. The continental masses, in a sense, float on the heavier asthenosphere.

Continents form when relatively light magma bursts from below to the surface, solidifying as rock. Plate movements that rub bits of crust together can cause continents to grow as the lightest material ends up staying on the surface.

Geologists believe that the early Earth had almost no continents or, at most, very small ones. Continents have generally been growing throughout time, because once the light rock reaches the surface it tends to stay there.

A distinctive feature of continents is mountain ranges, which form as plates crash together and then are eroded over tens of millions of years or more. Rocks on continents can be very old. Some of the oldest, more than three billion years old, are found in Canada and Australia.

3. Rocks and Minerals

a. Igneous

Igneous rock, which was once very hot and molten, makes up most of Earth's crust. Molten magma from under Earth's surface, when it cools and solidifies, becomes igneous rock. Volcanoes create igneous rock (extrusive igneous rock). Molten bodies of rock under the surface also create igneous rock (intrusive igneous rock). The base of the ocean's floor is igneous rock, having emerged at mid-ocean ridges. Types of igneous rock include granite, rhyolite, gabbro, and basalt.

Igneous rocks have crystals of minerals, which form when the magma cools and becomes rock. The slower the cooling, the larger the crystals. Therefore, crystals are larger in intrusive igneous rocks.

b. Sedimentary

Sedimentary rock is formed by sediments, which are either tiny particles physically deposited or chemicals precipitated from water. It makes up most of Earth's surface. Fossil evidence for the origin of life comes from sedimentary rocks (3.5–3.9 BYA).

Some types of sedimentary rock are made from physical particles cemented together: conglomerate (from sedimented gravel), sandstone (from sedimented sand), siltstone (from sedimented silt), and shale (from sedimented mud). Note that this sequence progresses from coarse to fine particles.

Some types of sedimentary rock are made primarily from chemical precipitation: limestone (from the mineral calcite) and dolostone (from the mineral dolomite). Calcite and dolomite are calcium carbonate and calcium-magnesium carbonate, respectively. These precipitates are usually biogenic, created by organisms that precipitate shells. The shells later were fused into rock. Examples of limestone are the white cliffs of Dover in England and much of Indiana, Illinois, and Florida. Sometimes limestone can be directly precipitated from water, such as stalactites and stalagmites that form in caves. Other types of sedimentary rock are created from precipitation during the evaporation of seawater: halite (salt) and gypsum (calcium sulfate).

c. Metamorphic

Metamorphic rock is created when either igneous or sedimentary rock is subjected to great heat and pressure. Rock already at Earth's surface can be buried deep, creating heat and pressure, or trapped in a mountain-building event, which squeezes the rock and twists the sediments. The mineral structure is changed though the rock is not melted (that would turn it back into igneous rock). Some types of metamorphic rock include slate (from shale), marble (from limestone), and quartzite (from sandstone).

d. Element Abundances
Minerals

What elements make up the crust of the continents? Here are the main elements and their percentages, rounded off to whole numbers: Oxygen (45%), silicon (27%), aluminum (8%), iron (6%), calcium

(5%), magnesium (3%), sodium (2%), potassium (2%), and titanium (1%). Hydrogen, manganese, phosphorus, and all the others make up the rest.

The large amount of oxygen and silicon in the crust means that many minerals are silicon oxides, or silicates. Other elements join in to create different kinds of silicates, such as magnesium-iron silicates, magnesium-aluminum silicates, and so forth.

Rocks are made of specific minerals, with definite chemical compositions and crystal structures. The minerals can be classed by hardness. Diamond, of course, is the hardest, with number ten on Mohs' Scale of Hardness. Talc is the softest, at number one on the scale. Other examples include calcite (hardness three) and quartz (hardness seven).

Rock Cycle

Elements are shifted from rock to the ocean by two processes. In physical weathering, bits of rock are sloughed off and transported by rivers to the ocean. In chemical weathering, minerals are actually dissolved or react with chemicals in water, and are then transported to the ocean. In this way, one kind of rock contributes to the chemistry of future kinds of rock. Rocks are thereby recycled and reformed.

4. Structure of the Biosphere

The biosphere is the thin, dynamic upper layer of our planet, which includes air, water, soil, and life.

a. Atmosphere

The atmosphere has a mixture of gases: nitrogen (N_2, 78.08%), oxygen (O_2, 20.95%), and argon (Ar, 0.93%). These three gases make up most of dry air; all the other gases are only 0.04% of the total. Of these, the most abundant is carbon dioxide or CO_2 (0.037%). Water vapor is not included in the dry air percentages, because it varies with the humidity, from 0.3% to 4%.

Clouds consist of huge numbers of condensed water droplets, microscopic aerosols. Clouds are important to climate, not only as the sources of precipitation but as reflectors of sunlight. Globally, clouds reflect about 30% of the sunlight back into space.

The atmosphere has four layers:

1. **Troposphere:** the lowest layer, about 15 km high (which varies with latitude and seasons). Weather takes place in the troposphere; almost all clouds are in the troposphere. Temperature decreases with height in the troposphere.
2. **Stratosphere:** next layer, up to about 50 km (between troposphere and stratosphere is a thin transition zone called the **tropopause**). Temperature increases with height in the stratosphere, primarily because in the upper regions the gas ozone (O_3) absorbs much of the ultraviolet energy in the Sun's spectrum.
3. **Mesosphere:** layer up to about 80 km (between stratosphere and mesosphere is a transition zone called the **stratopause**). Temperatures again drop with increasing altitude.
4. **Thermosphere:** in this layer, temperatures rise with altitude. The air in this zone is extremely thin.

Air pressure drops exponentially with altitude. For example, at the top of Mount Everest, it is only about 40% that of the pressure at sea level. If one were to compress the atmosphere all to a uniform pressure equal to that at sea level, the atmosphere would only be about 10 km thick (6 miles).

The winds, which move air from surface regions of high pressure to regions of low pressure, mix the entire atmosphere, even between northern and southern hemispheres, in about a year.

The spin of Earth creates the **Coriolis force**, which makes winds around low pressure systems in the northern hemisphere turn counterclockwise and winds around high pressure systems turn clockwise. The directions are reversed in the southern hemisphere.

b. Hydrosphere

The oceans are also mixed by surface currents, moved by the winds and tides. Large-scale, ocean-wide gyres (a circular ocean current) turn the water, and in places near certain western coasts of the ocean the flow intensifies to true currents: the Gulf Stream off the American Atlantic coast, the Pacific's Kuroshio Current off Japan, and the South Atlantic's Brazil Current off Brazil.

The large, basin-wide ocean gyres circulate clockwise in the northern hemisphere (North Pacific, North Atlantic) and counterclockwise in the southern hemisphere (South Pacific, South Atlantic). Again, Earth's spin and the resulting Coriolis force is the cause of these patterns.

The oceans have a second, different kind of circulation: the **thermohaline** ("temperature" [*thermo*] + "salt" [*haline*])—the factors that determine the density of water). When water gets cold, for example, in winter at high latitudes, it becomes more dense and will tend to sink. When sea ice forms, also in winter at high latitudes, the freezing of fresh water into ice leaves the remaining ocean water more salty. Saltier water is heavier water, and also tends to sink. These two factors create the densest water at certain high latitude regions, particularly in the north Atlantic and around Antarctica, in winter. This dense water plunges downward, flooding the deep basins of the world's oceans with cold water. Thus, surprisingly, if one goes downward from the hot water at the surface of the equator, one finds near the bottom a thick layer of water that is just a couple degrees above freezing. This cold water has come from the polar regions.

Considering the surface gyres and the deep thermohaline circulation, the world's oceans circulate in about 1,000 years. In that time period, all is mixed from surface to deep.

Oceans cover about 71% of Earth's surface.

The dominant ions in seawater are chloride (55% by weight), sodium (30%), sulfate (8%), magnesium (4%), and calcium (1%). When pre-cipitated, the sodium and chloride form salt, though the other elements are present as well.

c. Soil

Soil is derived from two factors: rock that has been physically weathered to small particles and biological material such as dead leaves. The amount of organic matter in the soil (from leaves and parts of organisms, for example) decreases with depth in the soil. Soil is typically about a meter thick, but this varies tremendously from place to place.

The amount of organic matter in the soil depends on the vegetation and, most crucially, on the temperature. Bacteria and fungi in the soil feed upon and thus break down the organic matter. This rate of breakdown changes with temperature. At higher temperatures, the bacteria are more active, at lower temperatures, less so. Very cold climates, then, tend to have thick soils with a high content of organic matter. Famous for this are the peats of northern Canada and Siberia. Tropical soils, despite the rich vegetation, tend to be thin with low amounts of organic matter, because the reuptake of nutrients by the vegetation is so rapid.

Soils hold water, to greater or lesser degrees. This water dissolves elements from the mineral grains in the soil (the material that came from parent rocks). The resulting dissolved ions serve as new sources of nutrients for the plants. The dissolved ions can also move away from the soil and into groundwater. These ions are carried by the flow of groundwater into streams and then rivers, eventually depositing them into the ocean.

The soil is key to the recycling of elements from vegetation to ions and then back to vegetation. As bacteria and fungi feed on the detritus from vegetation (leaves, dead roots, branches), they return elements to ionic forms in the soil water, making these nutrients again available for the plants.

Organisms in the soil must breathe. They can do so because air circulates between atmosphere and soil, via pores in the soil.

d. Life

Life is an active part of the biosphere, and it makes a huge difference to the surface state of the planet—to soil, ocean, and atmosphere.

Without life, there would be essentially no soil, only sand piles here and there between large zones of bedrock. The roots of plants and the organic matter from the detritus of plants create a matrix that holds soil together, a matrix that can retain water. Furthermore, the acids put forth by certain forms of soil life increase the rate of chemical weathering of soil minerals.

In the oceans, algae photosynthesize at the surface where the sunlight is. Other creatures feed on the algae. Their waste and also the dead bodies of algae sink downward. This removes elements from the surface of the ocean and places them into deep water. The elements circulate back up to the surface via the currents and the thermohaline circulation. Life, therefore, affects the chemistry of the ocean.

Life affects the atmosphere. Oxygen would be virtually nonexistent without photosynthesis. Other gases, such as carbon dioxide and methane are also altered by the presence of life. Compared to the CO_2-rich atmospheres of Mars and Venus (with hardly any oxygen), Earth's atmosphere is low in CO_2 and high in O_2.

You Should Review

- basic geological structure of Earth
- theory of plate tectonics
- geological time scale
- types of rocks
- structure and composition of atmosphere, ocean, and soil

Questions

41. The Atlantic Ocean is
   a. growing at several kilometers per year.
   b. shrinking at several kilometers per year.
   c. shrinking at several centimeters per year.
   d. growing at several centimeters per year.

42. The San Andreas fault in California is a
   a. subduction zone.
   b. spreading ridge.
   c. place of magnetic reversal.
   d. site of plate slippage.

43. Key evidence for the modern theory of plate tectonics came from
   a. the apparent fitting together of continents.
   b. mapping of depth contours on the ocean bottom.
   c. magnetic field stripes in the Atlantic Ocean's floor.
   d. chemical analysis of volcanoes.

44. Earth has layers because
   a. all planets have layers when they form.
   b. elements were in layers in the gas nebula that formed the solar system.
   c. it was once molten.
   d. plate tectonics causes geological shifts.

45. Which of Earth's layers is liquid?
   a. inner core
   b. outer core
   c. mantle
   d. crust

46. Which class(es) of rocks contain(s) fossil evidence?
   a. sedimentary
   b. igneous
   c. metamorphic
   d. all of the above

47. Which event would most likely create metamorphic rocks?
   a. seafloor spreading
   b. volcanic eruption
   c. mineral precipitation from water
   d. mountain building

48. When magma cools slowly,
   a. its mineral crystals are small.
   b. it has streaks.
   c. its mineral crystals grow large.
   d. it has bubbles.

49. Which is the second most abundant gas in Earth's atmosphere?
   a. carbon dioxide
   b. oxygen
   c. nitrogen
   d. water vapor

50. The thermohaline circulation is
   a. the way the polar atmosphere mixes.
   b. the way the deep ocean mixes.
   c. the way the lithosphere mixes.
   d. the way the soil mixes.

Answers

41. d. The Atlantic Ocean is growing in width, as magma at the mid-ocean ridge spreads the ocean floor, at a very slow rate.

42. d. At the San Andreas fault, two continental plates are slipping past each other. This happens in occasional jolts, causing the earthquakes in that region.

43. c. Magnetic field stripes in the Atlantic Ocean's floor showed that the floor was growing in size, spreading away from the Mid-Atlantic Ridge.

44. c. Earth, in its early "years," was molten, which caused heavier materials to sink toward the center, segregating Earth into layers.

45. b. Earth's outer core is molten iron and nickel. The flow of this liquid metal creates Earth's magnetic field. Although comprised of the same material, Earth's inner core is solid because of the greater pressure at the very center of the Earth.

46. a. Sedimentary rocks form on Earth's surface, where life is found. Plant and animal remains become fossilized in the sedimentary rocks as the rocks form. Fossils are not found in igneous or metamorphic rocks since they form under conditions of intense heat and pressure.

47. d. Metamorphic rocks form under conditions of heat and pressure that changes rock minerals without melting them. Mountain-building events commonly form large-scale regions of metamorphic rocks. Seafloor spreading and volcanic eruption form igneous rocks, and sedimentary rocks can form from mineral precipitation from water.

48. c. The crystals grow relatively large when the magma cools slowly. Whether it has streaks or bubbles cannot be determined from the information given.

49. b. At about 21%, oxygen is number two in abundance, after nitrogen. Even under moist conditions, water vapor concentration does not become as high as oxygen.

50. b. The thermohaline (referring to temperature and salt) creates dense water that sinks in the polar regions of the ocean, thereby mixing the deep ocean.

F. Biodiversity and Ecology

1. Species and Biodiversity

One can note biodiversity on a number of scales, from genes to ecosystems. But the focus at some point always comes down to that of species.

a. What Is a Species?

In its classic sense, a **species** is a group of genetically related organisms with the potential for mating and producing offspring who are themselves capable of successfully mating. For example, robins can reproduce only with other robins. A species is thus reproductively isolated.

Reproductive isolation is brought about by any number of evolved mechanisms: physical mating apparatus, mating rituals, genetic compatibility. Geographical separation often plays a role in allowing different populations of a species to genetically diverge and separate into two different species over time.

A **subspecies** is a taxonomic level within a species that is genetically distinct but not reproductively isolated. In other words, members of different subspecies can reproduce. For example, the Florida panther is a subspecies of the mountain lion, which lives in the western United States (but formerly lived all across the United States).

In 1973, the Endangered Species Act was passed to protect any species whose population is declining to such a level that the existence of the species is threatened.

b. How Many Species?

Today, we have catalogued and defined about 1.8 million species. Total species estimates range from 3–30 million. Most ecologists think the number is somewhere in between, perhaps 10 or more million. Occasionally, a new primate is discovered (for example, a new monkey was discovered recently in South America), but most undiscovered animal species are insects.

Estimates are made by surveying regions where new species are found. One technique kills all the insects on a specific tree. The insects are surveyed for new species that seem to be specific for that tree. Then, knowing how many trees are in the area, one can estimate the number of unknown insects in that area.

Here are some different groups of organisms and the number of species currently known: plants (300,000), insects (1,000,000), fungi (100,000), mammals (5,400), and birds (9,900).

c. Classification

Organisms are classified according to a nested hierarchy of named groups. Each species has a double name of genus and species. Humans are *Homo sapiens*. The word **species** gets applied in two different ways: The species is *Homo sapiens*, which consists of a genus (*Homo*) and the species name (*sapiens*). Within any genus, there can be many species. The ancient Neanderthals, *Homo neanderthalensis*, are the same genus as modern humans, but a different species.

Levels of classification (in increasing levels of inclusivity):

> family (more inclusive than genus)
> order
> class
> phylum
> kingdom

d. Tropical Biodiversity

The tropics, in particular the rain forests, are famed for their biodiversity. Maps of the numbers of species, from poles to tropics, for amphibians, trees, and others show species diversity increasing in almost all cases toward the tropics. A single forest plot in South America could have as many species of butterfly or tree as all of England. There are many possible reasons for the high diversity in the tropics.

The high amount of incoming sunlight in the tropics supplies energy to the plants, which, in turn, supports more animals. The larger the amount of biomass that can be supported, the larger the potential number of species.

Stability of climate allows species to enter into highly specific arrangements with each other. Species of fig tree, for instance, are pollinated with a single species of fig wasp. Both depend on each other. Also, during the recent ice ages, the tropical rain forests might have dried up into zones called **refugia**, where pressures to evolve made many new species.

The high latitudes experience large seasonal changes, which makes those species more adapted to wide geographical ranges, creating less diversity.

e. Biomes

Biomes are large geographical regions within which are located relatively similar basic types of plant and animals. A biome is larger than an ecosystem. The main determining factors that give shape to biomes are temperature and rainfall.

Tundra is characterized by polar regions with tiny plants produced during short summer growing seasons. It has thick soils of peat because of slow decomposition.

Boreal forest is characterized by evergreen trees such as spruce and fir across Canada and Russia. It has cold winters but warm summers.

Temperate deciduous forest is characterized by trees such as maple, birch, and oak, which lose their leaves each winter. It has cold winters and hot summers with adequate rainfall for trees. Despite the loss of the leaves, deciduous trees in these regions fare better than evergreen trees because flat leaves are more efficient solar collectors than needles.

Prairies and grasslands are characterized by warmer summers than areas of deciduous forests, but less rainfall. Hot dry summers create conditions for fires, which is often an important part of the structure of these biomes. Clearing native grasslands has created some of the great "breadbasket" farmlands of the world.

Deserts are very dry biomes with little rain. Plants and animals have special adaptations. Many plants are bulbous (cacti) to store water in their bodies for times of extended drought.

Tropical seasonal forests and rain forests: Some areas of the tropics have wet and dry seasons. In these areas, many trees can also be deciduous because they lose their leaves during the dry seasons. In the rain forests, enough year-round moisture supports green vegetation all year. Species diversity is at a maximum.

2. Principles of Biodiversity
a. Island Biogeography
In the 1960s, MacArthur and Wilson developed the theory of island biogeography by studying the relationship between numbers of species and areas of islands. They found that larger islands held a greater number of species, when specific groups were examined, such as birds or amphibians.

The theorists went farther. What determines the number of species on islands? Species die (go locally extinct) and species originate (they migrate from the mainland, fly over in the case of insects and birds, are blown over by the winds in the case of small insects, and come aboard from floating logs and other debris, in the case of lizards).

For islands of the same size, islands closer to the mainland have a greater number of species because the immigration rate is higher. Islands with diverse habitats (such as mountains and swamps) have a great number of species. For all else equal, smaller islands have a greater rate of extinctions, because the smaller populations are more susceptible to environmental stressors or disease, which leads to a smaller number of species.

For example, in the Caribbean, Cuba, the largest island, has the greatest number of species of reptiles and amphibians. Furthermore, plotting the sizes of islands versus their number of species shows a mathematical law, allowing scientists to count on some theory behind the distributions.

Data roughly along lines compatible with the theory of island biogeography from other regions on continents show that the theory has some applicability to what will happen to species as humans fragment the landscape more and more. The theory will help in the design of nature preserves. For example, butterflies increase in English woodlands as the sizes of the woodlands increase.

b. Predators and Prey
A key kind of interaction in nature is the **food chain**, the chain of eating: mouse eats seed, snake eats mouse, hawk eats snake. In real nature, we find not simple chains but webs, more complex networks because predators often (not always) feed upon many different kinds of prey, and prey often can be fed upon by many different kinds of predators.

Trophic levels describe the position on the food chain that an organism occupies. There are four levels.

> Level 1 (Primary producers)—autotrophs, producers such as plants and algae that turn sunlight, carbon dioxide, and nutrients into their bodies upon which all other terrestrial life depends.
>
> Level 2 (Primary consumers)—herbivores, creatures such as deer and many insects that feed on plants
>
> Level 3 (Secondary consumers)—carnivores that prey on the herbivores
>
> Level 4 (Tertiary consumers)—also carnivores, which in the idealized situation feed on other carnivores of level 3

As food passes from trophic level to trophic level (from gut to gut), it is converted into new organism bodies with an efficiency that is typically about 10%. In other words, it might take 10 kg of plant matter to make 1 kilogram of herbivore, and then 10 kg of herbivore to make 1 kg of carnivore. This is why the spectacular predators of ecosystems are rare and why there will always be far fewer eagles, for example, than mice.

c. Sex

Many creatures reproduce without sex between males and females. Bacteria, for instance, can reproduce by cell splitting, creating two clones in a process called **mitosis**. Each daughter cell has the same DNA as the mother cell.

Many plants can reproduce by **vegetation propagation** (for example, taking a cutting from a houseplant, rooting it in water, and then planting it in soil), making a clone of the original plant. Some trees, such as aspens, reproduce with underground runners. So what looks like a patch of individual trees is actually a family of clones. Certain invertebrates, such as hydra, can also reproduce asexually, by budding off small replicas, which fall off or swim away to form new individuals. Some insects and even some vertebrates (several species of lizards, for example) are capable of asexual reproduction in which the females lay eggs that are capable of growing into new adults.

For the individual of an asexual species, reproduction is less efficient than in the sexual mode, because, in sex, each parent is only putting half its genes into the offspring. In the asexual mode, the sole parent is putting one hundred percent of its genes into each offspring.

However, sexual reproduction has the benefit of mixing genes, which creates variation, one of the stages in the recipe for evolution. Mitosis relies on mutations for variation (except in some cases in which bacteria exchange genes)—but sex creates variation by its very nature. Parasites and diseases can evolve quickly, putting populations of clones at risk. But when sex mixes genes, offspring are all different. There is good evidence that sexual species can have lower susceptibility to parasites and other diseases. What is gained in producing lots of genetic variation seems to make up for what is lost in efficiency of gene transfer for each individual during sex.

In higher organisms, such as plants and animals, sex cells (pollen and egg in plants, sperm and egg in animals), receive half the chromosomes and therefore half the genes of the cells of the adults they derive from, in a special process of cell division called **meiosis**.

d. Invasive, Umbrella, and Keystone Species

Keystone species are species that play a key role (like the keystone in an arch) by holding the structure of the ecosystem together. Many top predators are keystone species because they affect the populations of their prey, which affects the populations lower in the trophic levels. For example, the starfish along rocky coastlines can be a keystone species because starfish affect the populations of many species of mollusks and barnacles.

Umbrella species are species that have a role in conservation. Preserving an umbrella species that needs a particular habitat will automatically act like an umbrella to save many other species that also use that habitat. A classic example is the northern spotted owl of the old-growth forests of the Pacific Northwest. (An old-growth forest is forest that has never been cut.) The owl requires holes in old growth trees for its nests and will not nest elsewhere.

A **poster** or **flagship species** is a particularly charismatic species that people tend to naturally rally around for its preservation. The giant panda of China is an example.

Invasive species are also called **alien** or **introduced species**, because they come from other regions of the world, transported by humans. The introduction is sometimes intentional, but is often unintentional, as species hitch rides on ships or even in airplane wheel cases. A classic example is the zebra mussel, originally from waters in Russia, now found all over the Great Lakes of the United States and even up stretches of the Missouri River. Its huge, dense populations clog pipes of factories and power plants, and cause billions of dollars of damage each year.

Introduced species can be successful invaders when they come into an area with no natural predators and where the prey lacks evolved defenses against the new species. Invasive species are a serious problem for the world's healthy maintenance of biodiversity and economies.

Extinct species are a natural part of Earth's past. But humans are causing extinctions at a far greater rate than the "background" rate of nature (not counting mass extinctions from impacts, for instance, like the one that took out the dinosaurs). The passenger pigeon and the dodo bird are two bird species that humans (or the animals humans introduced) caused to go extinct.

Endemic species are species that occur in a rather small region and nowhere else. Islands often have large numbers of endemic species. Lemurs, for example, are endemic to the island of Mada-gascar. Special regions where there are a large number of endemic species that are under threat (and which are unusually rich in overall biodiversity) are called hotspots.

3. Basics of Ecology

Ecology is the study of the interactions of organisms with each other and with their physical and chemical environments.

a. Definitions

A **population** is the system of locally interacting members of the same species. When individuals in a local population have substantial interaction among them (say, as potential mates) but only occasional links to other populations (say, in another valley), the populations are then said to be **metapopulations** in the context of the larger, more loosely linked species system.

A **community** is the locally interacting system of organisms of different species, usually considered as the plants, animals, and fungi. But there can also be soil communities that include species of bacteria.

An **ecosystem** can be a pond, swamp, local area of prairie, local woods, and so forth. It usually does not have defined boundaries (except in cases like ponds), but consists of the community or communities of creatures and the nonliving parts of the environment they are in contact with, such as water and soil.

Ecosystems can become disturbed, either by natural events such as volcanoes or by humans. If left to restore themselves, they undergo a process of succession. Early, colonizing species come in first, followed by later species that often require the conditions created by the earlier species. Eventually, a stable endpoint community of organisms is reached, called a **climax community**.

Carrying capacity is the maximum number of organisms of a particular species that an ecosystem can support.

Reserves are parts of nature set aside by humans for the preservation of species or wilderness in general. Reserves include National Parks and National Wildlife Refuges in the United States and various regions with different names in other countries.

Fragmentation occurs when a force (primarily human) fragments the natural landscape into patches (examples: construction of interstate highways and other roads, housing and urban developments, draining parts of wetlands, or cutting down parts of forests for farmlands).

A **watershed** is a region that includes all the drainage of tributaries that feed a larger stream or river. For example, the very large Mississippi watershed would include the watershed of the Missouri River, because the Missouri River empties into the Mississippi.

b. Soil Ecology

When leaves die from trees in autumn or grasses die for winter, they fall to the ground. This material contains carbon and other elements that start to decompose and become part of the soil.

The new material is called **detritus**. Organisms in the soil that perform decomposition are called **detritus feeders,** and include various insects, worms, fungi, and bacteria. Though we normally know fungi as their visible forms of mushrooms (the reproductive bodies), they normally occur as invisible threads (called **hyphae**) throughout the soil.

Organisms in the soil breathe because air enters and leaves the soil through openings between its grains. The deeper one goes in the soil, the air has less oxygen, because the oxygen has been used by the soil organisms.

Soil has layers. The uppermost, rich layer is topsoil, which is important to preserve in farmlands. Farmers must beware of losing topsoil to erosion by wind and water.

c. Marine Ecology

The continental shelf regions of oceans tend to be richer in life because they obtain increased nutrients from rivers and from the winds and tides that stir the shallow water, thereby mixing up nutrients from below to the surface. The open ocean is sometimes considered a marine desert; life is more sparse there.

At the top of the ocean is a zone called the **mixed layer**, varying in depth but usually about 100 meters thick. It is well mixed, having been stirred by the winds. The upper part that receives light is called the **pelagic zone**, which varies depending on how far light penetrates down. The deep parts are called the **benthos**. Thus, marine biologists distinguish organisms as pelagic species and benthic species.

Special areas called **upwelling zones** occur off certain coasts, such as Chile and the coast of northwest Africa. Here, deep, nutrient-rich waters are brought up and fish are hugely abundant.

Tiny organisms in the ocean constitute the **plankton**, which generally drift with the currents. There are **phytoplankton**, which are green because they have chlorophyll and perform photosynthesis (eukaryotic algae and prokaryotic cyanobacteria), and **zooplankton** ("animal-plankton"). Zooplankton include tiny multicellular swimming crustaceans as well as the swimming larvae of creatures that will grow to adult sizes out of the plankton range, such as jellyfish and mollusks. Zooplankton feed on phytoplankton, and all are fed upon by a variety of fish and other organisms, making a marine food web.

A **fishery** is a commercial entity engaged in harvesting fish in a particular region (examples: northwest salmon fishery, the New England cod fishery). Many fisheries are in decline as the stocks of fish have been depleted.

Aquaculture is the commercial raising of fish, shrimp, or oysters in tanks or fenced off areas of the ocean.

d. Ecology and Energy

Sunlight is captured by plants using the pigment molecule chlorophyll. Plants are green because chlorophyll absorbs the red and blue wavelengths of light, reflecting some of the green. The energy thus captured is used to drive the process of photosynthesis, which creates simple sugar molecules from carbon dioxide and water. Plants get water from the soil (through their **xylem**) and carbon dioxide from the air, through pores in their leaves called **stomata** (or stomates). Marine algae are also green because of chlorophyll, but they get the carbon dioxide from the water.

Terrestrial plants and marine algae are called **autotrophs**, for "self-feeders," because they create their own food, in a sense, from inorganic molecules. Insects and humans are **heterotrophs**, requiring autotrophs for food.

The molecules of organisms are high energy molecules, because they can be "burned" by the metabolisms of organisms to maintain their bodies and exert force upon the environment for movement and food capture. The energy comes from the Sun. Thus, when we walk, we are using transformed and stored solar energy. Life runs on solar energy.

The mass of a living thing or a collection of living things is called **biomass**, or biological mass. One can ask about the biomass of trees in a forest, or the insect biomass of an ecosystem.

When plants convert their simple sugars made by photosynthesis into more complex organic molecules that they need, such as proteins and starches, they use some of the sugar as a source of carbon for this next generation of organic molecules. They also "burn" some of the sugar for energy, to drive the chemical reactions inside their cells that create the next generations of molecules. This burning uses up some of the sugars and requires oxygen, and results in the chemical products of carbon dioxide and water, thus reversing the process of photosynthesis. This is called **respiration**. Heterotrophs perform respiration, too (but not photosynthesis).

The amount of biomass created by the photosynthesis in a plant is called **gross primary production (GPP)**. It is usually expressed in terms of carbon. The carbon that actually goes into the full metabolism of molecules inside a plant is less—that is called **net primary production (NPP)**.

$$GPP = NPP - \text{respiration}$$

NPP can be calculated at the level of ecosystem and biome, as well. It varies across ecosystems and biomes, being highest in tropical rain forests and lowest in deserts.

Limiting factors limit the amount of net primary production. Depending on the ecosystem or biome, limiting factors could include water, nitrate, phosphate, and other nutrients. Farmers overcome limiting factors in soils by adding fertilizers.

4. Biogeochemical Cycles

Biogeochemical cycles are the cycles of elements essential to life. These cycles are thus biological (*bio*) and include geological processes (*geo*) and chemical reactions (*chemical*).

a. Carbon on Land

The most important biogeochemical cycle is that of carbon, the essential element in the organic molecules of life. Carbon moves in and out of various forms. Photosynthesis and respiration form a coupled pair of processes that convert carbon dioxide into organic molecules (carbohydrates) and back again. Most respiration takes place in the soil, as respiration from bacteria and fungi releases carbon dioxide. The cycle is more complex with other forms of carbon as well. Some bacteria release waste carbon in the form of methane (CH_4). Other types of bacteria consume methane.

b. Carbon in the Biosphere

The atmosphere contains about 700 billion tons of carbon, primarily in the form of carbon dioxide. The carbon in all biomass is about the same amount. The carbon in the world's soils is about three times that amount. The oceans contain the largest pool or reservoir of carbon, because seawater has carbon in yet other forms: bicarbonate and carbonate ions. Atmosphere, plants, algae, soil, and ocean—these are all considered **pools**, between which carbon is shuffled in and out of various forms, in amounts known as **fluxes**. Global net primary productivity is the flux of carbon from the atmosphere into all photosynthesizers, for example.

c. Nitrogen in the Biosphere

Nitrogen, which is important in protein synthesis, is another element that has a biogeochemical cycle. Like carbon, there are pools (or reservoirs) of nitrogen, in the atmosphere (as N_2 gas), in organisms (primarily in proteins), in the soil (in the detritus), and in water (as nitrate and ammonium ions). Fluxes describe the conversion of nitrogen from one form to another.

Nitrogen fixation occurs when soil or marine bacteria take nitrogen gas and convert it into the useful ammonium ion for their bodies. Some ecologically and agriculturally important soil bacteria live within the roots of plants, in a symbiotic relationship. When we say that bean plants or clover can fix nitrogen, it is really the bacteria in the nodules on their roots that perform that function, not the plants themselves.

Ammoniafication is also done by bacteria, in the soil, as the bacteria process proteins in detritus and converts the organic nitrogen into ammonium ions.

Nitrogen assimilation occurs when organisms take up nitrogen as ammonium ions or nitrate ions from the environment of soil or water.

In **denitrification**, other kinds of bacteria convert nitrate ions in soil or water into nitrogen gas. Denitrifiers live in places of no or little oxygen. Finally, nitrifying bacteria take ammonium ions and make nitrate ions.

d. Phosphorus in the Biosphere

Phosphorus is another crucial element for all living things. It has a cycle, too, which is relatively simpler than the cycles of carbon and nitrogen, because phosphorus does not have a gaseous form. It primarily cycles between its ion (phosphate ions in soil and water) and its form in life (various molecules inside cells). Phosphorus is used as part of the ladder of DNA and is essential for energy molecules inside cells, such as ATP.

e. Bioessential Elements

All the dozen or so elements that are essential to living things have their biogeochemical cycles. The major elements and their approximate mass percentages in a typical plant are carbon (C, 45%), oxygen (O, 45%), hydrogen (H, 6%), nitrogen (N, 1.6%), sulfur (S, 0.1%), phosphorus (P, 0.2%), potassium (K, 1%), calcium (Ca, 0.5%), magnesium (Mg, 0.2%), and iron (Fe, 0.01%). The elements N, S, P, K, Ca, and Mg are the macronutrients, because they occur in relatively large amounts. Iron and other elements not listed, such as manganese, molybdenum, and copper, are micronutrients. Hydrogen and oxygen, though essential elements, are not considered nutrients because they occur abundantly in water. In humans, the percentages change somewhat but not drastically (not so much that iron is larger than phosphorus, for example). More proteins in humans means more nitrogen, to cite one element's differences between humans and plants.

You Should Review

- principles of biodiversity and ecology
- numbers of species
- classification system
- biome types
- food webs in ocean and on land
- interaction of predators and prey
- asexual versus sexual reproduction
- biogeochemical cycles of carbon and nitrogen

Questions

51. According to biological classification, which group has the potential for mating and producing offspring?
  a. family
  b. species
  c. kingdom
  d. class

52. The high diversity in the tropics occurs because these regions
  a. receive high levels of solar energy.
  b. are closest to the oceans.
  c. have high seasonal variability.
  d. contain more land area.

53. Fire can be an important part in the structure of an ecosystem. This is particularly true in which of the following biomes?
  a. tundra
  b. chaparral
  c. boreal forest
  d. prairie

54. Food chains are parts of food webs, in which we go from plants at the first trophic level (primary producers) to a second trophic level, and so on. Why do food chains in nature rarely exceed four or five levels?
  a. because evolution has not yet created that degree of complexity
  b. because organisms die more easily at the higher levels
  c. because of inefficiencies; the available energy becomes less and less at higher levels
  d. because food chains limit the levels of food webs

55. The California sea otter, native to the coast, controls the populations of starfish, which control the populations of many other marine creatures among the kelp beds. The otter is an example of a(n)
  a. umbrellate species.
  b. invasive species.
  c. keystone species.
  d. mammal species.

56. Consider the following food web: oak seedlings eaten by rabbits; rabbits eaten by wolves. What happens to the oak seedlings if the wolf population suddenly declines from a disease?
  a. Seedlings decrease.
  b. Seedlings are eaten by something else.
  c. Seedlings increase.
  d. Seedlings are also hit by a disease.

57. Which organisms are at the base of the marine food web?
  a. crustaceans
  b. jellyfish
  c. phytoplankton
  d. zooplankton

58. The term *fragmentation* refers to which of the following?
  a. invasive species that divide the structure of ecosystems
  b. the dispersed nature of marine food webs
  c. successive waves of species as an ecosystem develops
  d. humans segregating up nature into chunks

59. In considering the pools of the biogeochemical carbon cycle, which has the most carbon in it?
  a. ocean
  b. soil
  c. plants
  d. atmosphere

60. The process by which bacteria convert nitrogen gas into useful compounds like ammonia is
   a. denitrification.
   b. nitrogen assimilation.
   c. nitrogen fixation.
   d. ammoniafication.

Answers

51. b. In a basic sense, species are genetically related organisms able to produce offspring. Biological classification, in decreasing order of inclusivity, is: kingdom, phylum, class, order, family, genus, and species.

52. a. Tropical regions receive a high amount of sunlight year-round, which supports the year-round growth of a greater number of plants. This in turn supports a larger population of animals, increasing biodiversity further.

53. d. Prairies have dense vegetation and often long intervals of summer drought. Fires started by lightning are a natural part of these grasslands, and many plants have even become evolutionarily adapted by having seeds that germinate after a fire.

54. c. Typically, each level only converts 10% of the energy of the previous level. As the levels progress, the energy available is very small, thus limiting the levels reached.

55. c. The otter is a keystone species, because like the top stone in an arch, it holds much of the rest of the ecosystem in its structure.

56. a. If the wolves decline, the rabbits increase in population. If the rabbits increase, they eat more seedlings, so the seedlings decline.

57. c. Phytoplankton are photosynthetic organisms like algae and cyanobacteria that produce their own food using energy from sunlight. Thus, they are primary producers at the lowest level of the marine food web.

58. d. Human activities fragment nature.

59. a. The ocean has about 10–50 times more carbon than any of the other pools. In the ocean, carbon is found mostly in the form of the bicarbonate ion (with the carbonate ion second).

60. c. Nitrogen fixation occurs when bacteria convert atmospheric nitrogen into ammonium ions and turn them into useful compounds like ammonia for their bodies. Ammoniafication involves the conversion of organic nitrogen in detritus material into ammonium ions. Organisms that cannot independently perform nitrogen fixation may use the process of nitrogen assimilation.

G. Global Environmental Challenges
1. Population and Land Use
a. Population

Prior to the invention of agriculture, some 10,000 years ago, humans in their hunting and gathering phase were limited to about ten million people worldwide. But by the pyramid days of ancient Egypt, 5,000 years ago, global population had grown tenfold, to about 100 million, an increase due to agriculture.

By 1830, the population had reached the first billion.

By the late 1950s, the world held two billion people.

The third, fourth, and fifth billion marks were reached by the late 1950s, the early 1970s, and the mid-1980s, respectively.

The six-billion mark was reached in the late 1990s, and seven billion in 2011, due to a growth rate of about 85 million people a year (10 times the population of New York or Los Angeles). However, while the population continues to grow, the growth rate is starting to decline. Factors that cause the growth rate to decline include a higher standard of living and better education (for women, in particular). Scientists expect the world population to reach at least eight billion, but variables may influence how high the population climbs.

b. Land Use

Global land = 140 million square kilometers = 14 billion hectares (about five acres per person).

Usable land: 31% of the world's land (4.4 billion hectares) is unusable, because it is rock, ice, tundra, or desert, leaving 9.6 billion hectares for potential human use.

Agricultural use: The major human land use is for agricultural production, which is currently 4.7 billion hectares. Of that, 70% is permanent pasture and 30% is crop land. So agriculture (pasture + crops) takes 34% of the world's land.

Urbanized land: Globally, only about 1% of land (about 140 million hectares) is considered urbanized, including highways. In some local areas, the urbanized land approaches 100% of coverage.

Therefore, 14 billion hectares – 4.4 billion (unusable) – 4.7 billion (agriculture) – 0.14 billion (urbanized) = 4.8 billion hectares of potential usable land remains.

This is about 34% of the total land, or about as much as humans currently use for all agriculture. However, much of the prime land for agriculture is already in use, so what remains is not as high in quality.

2. Humans Alter the Biosphere

Unlike other species, humans deploy vast arrays of chemical processes (factories, residences, and forms of transportation). In our use of energy and in the ways we process matter, we create substances that alter the chemistry of the biosphere.

a. Carbon Dioxide and the Greenhouse Effect

Carbon dioxide (CO_2) is typically measured in units of ppm (parts per million), because there are only small amounts of it in the atmosphere. *Million* refers to a million randomly selected molecules of air (such as N_2, O_2, and so forth). Today, CO_2 is somewhat more than 400 ppm (which is equal to 0.040%).

CO_2, though such a small amount of the atmosphere, is of critical importance because it is a greenhouse gas. Oxygen and nitrogen gases are not. A greenhouse gas lets in visible radiation (light, short-wave radiation) from the Sun, which enters the atmosphere, and passes directly through to the ground (therefore we can't see the CO_2). But a greenhouse gas absorbs infrared radiation. Infrared radiation (long-wave radiation) is what the Earth emits to outer space to cool its surface and to balance the energy received from the Sun. Greenhouse gases are like one-way insulation, letting light in but blocking the escape of infrared radiation. Earth's surface will warm up as a result of any extra insulation in the atmosphere.

Without CO_2, Earth would be very cold, below the freezing point of water. So present conditions require CO_2.

But there can also be too much: CO_2, emitted as a waste gas from the combustion of fossil fuels (coal, oil, natural gas), is rising. Data from bubbles trapped in ice at Antarctica show that for 10,000 years prior to the industrial revolution, CO_2 was fairly constant at about 280 ppm. Now it is above 400 ppm and rising from human activities at the rate of 1.5–2 ppm per year.

b. Ozone and Ultraviolet Radiation

Ozone (O_3) is a molecule with three oxygen atoms, unlike regular oxygen (O_2) that makes up 21% of Earth's atmosphere. Ozone is made naturally, by cosmic rays that cause chemical reactions in Earth's stratosphere. Ozone readily absorbs the ultraviolet portions of the Sun's spectrum that enters Earth's atmosphere. This absorption also destroys some of the ozone, so a balance is reached between creation and destruction, resulting in a natural amount of ozone that is constantly present.

Without this protective ozone layer, biologically damaging ultraviolet (UV) rays would reach the surface of the planet. UV exposure is a main cause of skin cancer.

Until recently, ozone was on a worrisome decline. Human-made gases called **chlorofluorocarbons** (CFCs, containing chlorine, fluorine, and carbon) used in refrigerators, air-conditioners, and some aerosol cans, when released, travel up into the stratosphere. There, the CFCs act as a catalyst to destroy the ozone at a rate much faster than its natural rate of destruction. Humans had altered the balance, and global ozone levels started dropping, particularly in the ozone "hole" area above Antarctica, endangering people in Australia and New Zealand.

In 1987, many nations signed the Montreal Protocol, a global agreement to phase out the production and use of CFCs. Substitute gases were invented to replace CFCs. As a result, the ozone decline has been halted. Over the coming decades, the ozone layer should be able to repair itself and return to its natural level.

c. Acid Rain

Acid rain is yet another human perturbation to the atmosphere, related to the combustion of fossil fuels, coal in particular. Coal, the remains of ancient plants from hundreds of millions of years ago, contains sulfur (one of the bio-essential elements). When the coal is burned in power plants to obtain energy (most of which comes from converting carbon to CO_2), the sulfur also combines with oxygen to create sulfur dioxide (SO_2), a gas that enters the atmosphere. The SO_2 further combines with water vapor and ultimately becomes sulfuric acid (H_2SO_4) in cloud droplets. The rain that falls from these clouds is acidic—acid rain.

Nitrogen also contributes to acid rain, as nitric acid, derived from nitrogen oxides created from the high temperature reactions with air in power plants and automobiles.

Acid rain falls mostly in the regions downwind of power plants. It has been responsible for ecological damage to many streams and lakes.

Laws governing the release of acids from power plants are in place, but could be strengthened further. Acid rain is a problem that potentially could be controlled, with adequate environmental regulation. Emissions of pollutants from automobiles have been improved, for example, with better technology.

d. Toxins

Primary pollutants are chemicals released directly into the atmosphere.

Besides some of the gases already discussed, primary pollutants include the following:

- *Suspended particulate matter* (PM) consists of all kinds of tiny particles from smog stacks and even from metals.
- *Volatile organic compounds* (VOC, hydrocarbons) are organic gases from a variety of sources, such as leaks into the air that you smell when you fill your car with gasoline and even gases from lighter fluids used to start barbecues.
- *Carbon monoxide* (CO) derives from incomplete combustion of fossil fuels (organic carbon is oxidized to CO, rather than CO_2 during complete combustion); an odorless gas, CO is the leading annual cause of death by poisoning in the United States.

Primary pollutants can be altered chemically by interactions with sunlight, and become **secondary** or **photochemical pollutants**.

- **Tropospheric ozone** is one such pollutant. Different from the natural, much-higher-up stratospheric ozone, tropospheric ozone is ozone or pollution in an urban area.
- **Photochemical smog**, another secondary pollutant, is created when car exhaust is acted

upon by sunlight to form a brown haze that is highly irritating to the lungs. Smog is particularly troublesome in cities that lie in valleys and are subject to air inversions, in which a lid of air sits over the city and does not move for a long period of time.

After cigarette smoke, **radon gas** is the second leading cause of lung cancer. Radon, a daughter product of uranium in Earth's rocks, is a radioactive gas that leaks from particular kinds of soils. It can accumulate indoors, for example, in basements. When breathed in, radon follows a nuclear decay pathway within the lungs, releasing radiation and ultimately leaving lead trapped within the lungs.

Scrap rocks from uranium mining are a form of radioactive waste. Of even more concern are the waste byproducts from nuclear power plants. These are daughter products of the process of controlled nuclear fission, which uses uranium but then creates radioactive iodine, cesium, plutonium, and other elements as waste. This material is secured and stored on the site of the nuclear power plants, but plans are being created for long-term, permanent storage. Many communities oppose nuclear waste storage in their areas due to fears of radioactive contamination. The most planning has been done for a site in Nevada, at which the material would have to be kept safe from earthquakes and groundwater for many thousands of years. However, most Nevadans oppose the construction of such a site, and political and technological difficulties have delayed the opening of this facility.

3. Energy Systems

Our lives are dependent on external sources of energy, as we burn fossil fuels at a total rate that is many times greater than the metabolisms of all humans.

a. Energy versus Power

Power is the rate of energy flow; unit is kilowatts ($1 \text{ kW} = 1 \frac{\text{kilojoule}}{\text{second}}$).

Energy is the summation of power over time; measured in kilowatt-hours or BTU (for British thermal unit, the energy it takes to raise 1 pound of water by 1 degree Fahrenheit).

b. Fossil Fuel Combustion

All fossil fuels contain carbon and hydrogen. When a fossil fuel is reacted (burned) with oxygen (from the air), the chemical products are carbon dioxide and water (as a vapor). Because the produced CO_2 and H_2O together have a lower molecular energy than the reactants of fossil fuel and oxygen, energy is released in the reaction. Fossil fuel energy is the main source of energy for all the processes of civilization.

Types of fossil fuels differ in their relative amounts of carbon and hydrogen. The more carbon a fossil fuel has, the more carbon dioxide it releases for a given amount of energy. In this regard, coal is the worst fuel and natural gas (which is primarily methane, CH_4) is the best fuel, with oil rating somewhere in the middle.

Fossil fuels come from biological sources of many millions of years ago. Oil is from marine algae, buried and transformed. Coal is from terrestrial plants that lived in vast swampy environments, buried and transformed. Natural gas (methane) is mostly derived as a breakdown product of either coal or oil. All occur underground and must be dug up or piped to the surface, transported, and processed for human use.

A significant factor in world politics is the uneven distribution of fossil fuels, especially oil. This shows how geological processes from hundreds of millions of years ago affect human life today.

c. Energy Today

The global primary energy supply consists of the following (total is 99% because numbers are rounded off):

- oil (31%)
- coal (29%)

- natural gas (21%)
- wood and combustible wastes (10%)
- nuclear (5%)
- hydroelectric (2%)
- other (renewable sources): 1%

How is energy used? Roughly one-third of it is used for industry, one-third for transportation, and one-third for residential (varies by country).

Hydroelectric energy uses vertical drops in rivers. Water is diverted, usually from behind dams, into turbines, which turn generators to produce electricity. (All mechanical electricity-generating power plants turn turbines to make electricity.)

Nuclear power plants generate intense heat from the controlled splitting (fission) of uranium atoms. The heat creates steam, which turns turbines to make electricity.

Fossil fuel power plants work the same way, except that the source of heat is the combustion of the fuel.

d. Efficiency from Supply to Use

Efficiency is output of useful work divided by the input energy, measured in percent. For example, how much of the energy in oil goes into making the automobile travel, and how much is wasted as heat in the exhaust system and from cooling the engine?

For fossil fuel power plants, a typical efficiency is about 33%. Although better engineering can improve this number, it cannot and will not ever be 100%, because the Second Law of Thermodynamics limits how much of one kind of energy can be converted into a different kind of energy.

All devices, from refrigerators to light bulbs to cars, can be quantified in terms of efficiency. Improvements in energy efficiency can cut down on pollutants and the use of fossil fuels, which not only are nonrenewable but produce the greenhouse gas carbon dioxide.

e. Future Energy Technologies

Research continues on future energy technologies, on sources of energy that do not emit carbon dioxide and are renewable.

Hydrogen can be burned with oxygen to produce harmless water (vapor). However, hydrogen does not occur naturally. To have a hydrogen economy in the future, therefore, we need to make hydrogen from the splitting of water, which requires an energy source, like fossil fuel or solar energy. (Hydrogen can also be made from natural gas [methane], but this creates CO_2, so to avoid the emission of CO_2, it would have to be sequestered.)

Carbon sequestration is a technology that stops the emission of CO_2 (by trapping and disposing of carbon dioxide waste) and would allow humans to continue burning fossil fuels, depending on supply. One possibility is to pipe carbon dioxide deep into the ocean (but this might make conditions intolerably acidic for some benthic marine life). Another possibility is to pipe it into deep aquifers of salty, unusable water far beneath the land surface. But would the CO_2 leak back up into the atmosphere? A small industrial project off the shores of Scandinavia is currently injecting CO_2 into the ocean. Much remains to be tested with these technologies.

Wind energy uses the pressure of moving air to turn turbines to make electricity. Many large wind turbines are going up all over the world, particularly in northern Europe. These have blades 100 feet or more in length. Wind energy is site-specific. In the United States, for example, states such as the Dakotas and the western part of Texas have particular potential for wind development. If set up in farm fields, only a small percent of the land is used, and farmers can still grow their crops under the turbines; the land would then do double duty.

Solar energy has two main types: **solar thermal energy** that uses sunlight to heat water or air for direct use, mainly for domestic water heating or wintertime home heating, but also for heating liquids into vapor to turn turbines and generate electricity; and **solar photovoltaic energy** that uses solar cells (silicon cells, originally perfected by NASA for space use) to create electricity directly from the photons of the Sun. Like wind electricity, photovoltaic electricity is increasing, especially as the cost of solar cells continues to drop.

Nuclear fusion would use energy released from fusing hydrogen into helium (which is the process that takes place in the center of the Sun). Fusion requires enormous temperatures and pressures in the fusion reactor's center, which will probably use incredibly high-tech magnetic "bottles" to hold the reactants (because nothing material could withstand those conditions). Fusion has been accomplished in high-energy physics labs, but no fusion energy plants exist yet.

4. Systems of Matter and Life

The biosphere is an interacting system of matter and energy, of humans and nature.

a. Waste Disposal

Municipal solid waste describes general garbage. Disposal methods include landfills, combustion, recycling, and the composting of organics.

Sewage describes liquid and solid body wastes treated in sewage treatment plants. A number of steps are involved: Preliminary and primary treatments remove debris and organic particles, respectively. Secondary treatment involves bacteria in aqueous slurries. The bacteria consume the dissolved organics in the sewage. Before the treated waste water is put back into a natural water system, it is disinfected. Many variations exist, and new technologies, often using more advanced biological processes to help, are being explored. In sewage treatment, we are mimicking (and using) the natural recycling capabilities of bacteria in nature, in the soil, and in the deep ocean.

b. Deforestation

Deforestation is the cutting of areas of forest. This occurs at a rate of 10 million hectares per year. Deforestation occurs to supply raw material for the lumber and paper industries, or it can also take place when trees are burned to create open land for pasture or crops.

Clear-cutting is the term used when patches of forest are completely cut for industrial use. The other approach is **selective cutting**, when only certain trees (such as large trees or a certain species) are harvested, leaving the rest to grow for future harvests or just remain as forest.

Certain regions, such as the New England states, are undergoing **reforestation**. Farming, which was a strong part of the region's economy up to a hundred years ago, eventually could not compete with the midwestern and western farms. Through reforestation, much land in New England is returning to forest.

Deforestation usually releases CO_2. If trees are burned, CO_2 goes right into the atmosphere. Even if the trees are to be used for paper or lumber, the twigs and dead roots decay fairly rapidly, and thus are a lesser, though still important, source of CO_2 from these areas of deforestation. Reforestation, on the other hand, removes CO_2 from the atmosphere, and thus can help mitigate the rising threat of a greenhouse effect.

c. Nature's Services

Nonrenewable resources are resources that cannot be renewed in anywhere close to the time in which we are depleting them. For example, though oil is formed continuously during the geological ages, the rate is infinitesimal compared to our rate of extraction and burning it. Minerals are also nonrenewable resources.

Renewable resources, on the other hand, can be regenerated by natural processes. For example, fresh water is reformed by the water cycle, in which water from the ocean is evaporated (leaving the salt behind), then forms droplets in clouds, which in turn rain over land. Thus, the fresh water in rivers is renewed. Of course, humans can still exert stress upon the water systems, when deep, underground aquifers are pumped faster than they are being renewed, or when water is drawn from watersheds at rates that do not allow enough water for the fish in the natural stream.

Trees would be considered a renewable resource, because they can regrow. However, old-growth forests are nonrenewable, because they take many hundreds of years to develop to the full climax state.

Nature is our basic life support system. It is important to preserve the services of nature. Much is not yet understood, but it is clear that biodiversity is crucial for the healthy continuation of most natural systems.

You Should Review

- human population
- land use
- greenhouse effect
- acid rain
- toxins
- ozone depletion
- energy technologies
- waste disposal and deforestation
- renewable versus nonrenewable resources

Questions

61. Based upon current population projections, what will be the approximate world population in 2025?
  a. five billion
  b. six billion
  c. seven billion
  d. eight billion

62. Which of the following statements about global land use is NOT true?
  a. Cropland is increasing.
  b. Old-growth forest is decreasing.
  c. Unusable land (rock, ice, desert) is greater than urbanized land area.
  d. Pasture is less than cropland.

63. Considering the unit *ppm* as parts per million, how many ppm is oxygen in Earth's atmosphere?
  a. 21 ppm
  b. 21,000 ppm
  c. 210,000 ppm
  d. 2,100 ppm

64. Stratospheric ozone absorbs
  a. infrared radiation.
  b. visible light.
  c. ultraviolet radiation.
  d. green radiation.

65. The Montreal Protocol limited
  a. the production of carbon dioxide.
  b. the production of acid rain.
  c. the production of dimethyl sulfide.
  d. the production of chlorofluorocarbons.

66. Place your hand on a running gas powered car engine, and it will feel hot. You will also hear the sound of the engine running and feel it vibrating. All of these are signs that
  a. the engine is not 100% efficient.
  b. the engine is releasing particulate matter.
  c. energy is not being conserved.
  d. the car is releasing carbon monoxide.

67. Which is mostly methane?
  a. oil
  b. natural gas
  c. coal waste
  d. propane

68. Which is not a future possibility as a primary source of energy?
   a. fusion
   b. hydrogen
   c. wind
   d. photovoltaic

69. A good future source of energy for farmers to consider as a source of profit is
   a. fission.
   b. fusion.
   c. wind.
   d. hydrogen.

70. Which is NOT a primary pollutant?
   a. carbon monoxide
   b. tropospheric ozone
   c. suspended particulate matter
   d. volatile organic compounds

Answers

61. d. The current human population is about seven billion people. Based upon current projections, the world population will be approximately eight billion in 2025.

62. d. Pasture is about twice the area of cropland, for the world average. The other statements are true.

63. c. Oxygen gas is 21% of Earth's atmosphere, which converts to 210,000 ppm; ($\frac{210,000}{1,000,000} = 0.21 = 21\%$).

64. c. Stratospheric ozone is a natural protective shield because it absorbs the ultraviolet wavelengths of solar radiation that would otherwise cause great damage to living things at the surface.

65. d. The Montreal Protocol was a global agreement to phase out the production and release of the ozone-destroying chlorofluorocarbons.

66. a. Based on the Second Law of Thermodynamics, no machine can be 100% efficient in converting energy to work (in this case, gas making the car move). Rather, energy is converted into other forms of energy, such as heat and sound.

67. b. Natural gas is predominantly methane, piped up from underground reservoirs, sometimes from gas domes at the top of oil pools under the earth.

68. b. Hydrogen cannot be a primary source of energy because there are no natural supplies of hydrogen. Hydrogen must be made from water, by splitting water (or using methane) via a primary energy source. Hydrogen is therefore best considered a possible energy storage material.

69. c. Wind energy could be particularly attractive to farmers because the wind turbines take up little space and thus the land can still be used for farming as well. Thus, the land does double duty.

70. b. Primary pollutants are released directly from a polluting source. They can be altered by reactions that are catalyzed by sunlight, creating secondary pollutants (also known as photochemical pollutants) such as tropospheric ozone.

10 ▶ PRACTICE EXAM II

CHAPTER SUMMARY

This is the second of three practice exams based on actual health occupations entrance exams used today. Take this test to see how much you have improved since you took the first exam.

The practice test that follows is closely modeled after real entrance exams used to admit candidates to health education programs throughout the country. This test will help prepare you for admissions tests like the HOAE, the TEAS, and other entrance tests. As with the first practice test in Chapter 3, it covers six essential topics—Verbal Ability, Reading Comprehension, Math, General Science, Biology, and Chemistry—and uses a multiple-choice format, with four answer choices, **a–d**. Although the practice tests in this book will prepare you for *any* health occupations entrance exam, be sure to learn the specifics about the exam that you are facing—it may vary somewhat in content and format (number of questions or sections) from this practice test.

For this second exam, simulate an actual test-taking experience as much as possible. First, find a quiet place where you can work undisturbed for four hours. Keep a timer or alarm clock on hand to observe the time limits specified in the directions. Time each section separately, according to the directions set out at the beginning of each segment. Stop working when the alarm goes off, even if you have not completed the section. Between sections, take five minutes to clear your mind, and take a 15-minute break after Section 3. These breaks, and the time limits given for each section, approximate the testing schedule of commonly used entrance exams, such as the HOAE and TEAS.

Using a number 2 pencil, mark your answers on the answer sheet on the following pages. The answer key is located on page 316—of course, you should not refer to it until you have completed the test. A section about how to score your exam follows the answer key.

Section 1: Verbal Ability

	a	b	c	d		a	b	c	d		a	b	c	d
1.	ⓐ	ⓑ	ⓒ	ⓓ	18.	ⓐ	ⓑ	ⓒ	ⓓ	35.	ⓐ	ⓑ	ⓒ	ⓓ
2.	ⓐ	ⓑ	ⓒ	ⓓ	19.	ⓐ	ⓑ	ⓒ	ⓓ	36.	ⓐ	ⓑ	ⓒ	ⓓ
3.	ⓐ	ⓑ	ⓒ	ⓓ	20.	ⓐ	ⓑ	ⓒ	ⓓ	37.	ⓐ	ⓑ	ⓒ	ⓓ
4.	ⓐ	ⓑ	ⓒ	ⓓ	21.	ⓐ	ⓑ	ⓒ	ⓓ	38.	ⓐ	ⓑ	ⓒ	ⓓ
5.	ⓐ	ⓑ	ⓒ	ⓓ	22.	ⓐ	ⓑ	ⓒ	ⓓ	39.	ⓐ	ⓑ	ⓒ	ⓓ
6.	ⓐ	ⓑ	ⓒ	ⓓ	23.	ⓐ	ⓑ	ⓒ	ⓓ	40.	ⓐ	ⓑ	ⓒ	ⓓ
7.	ⓐ	ⓑ	ⓒ	ⓓ	24.	ⓐ	ⓑ	ⓒ	ⓓ	41.	ⓐ	ⓑ	ⓒ	ⓓ
8.	ⓐ	ⓑ	ⓒ	ⓓ	25.	ⓐ	ⓑ	ⓒ	ⓓ	42.	ⓐ	ⓑ	ⓒ	ⓓ
9.	ⓐ	ⓑ	ⓒ	ⓓ	26.	ⓐ	ⓑ	ⓒ	ⓓ	43.	ⓐ	ⓑ	ⓒ	ⓓ
10.	ⓐ	ⓑ	ⓒ	ⓓ	27.	ⓐ	ⓑ	ⓒ	ⓓ	44.	ⓐ	ⓑ	ⓒ	ⓓ
11.	ⓐ	ⓑ	ⓒ	ⓓ	28.	ⓐ	ⓑ	ⓒ	ⓓ	45.	ⓐ	ⓑ	ⓒ	ⓓ
12.	ⓐ	ⓑ	ⓒ	ⓓ	29.	ⓐ	ⓑ	ⓒ	ⓓ	46.	ⓐ	ⓑ	ⓒ	ⓓ
13.	ⓐ	ⓑ	ⓒ	ⓓ	30.	ⓐ	ⓑ	ⓒ	ⓓ	47.	ⓐ	ⓑ	ⓒ	ⓓ
14.	ⓐ	ⓑ	ⓒ	ⓓ	31.	ⓐ	ⓑ	ⓒ	ⓓ	48.	ⓐ	ⓑ	ⓒ	ⓓ
15.	ⓐ	ⓑ	ⓒ	ⓓ	32.	ⓐ	ⓑ	ⓒ	ⓓ	49.	ⓐ	ⓑ	ⓒ	ⓓ
16.	ⓐ	ⓑ	ⓒ	ⓓ	33.	ⓐ	ⓑ	ⓒ	ⓓ	50.	ⓐ	ⓑ	ⓒ	ⓓ
17.	ⓐ	ⓑ	ⓒ	ⓓ	34.	ⓐ	ⓑ	ⓒ	ⓓ					

Section 2: Reading Comprehension

	a	b	c	d		a	b	c	d		a	b	c	d
1.	ⓐ	ⓑ	ⓒ	ⓓ	18.	ⓐ	ⓑ	ⓒ	ⓓ	35.	ⓐ	ⓑ	ⓒ	ⓓ
2.	ⓐ	ⓑ	ⓒ	ⓓ	19.	ⓐ	ⓑ	ⓒ	ⓓ	36.	ⓐ	ⓑ	ⓒ	ⓓ
3.	ⓐ	ⓑ	ⓒ	ⓓ	20.	ⓐ	ⓑ	ⓒ	ⓓ	37.	ⓐ	ⓑ	ⓒ	ⓓ
4.	ⓐ	ⓑ	ⓒ	ⓓ	21.	ⓐ	ⓑ	ⓒ	ⓓ	38.	ⓐ	ⓑ	ⓒ	ⓓ
5.	ⓐ	ⓑ	ⓒ	ⓓ	22.	ⓐ	ⓑ	ⓒ	ⓓ	39.	ⓐ	ⓑ	ⓒ	ⓓ
6.	ⓐ	ⓑ	ⓒ	ⓓ	23.	ⓐ	ⓑ	ⓒ	ⓓ	40.	ⓐ	ⓑ	ⓒ	ⓓ
7.	ⓐ	ⓑ	ⓒ	ⓓ	24.	ⓐ	ⓑ	ⓒ	ⓓ	41.	ⓐ	ⓑ	ⓒ	ⓓ
8.	ⓐ	ⓑ	ⓒ	ⓓ	25.	ⓐ	ⓑ	ⓒ	ⓓ	42.	ⓐ	ⓑ	ⓒ	ⓓ
9.	ⓐ	ⓑ	ⓒ	ⓓ	26.	ⓐ	ⓑ	ⓒ	ⓓ	43.	ⓐ	ⓑ	ⓒ	ⓓ
10.	ⓐ	ⓑ	ⓒ	ⓓ	27.	ⓐ	ⓑ	ⓒ	ⓓ	44.	ⓐ	ⓑ	ⓒ	ⓓ
11.	ⓐ	ⓑ	ⓒ	ⓓ	28.	ⓐ	ⓑ	ⓒ	ⓓ	45.	ⓐ	ⓑ	ⓒ	ⓓ
12.	ⓐ	ⓑ	ⓒ	ⓓ	29.	ⓐ	ⓑ	ⓒ	ⓓ					
13.	ⓐ	ⓑ	ⓒ	ⓓ	30.	ⓐ	ⓑ	ⓒ	ⓓ					
14.	ⓐ	ⓑ	ⓒ	ⓓ	31.	ⓐ	ⓑ	ⓒ	ⓓ					
15.	ⓐ	ⓑ	ⓒ	ⓓ	32.	ⓐ	ⓑ	ⓒ	ⓓ					
16.	ⓐ	ⓑ	ⓒ	ⓓ	33.	ⓐ	ⓑ	ⓒ	ⓓ					
17.	ⓐ	ⓑ	ⓒ	ⓓ	34.	ⓐ	ⓑ	ⓒ	ⓓ					

Section 3: Math

	a	b	c	d			a	b	c	d			a	b	c	d
1.	ⓐ	ⓑ	ⓒ	ⓓ		18.	ⓐ	ⓑ	ⓒ	ⓓ		35.	ⓐ	ⓑ	ⓒ	ⓓ
2.	ⓐ	ⓑ	ⓒ	ⓓ		19.	ⓐ	ⓑ	ⓒ	ⓓ		36.	ⓐ	ⓑ	ⓒ	ⓓ
3.	ⓐ	ⓑ	ⓒ	ⓓ		20.	ⓐ	ⓑ	ⓒ	ⓓ		37.	ⓐ	ⓑ	ⓒ	ⓓ
4.	ⓐ	ⓑ	ⓒ	ⓓ		21.	ⓐ	ⓑ	ⓒ	ⓓ		38.	ⓐ	ⓑ	ⓒ	ⓓ
5.	ⓐ	ⓑ	ⓒ	ⓓ		22.	ⓐ	ⓑ	ⓒ	ⓓ		39.	ⓐ	ⓑ	ⓒ	ⓓ
6.	ⓐ	ⓑ	ⓒ	ⓓ		23.	ⓐ	ⓑ	ⓒ	ⓓ		40.	ⓐ	ⓑ	ⓒ	ⓓ
7.	ⓐ	ⓑ	ⓒ	ⓓ		24.	ⓐ	ⓑ	ⓒ	ⓓ		41.	ⓐ	ⓑ	ⓒ	ⓓ
8.	ⓐ	ⓑ	ⓒ	ⓓ		25.	ⓐ	ⓑ	ⓒ	ⓓ		42.	ⓐ	ⓑ	ⓒ	ⓓ
9.	ⓐ	ⓑ	ⓒ	ⓓ		26.	ⓐ	ⓑ	ⓒ	ⓓ		43.	ⓐ	ⓑ	ⓒ	ⓓ
10.	ⓐ	ⓑ	ⓒ	ⓓ		27.	ⓐ	ⓑ	ⓒ	ⓓ		44.	ⓐ	ⓑ	ⓒ	ⓓ
11.	ⓐ	ⓑ	ⓒ	ⓓ		28.	ⓐ	ⓑ	ⓒ	ⓓ		45.	ⓐ	ⓑ	ⓒ	ⓓ
12.	ⓐ	ⓑ	ⓒ	ⓓ		29.	ⓐ	ⓑ	ⓒ	ⓓ		46.	ⓐ	ⓑ	ⓒ	ⓓ
13.	ⓐ	ⓑ	ⓒ	ⓓ		30.	ⓐ	ⓑ	ⓒ	ⓓ		47.	ⓐ	ⓑ	ⓒ	ⓓ
14.	ⓐ	ⓑ	ⓒ	ⓓ		31.	ⓐ	ⓑ	ⓒ	ⓓ		48.	ⓐ	ⓑ	ⓒ	ⓓ
15.	ⓐ	ⓑ	ⓒ	ⓓ		32.	ⓐ	ⓑ	ⓒ	ⓓ		49.	ⓐ	ⓑ	ⓒ	ⓓ
16.	ⓐ	ⓑ	ⓒ	ⓓ		33.	ⓐ	ⓑ	ⓒ	ⓓ		50.	ⓐ	ⓑ	ⓒ	ⓓ
17.	ⓐ	ⓑ	ⓒ	ⓓ		34.	ⓐ	ⓑ	ⓒ	ⓓ						

Section 4: General Science

	a	b	c	d			a	b	c	d			a	b	c	d
1.	ⓐ	ⓑ	ⓒ	ⓓ		18.	ⓐ	ⓑ	ⓒ	ⓓ		35.	ⓐ	ⓑ	ⓒ	ⓓ
2.	ⓐ	ⓑ	ⓒ	ⓓ		19.	ⓐ	ⓑ	ⓒ	ⓓ		36.	ⓐ	ⓑ	ⓒ	ⓓ
3.	ⓐ	ⓑ	ⓒ	ⓓ		20.	ⓐ	ⓑ	ⓒ	ⓓ		37.	ⓐ	ⓑ	ⓒ	ⓓ
4.	ⓐ	ⓑ	ⓒ	ⓓ		21.	ⓐ	ⓑ	ⓒ	ⓓ		38.	ⓐ	ⓑ	ⓒ	ⓓ
5.	ⓐ	ⓑ	ⓒ	ⓓ		22.	ⓐ	ⓑ	ⓒ	ⓓ		39.	ⓐ	ⓑ	ⓒ	ⓓ
6.	ⓐ	ⓑ	ⓒ	ⓓ		23.	ⓐ	ⓑ	ⓒ	ⓓ		40.	ⓐ	ⓑ	ⓒ	ⓓ
7.	ⓐ	ⓑ	ⓒ	ⓓ		24.	ⓐ	ⓑ	ⓒ	ⓓ		41.	ⓐ	ⓑ	ⓒ	ⓓ
8.	ⓐ	ⓑ	ⓒ	ⓓ		25.	ⓐ	ⓑ	ⓒ	ⓓ		42.	ⓐ	ⓑ	ⓒ	ⓓ
9.	ⓐ	ⓑ	ⓒ	ⓓ		26.	ⓐ	ⓑ	ⓒ	ⓓ		43.	ⓐ	ⓑ	ⓒ	ⓓ
10.	ⓐ	ⓑ	ⓒ	ⓓ		27.	ⓐ	ⓑ	ⓒ	ⓓ		44.	ⓐ	ⓑ	ⓒ	ⓓ
11.	ⓐ	ⓑ	ⓒ	ⓓ		28.	ⓐ	ⓑ	ⓒ	ⓓ		45.	ⓐ	ⓑ	ⓒ	ⓓ
12.	ⓐ	ⓑ	ⓒ	ⓓ		29.	ⓐ	ⓑ	ⓒ	ⓓ		46.	ⓐ	ⓑ	ⓒ	ⓓ
13.	ⓐ	ⓑ	ⓒ	ⓓ		30.	ⓐ	ⓑ	ⓒ	ⓓ		47.	ⓐ	ⓑ	ⓒ	ⓓ
14.	ⓐ	ⓑ	ⓒ	ⓓ		31.	ⓐ	ⓑ	ⓒ	ⓓ		48.	ⓐ	ⓑ	ⓒ	ⓓ
15.	ⓐ	ⓑ	ⓒ	ⓓ		32.	ⓐ	ⓑ	ⓒ	ⓓ		49.	ⓐ	ⓑ	ⓒ	ⓓ
16.	ⓐ	ⓑ	ⓒ	ⓓ		33.	ⓐ	ⓑ	ⓒ	ⓓ		50.	ⓐ	ⓑ	ⓒ	ⓓ
17.	ⓐ	ⓑ	ⓒ	ⓓ		34.	ⓐ	ⓑ	ⓒ	ⓓ						

Section 5: Biology

1. ⓐ ⓑ ⓒ ⓓ	18. ⓐ ⓑ ⓒ ⓓ	35. ⓐ ⓑ ⓒ ⓓ
2. ⓐ ⓑ ⓒ ⓓ	19. ⓐ ⓑ ⓒ ⓓ	36. ⓐ ⓑ ⓒ ⓓ
3. ⓐ ⓑ ⓒ ⓓ	20. ⓐ ⓑ ⓒ ⓓ	37. ⓐ ⓑ ⓒ ⓓ
4. ⓐ ⓑ ⓒ ⓓ	21. ⓐ ⓑ ⓒ ⓓ	38. ⓐ ⓑ ⓒ ⓓ
5. ⓐ ⓑ ⓒ ⓓ	22. ⓐ ⓑ ⓒ ⓓ	39. ⓐ ⓑ ⓒ ⓓ
6. ⓐ ⓑ ⓒ ⓓ	23. ⓐ ⓑ ⓒ ⓓ	40. ⓐ ⓑ ⓒ ⓓ
7. ⓐ ⓑ ⓒ ⓓ	24. ⓐ ⓑ ⓒ ⓓ	41. ⓐ ⓑ ⓒ ⓓ
8. ⓐ ⓑ ⓒ ⓓ	25. ⓐ ⓑ ⓒ ⓓ	42. ⓐ ⓑ ⓒ ⓓ
9. ⓐ ⓑ ⓒ ⓓ	26. ⓐ ⓑ ⓒ ⓓ	43. ⓐ ⓑ ⓒ ⓓ
10. ⓐ ⓑ ⓒ ⓓ	27. ⓐ ⓑ ⓒ ⓓ	44. ⓐ ⓑ ⓒ ⓓ
11. ⓐ ⓑ ⓒ ⓓ	28. ⓐ ⓑ ⓒ ⓓ	45. ⓐ ⓑ ⓒ ⓓ
12. ⓐ ⓑ ⓒ ⓓ	29. ⓐ ⓑ ⓒ ⓓ	46. ⓐ ⓑ ⓒ ⓓ
13. ⓐ ⓑ ⓒ ⓓ	30. ⓐ ⓑ ⓒ ⓓ	47. ⓐ ⓑ ⓒ ⓓ
14. ⓐ ⓑ ⓒ ⓓ	31. ⓐ ⓑ ⓒ ⓓ	48. ⓐ ⓑ ⓒ ⓓ
15. ⓐ ⓑ ⓒ ⓓ	32. ⓐ ⓑ ⓒ ⓓ	49. ⓐ ⓑ ⓒ ⓓ
16. ⓐ ⓑ ⓒ ⓓ	33. ⓐ ⓑ ⓒ ⓓ	50. ⓐ ⓑ ⓒ ⓓ
17. ⓐ ⓑ ⓒ ⓓ	34. ⓐ ⓑ ⓒ ⓓ	

Section 6: Chemistry

1. ⓐ ⓑ ⓒ ⓓ	18. ⓐ ⓑ ⓒ ⓓ	35. ⓐ ⓑ ⓒ ⓓ
2. ⓐ ⓑ ⓒ ⓓ	19. ⓐ ⓑ ⓒ ⓓ	36. ⓐ ⓑ ⓒ ⓓ
3. ⓐ ⓑ ⓒ ⓓ	20. ⓐ ⓑ ⓒ ⓓ	37. ⓐ ⓑ ⓒ ⓓ
4. ⓐ ⓑ ⓒ ⓓ	21. ⓐ ⓑ ⓒ ⓓ	38. ⓐ ⓑ ⓒ ⓓ
5. ⓐ ⓑ ⓒ ⓓ	22. ⓐ ⓑ ⓒ ⓓ	39. ⓐ ⓑ ⓒ ⓓ
6. ⓐ ⓑ ⓒ ⓓ	23. ⓐ ⓑ ⓒ ⓓ	40. ⓐ ⓑ ⓒ ⓓ
7. ⓐ ⓑ ⓒ ⓓ	24. ⓐ ⓑ ⓒ ⓓ	41. ⓐ ⓑ ⓒ ⓓ
8. ⓐ ⓑ ⓒ ⓓ	25. ⓐ ⓑ ⓒ ⓓ	42. ⓐ ⓑ ⓒ ⓓ
9. ⓐ ⓑ ⓒ ⓓ	26. ⓐ ⓑ ⓒ ⓓ	43. ⓐ ⓑ ⓒ ⓓ
10. ⓐ ⓑ ⓒ ⓓ	27. ⓐ ⓑ ⓒ ⓓ	44. ⓐ ⓑ ⓒ ⓓ
11. ⓐ ⓑ ⓒ ⓓ	28. ⓐ ⓑ ⓒ ⓓ	45. ⓐ ⓑ ⓒ ⓓ
12. ⓐ ⓑ ⓒ ⓓ	29. ⓐ ⓑ ⓒ ⓓ	46. ⓐ ⓑ ⓒ ⓓ
13. ⓐ ⓑ ⓒ ⓓ	30. ⓐ ⓑ ⓒ ⓓ	47. ⓐ ⓑ ⓒ ⓓ
14. ⓐ ⓑ ⓒ ⓓ	31. ⓐ ⓑ ⓒ ⓓ	48. ⓐ ⓑ ⓒ ⓓ
15. ⓐ ⓑ ⓒ ⓓ	32. ⓐ ⓑ ⓒ ⓓ	49. ⓐ ⓑ ⓒ ⓓ
16. ⓐ ⓑ ⓒ ⓓ	33. ⓐ ⓑ ⓒ ⓓ	50. ⓐ ⓑ ⓒ ⓓ
17. ⓐ ⓑ ⓒ ⓓ	34. ⓐ ⓑ ⓒ ⓓ	

Section 1: Verbal Ability

Find the correctly spelled word in each of the following lists. You have 15 minutes to answer the 50 questions in this section.

1. a. commitment
   b. committent
   c. comittment

2. a. rediculous
   b. rediculus
   c. ridiculous

3. a. respatory
   b. respiratory
   c. respireatory

4. a. percise
   b. precize
   c. precise

5. a. asurrance
   b. assurance
   c. assurence

6. a. frequently
   b. frequintly
   c. frequentlly

7. a. developement
   b. develupment
   c. development

8. a. concede
   b. conceed
   c. consede

9. a. encouredging
   b. encouraging
   c. incurraging

10. a. phenomina
    b. phenominna
    c. phenomena

11. a. compatibel
    b. compatable
    c. compatible

12. a. clinician
    b. clinishan
    c. cliniachen

13. a. comencement
    b. commencement
    c. commencment
    d. comencment

14. a. superviser
    b. supervisor
    c. supervizor

15. a. neumonia
    b. pneumonia
    c. pnumonia

16. a. annoid
    b. anoyed
    c. annoyed

17. a. apperatus
    b. aparatus
    c. apparatus

18. a. coedeine
    b. codine
    c. codeine

19. a. accompany
    b. acommpany
    c. accompeny

20. **a.** incessent
  b. incessant
  c. incesant

21. **a.** delemma
  b. dilemma
  c. dilema

22. **a.** eficient
  b. eficeint
  c. efficient

23. **a.** therupy
  b. therapy
  c. thairapy

24. **a.** viewpoint
  b. veiwpoint
  c. viewpointe

25. **a.** agravated
  b. agravaeted
  c. aggravated

26. **a.** artieries
  b. artaries
  c. arteries

27. **a.** alumni
  b. alumnuses
  c. allumni

28. **a.** announcement
  b. anouncement
  c. announcemant

29. **a.** asle
  b. aisl
  c. aisle

30. **a.** sensable
  b. sensible
  c. sensibal

31. **a.** heifer
  b. hiefer
  c. heifre

32. **a.** association
  b. associacion
  c. associatione

33. **a.** rehearsel
  b. rehearsal
  c. reahearsal

34. **a.** fasinated
  b. facinated
  c. fascinated

35. **a.** destructive
  b. distructive
  c. destructiv

36. **a.** disolve
  b. dissollve
  c. dissolve

37. **a.** illuminate
  b. iluminate
  c. ilumminate

38. **a.** knowledje
  b. knowladge
  c. knowledge

39. **a.** metearology
  b. meteorology
  c. meterology

40. a. adjournment
   b. ajournment
   c. adjurnment

41. a. vengence
   b. vengance
   c. vengeance

42. a. tremendus
   b. tremendos
   c. tremendous

43. a. imortality
   b. immortality
   c. immortalaty

44. a. capitalizashion
   b. capitolization
   c. capitalization

45. a. brilliant
   b. brilleant
   c. briliant

46. a. parenthiseses
   b. parenthesis
   c. parenthesise

47. a. wierd
   b. werd
   c. weird

48. a. sonet
   b. sonnit
   c. sonnet

49. a. depot
   b. depo
   c. depote

50. a. presum
   b. presumme
   c. presume

Section 2:
Reading Comprehension

Read each passage and answer the questions based on the information in the text. You have 45 minutes to complete this section.

Millions of people in the United States are affected by eating disorders. More than 90% of those afflicted are adolescent or young adult women. While all eating disorders share some common manifestations, anorexia nervosa, bulimia nervosa, and binge eating each have distinctive symptoms and risks.

People who intentionally starve themselves (even while experiencing severe hunger pains) suffer from *anorexia nervosa*. The disorder, which usually begins around the time of puberty, involves extreme weight loss to at least 15% below the individual's normal body weight. Many people with the disorder look emaciated but are convinced they are overweight. In patients with anorexia nervosa, starvation can damage vital organs such as the heart and brain. To protect itself, the body shifts into slow gear: Menstrual periods stop, blood pressure rates drop, and thyroid function slows. Excessive thirst and frequent urination may occur. Dehydration contributes to constipation, and reduced body fat leads to lowered body temperature and the inability to withstand cold. Mild anemia, swollen joints, reduced muscle mass, and light-headedness also commonly occur in those with anorexia nervosa.

Anorexia nervosa sufferers can exhibit sudden angry outbursts or become socially withdrawn. One in ten cases of anorexia nervosa leads to death from starvation, cardiac arrest, other medical complications, or suicide. Clinical depression and anxiety place many individuals with eating disorders at risk for suicidal behavior.

People with *bulimia nervosa* consume large amounts of food and then rid their bodies of the excess calories by vomiting, abusing laxatives or diuretics, taking enemas, or exercising obsessively. Some use a combination of all these forms of purging. Individuals with bulimia who use drugs to stimulate vomiting, bowel movements, or urination may be in considerable danger, as this practice increases the risk of heart failure. Dieting heavily between episodes of binging and purging is common.

Because many individuals with bulimia binge and purge in secret and maintain normal or above-normal body weight, they can often successfully hide their problem for years. But bulimia nervosa patients—even those of normal weight—can severely damage their bodies by frequent binge eating and purging. In rare instances, binge eating causes the stomach to rupture; purging may result in heart failure due to loss of vital minerals such as potassium. Vomiting can cause the esophagus to become inflamed and glands near the cheeks to become swollen. As in anorexia nervosa, bulimia may lead to irregular menstrual periods. Psychological effects include compulsive stealing as well as possible indications of obsessive-compulsive disorder, an illness characterized by repetitive thoughts and behaviors. Obsessive-compulsive disorder can also accompany anorexia nervosa. As with anorexia nervosa, bulimia typically begins during adolescence. Eventually, half of those with anorexia nervosa will develop bulimia. The condition occurs most often in women but is also found in men.

Binge-eating disorder is found in about 2% of the general population. As many as one-third of this group are men. It also affects older women, though with less frequency. Recent research shows that binge-eating disorder occurs in about 30% of people participating in medically supervised weight-control programs. This disorder differs from bulimia because its sufferers do not purge. Individuals with binge-eating disorder feel that they lose control of themselves when eating. They eat large quantities of food and do not stop until they are uncomfortably full. Most sufferers are overweight or obese and have a history of weight fluctuations. As a result, they are prone to the serious medical problems associated with obesity, such as high cholesterol, high blood pressure, and diabetes. Obese individuals also have a higher risk for gallbladder disease, heart disease, and some types of cancer. Usually, they have more difficulty losing weight and keeping it off than do people with other serious weight problems. Like anorexics and bulimics who exhibit psychological problems, individuals with binge-eating disorder have high rates of simultaneously occurring psychiatric illnesses—especially depression.

1. Fatalities occur in what percent of people with anorexia nervosa?
   a. 2%
   b. 10%
   c. 15%
   d. 30%

2. Which of the following consequences do all the eating disorders mentioned in the passage have in common?
   a. heart ailments
   b. stomach rupture
   c. swollen joints
   d. diabetes

3. Which of the following best describes the word *withdrawn* as it is used in the third paragraph of the passage?
   a. pulled
   b. taken
   c. introverted
   d. undone

4. People usually begin suffering from anorexia nervosa when they are in
   a. childhood.
   b. adolescence.
   c. late teens.
   d. adulthood.

5. People who have an eating disorder but nevertheless appear to be of normal weight are most likely to have
   a. obsessive-compulsive disorder.
   b. bulimia nervosa.
   c. binge-eating disorder.
   d. anorexia nervosa.

6. Which paragraph explains why glandular functions of anorexia patients slow down?
   a. Paragraph 1
   b. Paragraph 2
   c. Paragraph 3
   d. Paragraph 4

7. Recent research shows that binge-eating disorder occurs in about 30% of
   a. people participating in medically supervised weight-control programs.
   b. people participating in marathon running.
   c. people between the ages of 60 and 75.
   d. people who had recently moved higher on the corporate ladder.

8. Which of the following is true of bulimia patients?
   a. They may demonstrate unpredictable social behavior.
   b. They often engage in compulsive exercise.
   c. They are less susceptible to dehydration than are anorexia patients.
   d. They frequently experience stomach ruptures.

9. The passage is chiefly concerned with the similarities and differences between different kinds of
   a. individuals.
   b. diseases.
   c. diets.
   d. disorders.

The U.S. population is going gray. A rising demographic tide of aging baby boomers—those born between 1946 and 1964—and increased longevity have made adults age 65 and older the fastest growing segment of today's population. In thirty years, this segment of the population will be nearly twice as large as it is today. By then, an estimated 70 million people will be over age 65. The number of "oldest old"—those age 85 and older—is 34 times greater than in 1900 and likely to expand five-fold by 2050.

This unprecedented "elder boom" will have a profound effect on American society, particularly the field of healthcare. Is the U.S. health system equipped to deal with the demands of an aging population? Although we have adequate physicians and nurses, many of them are not trained to handle the multiple needs of older patients. Today, we have about

9,000 *geriatricians* (physicians who are experts in aging-related issues). Some studies estimate a need for 36,000 geriatricians by 2030.

Many doctors today treat a patient of 75 the same way they would treat a 40-year-old patient. However, although seniors are healthier than ever, physical challenges often increase with age. By age 75, adults often have two to three medical conditions. Diagnosing multiple health problems and knowing how they interact is crucial for effectively treating older patients. Healthcare professionals—often pressed for time in hectic daily practices—must be diligent about asking questions and collecting "evidence" from their elderly patients. Finding out about a patient's over-the-counter medications or living conditions could reveal an underlying problem.

Lack of training in geriatric issues can result in healthcare providers overlooking illnesses or conditions that may lead to illness. Inadequate nutrition is a common, but often unrecognized, problem among frail seniors. An elderly patient who has difficulty preparing meals at home may become vulnerable to malnutrition or another medical condition. Healthcare providers with training in aging issues may be able to address this problem without the costly solution of admitting a patient to a nursing home.

Depression, a treatable condition that affects nearly five million seniors, also goes undetected by some healthcare providers. Some healthcare professionals view depression as "just part of getting old." Untreated, this illness can have serious, even fatal consequences. According to the National Institute of Mental Health, older Americans account for a disproportionate share of suicide deaths, making up 18% of suicide deaths in 2000.

Healthcare providers could play a vital role in preventing this outcome—several studies have shown that up to 75% of seniors who die by suicide visited a primary care physician within a month of their death.

Healthcare providers face additional challenges to providing high-quality care to the aging population. Because the numbers of ethnic minority elders are growing faster than the aging population as a whole, providers must train to care for a more racially and ethnically diverse population of elderly patients. Respect and understanding of diverse cultural beliefs is necessary to provide the most effective healthcare to all patients. Providers must also be able to communicate complicated medical conditions or treatments to older patients who may have a visual, hearing, or cognitive impairment.

As older adults make up an increasing proportion of the healthcare caseload, the demand for aging specialists must expand as well. Healthcare providers who work with the elderly must understand and address not only the physical but mental, emotional, and social changes of the aging process. They need to be able to distinguish between "normal" characteristics associated with aging and illness. Most crucially, they should look beyond symptoms and consider ways that will help a senior maintain and improve his or her quality of life.

10. The author uses the phrase *going gray* in order to
   a. maintain that everyone's hair loses its color eventually.
   b. suggest the social phenomenon of an aging population.
   c. depict older Americans in a positive light.
   d. demonstrate the normal changes of aging.

11. In the third paragraph, the author implies that doctors who treat elderly patients as they would a 40-year-old patient
   a. provide equitable, high-quality care.
   b. avoid detrimental stereotypes about older patients.
   c. encourage middle-age adults to think about the long-term effects of their habits.
   d. do not offer the most effective care to their older patients.

12. The number of senior citizens who suffer from depression is approximately
   a. 9,000.
   b. 36,000.
   c. 5 million.
   d. 70 million.

13. The sixth paragraph is chiefly concerned with
   a. race.
   b. ethnicity.
   c. diversity.
   d. communication.

AVERAGE LIFE EXPECTANCY FROM 1880 TO 2080	
YEAR	AVERAGE LIFE EXPECTANCY
1880	39
1940	62
1980	73
2020	81
2080	100

14. Which of the following is true based on the table?
   a. The average life expectantly has risen consistently since 1880.
   b. An average life expectancy of 100 is only speculation.
   c. The average life expectancy will eventually fall again.
   d. The average life expectancy will never rise above 100.

Scientists have been studying radon and its effects since the turn of the century. This inert gas has been proven to cause lung cancer and is suspected of being responsible for a range of other serious illnesses.

Radon gas is created as the result of the decaying of uranium and radium. At the culmination of this lengthy process, the disintegrating matter becomes radon, which then decays further, releasing additional radiation and transforming into what are known as radon daughters. Unlike radon, the daughters are not inert because they are highly sensitive to their surroundings and are chemically active. Thus, when the daughters enter buildings, attach to clothing, mingle with dust particles, or are inhaled, health risks increase dramatically. Radon exists across the United States, with somewhat higher amounts located in areas where granite is common.

Radon gas released directly into the atmosphere poses slight health risks. Conversely, when it is trapped and has the opportunity to accumulate, such as beneath houses and other structures, risks increase significantly. This colorless, tasteless, and odorless element can seep into buildings through walls, soil, water supplies, and natural gas pipelines. It can also be part of the properties of materials such as brick, wallboard, and concrete. When radon is prevalent in a building, it circulates in that building's air exchange and is inhaled by humans.

The majority of the radon daughters exhibit electrostatic qualities as they attach to items such as clothing, furniture, and dust, a magnetic process known as *plating out*. The remainder of the daughters do not attach to anything. As an individual breathes the potentially damaging air, the attached and unattached daughters enter the body. As the daughters travel through the body, particles become attached to the respiratory tract, the bronchial region, the nose, and the throat. Some particles are expelled during exhalation, but most remain within the individual.

The unattached daughters are the most dangerous as their untethered route often carries them directly to the lungs. They deposit significantly more radioactivity than the attached daughters—indeed, up to 40 times as much. Research indicates that those individuals who breathe primarily through their noses receive fewer doses than those who breathe primarily through their mouths.

Alpha radiation begins penetrating the lungs and other organs after radon daughters settle there. Penetration and the subsequent depositing of radiation are the result of a continuation of the decaying process. An appreciable dose of alpha particles can lead to cell destruction. Higher doses can be fatal. One comparative study analyzed similar doses from radon, X-rays, and atom bombs, and concluded that the chances of developing lung cancer from radon were equal to those from the other two radiation sources. In the United States, most incidences involve lower-level doses, which destroy a relatively low number of cells. The body will regenerate lost cells, so serious health problems become less likely.

Serious problems materialize when cells are exposed repeatedly. The cycle of exposure-damage-regeneration-exposure can weaken cells and ultimately change their makeup. Cell alteration can lead to lung cancer, genetic changes, and a host of other medical problems.

15. As radon decays, it transforms into
   a. uranium.
   b. radium.
   c. daughters.
   d. radiation.

16. It can be inferred from the passage that an inert gas such as radon is
   a. unusually likely to decay.
   b. dormant in terms of chemical reactions.
   c. more dangerous than radon daughters.
   d. created as the result of a distinct series of events.

17. One reason unattached daughters are more dangerous than attached daughters is that they
   a. demonstrate electrostatic qualities.
   b. are less likely to be expelled.
   c. regenerate after entering the lungs.
   d. have a free path toward internal organs.

18. *Plating out* is a term for a process of
   a. cohering.
   b. disseminating.
   c. deteriorating.
   d. permeating.

19. A study comparing similar doses from radon, X-rays, and atom bombs found that the chances of developing lung cancer
   a. were equal from all three sources.
   b. were greatest from an atom bomb.
   c. were significantly less from radon.
   d. were higher from X-rays.

20. Radon is formed as a consequence of
   a. the alteration of cells.
   b. the breakdown of elements.
   c. exposure to the atmosphere.
   d. an electrostatic process.

21. Radon released into the atmosphere is mostly
   a. deadly.
   b. visible.
   c. dangerous.
   d. harmless.

The *dystonias* are movement disorders in which sustained muscle contractions cause twisting and repetitive movements or abnormal postures. The movements, which are involuntary and sometimes painful, may affect a single muscle; a group of muscles such as those in the arms, legs, or neck; or the entire body. Diminished intelligence and emotional imbalance are not usually features of the dystonias.

Generalized dystonia affects most or all of the body. *Focal dystonia* is localized to a specific body part. *Multifocal dystonia* involves two or more unrelated body parts. *Segmental dystonia* affects two or more adjacent parts of the body. *Hemidystonia* involves the arm and leg on the same side of the body.

Early symptoms may include a deterioration in handwriting after writing several lines, foot cramps, and a tendency of one foot to pull up or drag after running or walking some distance. The neck may turn or pull involuntarily, especially when the person is tired. Other possible symptoms are tremor and voice or speech difficulties. The initial symptoms can be very mild and may be noticeable only after prolonged exertion, stress, or fatigue. Over a period of time, the symptoms may become more noticeable and widespread and may be unrelenting; however, sometimes, there is little or no progression.

Torsion dystonia, previously called *dystonia musculum deformans* or DMD, is a rare, generalized dystonia that may be inherited, usually begins in childhood, and becomes progressively worse. It can leave individuals seriously disabled and confined to a wheelchair.

Spasmodic torticollis, or *torticollis*, is the most common of the focal dystonias. In torticollis, the muscles in the neck that control the position of the head are affected, causing the head to twist and turn to one side. In addition, the head may be pulled forward or backward. Torticollis can occur at any age, although most individuals first experience symptoms in middle age. It often begins slowly and usually reaches a plateau. About 10% to 20% of those with torticollis experience a spontaneous remission; however, the remission may not be lasting.

Blepharospasm, the second most common focal dystonia, is the involuntary, forcible closure of the eyelids. The first symptoms may be uncontrollable blinking. Only one eye may be affected initially, but eventually both eyes are usually involved. The spasms may leave the eyelids completely closed, causing functional blindness even though the eyes and vision are normal.

Cranial dystonia is a term used to describe dystonia that affects the muscles of the head, face, and neck. *Oromandibular dystonia* affects the muscles of the jaw, lips, and tongue. The jaw may be pulled either open or shut, and speech and swallowing can be difficult. *Spasmodic dysphonia* involves the muscles of the throat that control speech. Also called *spastic dysphonia* or *laryngeal dystonia*, it causes strained and difficult speaking or breathy and effortful speech. *Meige's syndrome* is the combination of blepharospasm and oro-mandibular dystonia and sometimes spasmodic dysphonia.

   Dopa-responsive dystonia (DRD) is a condition successfully treated with drugs. Typically, DRD begins in childhood or adolescence with progressive difficulty in walking and, in some cases, spasticity. In *Segawa's dystonia*, the symptoms fluctuate during the day from relative mobility in the morning to increasingly worse disability in the afternoon and evening as well as after exercise. Some scientists feel DRD is not only rare but also rarely diagnosed since it mimics many of the symptoms of cerebral palsy.

22. Which is true about torticollis?
   a. It is the rarest of all the types of focal dystonias.
   b. About 10% to 20% of patients have a spontaneous remission, but it may not last.
   c. It affects only people in their teens.
   d. It affects only the muscles of the hand, making it hard to write.

23. One symptom not typically experienced by dystonia patients is
   a. enunciation difficulties.
   b. hampered mobility.
   c. optical deficiencies.
   d. emotional instability.

24. Genetics may be implicated in
   a. torsion dystonia.
   b. torticollis.
   c. oromandibular dystonia.
   d. DRD.

25. Meige's syndrome directly affects both
   a. speech and mobility.
   b. mobility and vision.
   c. vision and speech.
   d. hearing and vision.

26. The symptoms of torticollis are most similar to those of
   a. cranial dystonia.
   b. DRD.
   c. blepharospasm.
   d. oromandibular dystonia.

27. A person with DRD usually
   a. has difficulty verbalizing.
   b. experiences writer's cramp.
   c. improves following exercise.
   d. responds well to medication.

28. All dystonia patients experience
   a. uncontrolled movement.
   b. progressive deterioration.
   c. symptoms at an early age.
   d. incessant discomfort.

29. Cranial dystonia is an example of a
   a. hemidystonia.
   b. multifocal dystonia.
   c. segmental dystonia.
   d. generalized dystonia.

30. Which of the following describes the word *progressive* as it is used in the final paragraph of the passage?
   a. improved
   b. futuristic
   c. liberal
   d. increased

Lyme disease is sometimes called the "great imitator" because its many symptoms mimic those of other illnesses. When treated, this disease usually presents few or no lingering effects. Left untreated, however, it can be extremely debilitating and sometimes fatal.

Lyme disease is caused by a bacterium carried and transmitted by the *Ixodes dammini* family of ticks. In 1982, the damaging microorganism was identified as *Borrelia burgdorferi*. Ticks are parasites that require blood for sustenance. They feed three times during a two-year life cycle (the larva, nymph, and adult stages), and feedings can last up to several days. As many as 3,000 eggs hatch into larvae, the first stage of the life cycle. The larvae then attach to host organisms, such as mice. Human infection by a tick at this stage is a rare occurrence.

Following the first blood meal, larvae molt into nymphs. These transformed organisms are about the size of a bread crumb. During this and subsequent stages of the life cycle, the tick chooses larger hosts on which to feed, including humans. Because of their tiny size, nymphs present the greatest danger to humans. Some studies indicate that as many as 80% of human hosts are infected by nymphs. As the life cycle progresses, nymphs engorged with blood become adults. During this stage, adults will mate, assuring continuance of the life cycle. Ticks generally rely on humid conditions and temperatures above 40° Fahrenheit.

Human infection occurs when the tick attaches itself to the body, feeding on blood while transmitting the bacteria. Since this process can take up to 48 hours, it is possible for an individual to remove the tick before infection occurs. When infection does occur, one of the early visible signs is a rash called *erythema migrans*, although in some cases, there is no rash at all. The mark left by the tick, often taking a bull's-eye shape, can range from the size of a quarter to one foot across. Some rashes disappear temporarily and then return. This inconsistent symptom adds to the perplexing nature of the disease.

Symptoms can materialize within a few days to a few weeks following bacterial transmission and include flu-like aches and pains, fever, and weakness. As the illness progresses, problems such as respiratory distress, irregular heartbeat, liver infection, bladder discomfort, and double vision can occur. Infected individuals may experience all, none, or a combination of symptoms.

Early diagnosis and antibiotic treatment of the earliest acute stage of Lyme disease generally leads to rapid recovery. An inaccurate diagnosis or lack of early treatment can lead to health problems such as heart muscle damage, severe joint pain, and meningitis. Lyme disease that reaches a chronic stage can lead to severe arthritis, paralysis, brain infection, and nervous system disorders; however, symptoms of chronic Lyme disease, despite lasting six months or longer, are generally treatable with antibiotics, and long-term illness is rare. Researchers are working on a vaccine, but its completion remains uncertain.

31. Which is a fact about ticks that transmit Lyme disease?
   a. They are parasites that feed on blood.
   b. They have a two-year life cycle.
   c. A female may lay as many as 3,000 eggs.
   d. all of the above

32. Lyme disease that reaches the chronic stage tends to exhibit symptoms for
  a. 48 hours or less.
  b. a few days.
  c. six months or more.
  d. at least two years.

33. The third paragraph is chiefly concerned with
  a. molting.
  b. hosts.
  c. mating.
  d. nymphs.

34. Diagnosis of Lyme disease is made difficult by the
  a. similarities between it and other ailments.
  b. changing shape of the erythema migrans.
  c. unpredictable life cycle of the tick.
  d. lack of prolonged effects produced.

35. Transmission of *Borrelia burgdorferi* to humans during the larva stage
  a. accounts for the majority of infections.
  b. is a relatively infrequent phenomenon.
  c. generally occurs at temperatures below 40°F.
  d. lasts up to several days.

36. One early symptom of Lyme disease is
  a. arthritis.
  b. meningitis.
  c. fever.
  d. difficulty breathing.

There are two types of diabetes, insulin-dependent and non-insulin-dependent. Between 90% and 95% of the estimated 13 to 14 million people in the United States with diabetes have non-insulin-dependent, or Type II, diabetes. Because this form of diabetes usually begins in adults over the age of 40 and is most common after the age of 55, it used to be called *adult-onset* diabetes. Its symptoms often develop gradually and are hard to identify at first; therefore, nearly half of all people with diabetes do not know they have it. For instance, someone who has developed Type II diabetes may feel tired or ill without knowing why. This can be particularly dangerous because untreated diabetes can cause damage to the heart, blood vessels, eyes, kidneys, and nerves. While the causes, short-term effects, and treatments of the two types of diabetes differ, both types can cause the same long-term health problems.

Most important, both types affect the body's ability to use digested food for energy. Diabetes does not interfere with digestion, but it does prevent the body from using an important product of digestion, *glucose* (commonly known as sugar), for energy. After a meal, the normal digestive system breaks some food down into glucose. The blood carries the glucose or sugar throughout the body, causing blood glucose levels to rise. In response to this rise, the hormone *insulin* is released into the bloodstream and signals the body tissues to metabolize or burn the glucose for fuel, which causes blood glucose levels to return to normal. The glucose that the body does not use right away is stored in the liver, muscle, or fat.

In both types of diabetes, however, this normal process malfunctions. A gland called the *pancreas*, found just behind the stomach, makes insulin. In people with insulin-dependent diabetes, the pancreas does not produce insulin at all. This condition usually begins in childhood and is known as Type I (formerly called *juvenile-onset*) diabetes. These patients must have daily insulin injections to survive. People with non-insulin-dependent diabetes usually produce some insulin in their pancreas, but the body's tissues do not respond very well to the insulin signal and therefore do not metabolize the glucose properly, a condition known as *insulin resistance*.

Insulin resistance is an important factor in non-insulin-dependent diabetes, and scientists are searching for the causes of insulin resistance. They have identified two possibilities. The first is that there could be a defect in the insulin receptors on cells. Like an appliance that needs to be plugged into an electrical outlet, insulin has to bind to a receptor in order to function. Several things can go wrong with receptors. For example, there may not be enough receptors for insulin to bind to, or a defect in the receptors may prevent insulin from binding. The second possible cause of insulin resistance is that, although insulin may bind to the receptors, the cells do not read the signal to metabolize the glucose. Scientists continue to study these cells to see why this might happen.

A National Institutes of Health panel of experts recommends that the best treatment for non-insulin-dependent diabetes is a diet that helps one maintain a normal weight and pays particular attention to a proper balance of the different food groups. Many experts, including those in the American Diabetes Association, recommend that 50% to 60% of daily calories come from carbohydrates, 12% to 20% from protein, and no more than 30% from fat. Foods that are rich in carbohydrates, like breads, cereals, fruits, and vegetables, break down into glucose during digestion, causing blood glucose to rise. Additionally, studies have shown that cooked foods raise blood glucose higher than raw, unpeeled foods. A doctor or nutritionist should always be consulted for more information and for help in planning a diet to offset the effects of this form of diabetes.

37. The second paragraph is chiefly concerned with how diabetes affects the body's ability to use
  a. energy.
  b. blood.
  c. insulin.
  d. sugar.

38. Which of the following are the same for Type I and Type II diabetes?
  a. treatments
  b. long-term health risks
  c. short-term effects
  d. causes

39. Blood glucose rises after eating food rich in
  a. protein.
  b. calories.
  c. vitamins.
  d. carbohydrates.

40. A diet dominated by which of the following is recommended for non-insulin-dependent diabetics?
  a. protein
  b. fat
  c. carbohydrates
  d. raw foods

41. Which of the following is the main function of insulin?
  a. It signals tissues to metabolize sugar.
  b. It breaks down food into glucose.
  c. It carries glucose throughout the body.
  d. It binds to receptors.

42. Which of the following statements best summarizes the main theme of the passage?
   a. Type I and Type II diabetes are best treated by maintaining a high protein diet.
   b. Type II diabetes is a distinct condition that can be managed by maintaining a healthy diet.
   c. Type I diabetes is an insidious condition most harmful when the patient is not taking daily insulin injections.
   d. Adults who suspect they may have Type II diabetes should immediately adopt a high carbohydrate diet.

43. Which of the following is mentioned in the passage as a possible problem with insulin receptors in insulin-resistant individuals?
   a. Overeating causes the receptors not to function properly.
   b. There may be an overabundance of receptors present.
   c. A defect causes the receptors to bind with glucose.
   d. A defect hinders the receptors from binding with insulin.

YEAR	NUMBER OF DIABETES SUFFERERS IN THE U.S.
1995	7,765,000
1996	8,147,000
1997	8,462,000
1998	8,876,000
1999	9,269,000
2000	9,952,000
2001	10,699,000
2002	11,533,000
2003	12,466,000
2004	13,417,000
2005	14,473,000

44. Which of the following is true based on the table?
   a. Most of the people in the table have Type I diabetes.
   b. There will be fewer cases of diabetes as diabetes education increases.
   c. The passage was likely written in 2004.
   d. The U.S. has the highest population of diabetes sufferers in the world.

45. Based on the information in the passage, which of the following best describes people with Type I diabetes?
   a. They do not need to be treated with injections of insulin.
   b. They comprise the majority of people with diabetes.
   c. Their pancreases do not produce insulin.
   d. They are usually diagnosed as adults.

Section 3: Math

There are 50 questions in this section. You have 45 minutes to complete this section.

1. $4\frac{2}{5} + 3\frac{1}{2} + \frac{3}{8}$ is equal to
   a. $7\frac{3}{20}$.
   b. $7\frac{2}{5}$.
   c. $8\frac{11}{40}$.
   d. $8\frac{7}{8}$.

2. A doctor works nine hours and sees 32 patients. What is the average amount of time, to the nearest minute, that he spent with each patient?
   a. 170
   b. 17
   c. 28
   d. 225

3. A licensed practical nurse has to lift four patients during his eight-hour shift. The patients weigh 152 pounds, 168 pounds, 182 pounds, and 201 pounds. Approximately how many pounds will the nurse have to lift during his shift?
   a. 690 pounds
   b. 700 pounds
   c. 710 pounds
   d. 750 pounds

4. If $x = 6$, $y = -2$, and $z = 3$, what is the value of the following expression?
   $$\frac{xz - xy}{z^2}$$
   a. 5
   b. $3\frac{1}{3}$
   c. $\frac{2}{3}$
   d. $-\frac{2}{3}$

5. What is the area of a triangle with a height of 10 inches and a base of 2 inches?
   a. 10 square inches
   b. 12 square inches
   c. 20 square inches
   d. 22 square inches

6. It takes a medical transcriptionist 0.75 seconds to transcribe one word. At this rate, how many words can be transcribed in 60 seconds?
   a. 4.5
   b. 8
   c. 45
   d. 80

7. If $\frac{x}{2} + \frac{x}{6} = 4$, what is x?
   a. $\frac{1}{24}$
   b. $\frac{1}{6}$
   c. 3
   d. 6

8. $10^5 \div 10^2$ is equal to
   a. 10.
   b. 10^3.
   c. 10^7.
   d. 10^{10}.

9. $3.16 \div 0.079$ is equal to
   a. 0.025.
   b. 2.5.
   c. 4.0.
   d. 40.0.

10. $2\frac{5}{8} \div \frac{1}{3}$ is equal to
    a. $8\frac{1}{3}$.
    b. $7\frac{7}{8}$.
    c. $5\frac{11}{24}$.
    d. $\frac{7}{8}$.

11. What is the area of the following figure?

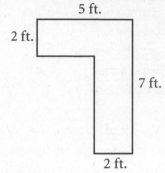

5 ft.

2 ft.

7 ft.

2 ft.

   a. 19 square feet
   b. 20 square feet
   c. 24 square feet
   d. 38 square feet

12. What is $7\frac{1}{5}\%$ of 465, rounded to the nearest tenth?
   a. 32.5
   b. 33
   c. 33.5
   d. 34

13. At a hospital 855 nurses, or 57% of all the nurses, are bilingual. How many nurses does the hospital have?
   a. 86
   b. 488
   c. 1,500
   d. 15,000

14. On the following number line, point L is to be located halfway between points M and N. What number will correspond to point L?

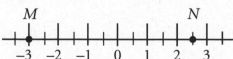

M   N

−3 −2 −1 0 1 2 3

   a. $-\frac{1}{4}$
   b. $-\frac{1}{2}$
   c. $-1\frac{1}{4}$
   d. 0

15. What kind of polygon is the following figure?

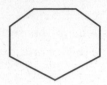

   a. pentagon
   b. octagon
   c. hexagon
   d. heptagon

16. Which of the following is equivalent to $2y^2$?
   a. $2y(y)$
   b. $2(y + y)$
   c. $y^2 + 2$
   d. $y + y + y + y$

17. 367.08×0.15 is equal to
   a. 22.0248.
   b. 55.051.
   c. 55.062.
   d. 540.62.

18. $(-10) + (-4) + (\frac{1}{2}) - (-\frac{1}{4})$ is equal to
   a. $-5\frac{3}{4}$.
   b. $-6\frac{1}{4}$.
   c. $-13\frac{1}{4}$.
   d. $-13\frac{3}{4}$.

19. Solve the equation $2(x - 14) = -6(-3x - 4)$ for x.
   a. $x = -\frac{13}{4}$
   b. $x = \frac{13}{4}$
   c. $x = 13$
   d. $x = -\frac{1}{4}$

20. What is the volume of a pyramid that has a rectangular base 5 feet by 3 feet and a height of 8 feet? ($V = \frac{1}{3}lwh$)
   a. 16 cubic feet
   b. 30 cubic feet
   c. 40 cubic feet
   d. 120 cubic feet

21. What is another way to write 7.25×10^3?
   a. 72,500
   b. 7,250
   c. 725
   d. 72.5

22. If $8n + 25 = 65$, then n is
   a. 5.
   b. 10.
   c. 40.
   d. 90.

23. What is the reciprocal of $3\frac{7}{8}$?
   a. $\frac{8}{31}$
   b. $\frac{31}{8}$
   c. $\frac{8}{2}$
   d. $-\frac{31}{8}$

24. Evaluate the expression $z(x^2 - y)$ for $x = 3$, $y = 2$, and $z = -5$.
   a. 35
   b. 10
   c. −10
   d. −35

25. $\sqrt{400} + \sqrt{625}$ is equal to
   a. 20.
   b. 45.
   c. 40.
   d. 30.

26. A hospital emergency room receives an admission on August 3 at 10:42 P.M. and another admission at 1:19 A.M. on August 4. How much time has elapsed between admissions?
   a. 1 hour 37 minutes
   b. 2 hours 23 minutes
   c. 2 hours 37 minutes
   d. 3 hours 23 minutes

27. A nurse currently receives a yearly salary of $69,000. He will make $72,450 next year. What percent increase did he receive?
   a. 5%
   b. 2.5%
   c. 15%
   d. 10%

28. Which of the following hospital rooms has the greatest perimeter?
   a. a rectangular room 12 feet × 8 feet
   b. a rectangular room 14 feet × 7 feet
   c. a square room 10 feet × 10 feet
   d. a square room 11 feet × 11 feet

29. A person can be scalded by hot water at a temperature of about 122°F. At about what temperature Centigrade could a person be scalded?
$C = \frac{5}{9}(F - 32)$
   a. 35.5°C
   b. 50°C
   c. 55°C
   d. 216°C

30. New nursing staff have to buy shoes to wear on duty at the full price of $84.50, but nurses who have worked in the hospital at least a year can get a 15% discount at a local shoe store, and nurses who have worked at least three years get an additional 10% off the discounted price. How much does a nurse who has worked at least three years have to pay for shoes?
a. $63.78
b. $64.65
c. $71.83
d. $72.05

31. There are 176 men and 24 women serving in a U.S. Army hospital. What percentage of the hospital's staff is women?
a. 12%
b. 14%
c. 16%
d. 24%

32. Body mass index (BMI) is equal to weight in kg divided by (height in m)^2. A man who weighs 64.8 kg has a BMI of 20. How tall is he?
a. 0.9 m
b. 1.8 m
c. 2.16 m
d. 3.24 m

33. Write an algebraic expression for the following phrase.
The cost of the surgery, x, is three times the sum of $4,000 and the cost of materials, y.
a. $x = 3(4,000 + y)$
b. $x = 3(4,000)$
c. $x = 3(4,000 + x)$
d. $x = 4,000 + y$

34. An insurance policy pays 80% of the first $20,000 of a certain patient's medical expenses, 60% of the next $40,000, and 40% of the $32,000 after that. If the patient's total medical bill is $92,000, how much will the policy pay?
a. $36,800
b. $49,600
c. $52,800
d. $73,600

35. A doctor can treat four Alzheimer's patients per hour; however, stroke patients need three times as much of the doctor's time. If the doctor treats patients six hours per day and has already treated ten Alzheimer's patients and three stroke patients today, how many more stroke patients will she have time to treat today?
a. one
b. two
c. three
d. five

36. If an ambulance travels at the speed of 62 mph for 15 minutes, how far will it travel?
a. 9.3 miles
b. 15.5 miles
c. 16 miles
d. 24.8 miles

37. What is the value of x in the following figure?

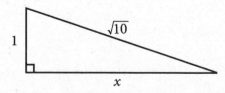

a. 2
b. 3
c. 5
d. 9

38. A-1 Painting was hired to paint a circular area in the entrance of a hospital. The diameter of the circle is 6 feet. What is the area of the circle? Use 3.14 for π.
   a. 452.16 square feet
   b. 37.68 square feet
   c. 18.84 square feet
   d. 113.04 square feet

39. Ron is half as old as Sam, who is three times as old as Ted. The sum of their ages is 55. How old is Ron?
   a. 5
   b. 10
   c. 15
   d. 30

40. The area of a triangle is 45 square feet. The length of the base of the triangle is 5 feet. What is the height of the triangle?
   a. 9 feet
   b. 10 feet
   c. 18 feet
   d. 5 feet

41. A floor plan is drawn to scale so that $\frac{1}{4}$ inch represents 2 feet. If a hall on the plan is 4 inches long, how long will the actual hall be when it is built?
   a. 2 feet
   b. 8 feet
   c. 16 feet
   d. 32 feet

42. 160% is equal to
   a. $\frac{4}{25}$.
   b. $\frac{3}{5}$.
   c. $\frac{6}{5}$.
   d. $\frac{8}{5}$.

43. What is the surface area of a cylinder that is 0.8 meters wide and 2 meters tall?
   a. 0.48π
   b. 0.96π
   c. 1.92π
   d. 3.84π

44. What is the value of x in the following figure?

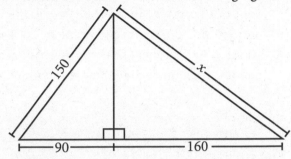

   a. 200
   b. 210
   c. 240
   d. 270

45. If the following figure is a regular decagon with a center at Q, what is the measure of the indicated angle?

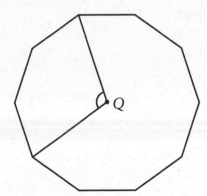

   a. 36°
   b. 45°
   c. 90°
   d. 108°

46. Which number is read as seven and ninety-one thousandths?
  a. 7.91
  b. 791.91
  c. 7.091
  d. 7.0091

47. If no treatment has been given within three hours after injury to a certain organ, the organ's function starts decreasing by 20% each hour. If no treatment has been given within six hours after injury, about how much function will remain?
  a. 50%
  b. 60%
  c. 70%
  d. 80%

48. A study shows that 600,000 women die each year in pregnancy and childbirth, one-fifth more than scientists previously estimated. How many such deaths did the scientists previously estimate?
  a. 120,000
  b. 300,000
  c. 480,000
  d. 500,000

49. To lower a fever of 105°, ice packs are applied for 1 minute and then removed for 5 minutes before being applied again. Each application lowers the fever by half a degree. How long will it take to lower the fever to 99°?
  a. 1 hour
  b. 1 hour 12 minutes
  c. 1 hour 15 minutes
  d. 1 hour 30 minutes

50. Fifteen milliliters of a solution separates into two liquids as shown in the following figure. The lighter liquid makes up what percentage of the total solution?

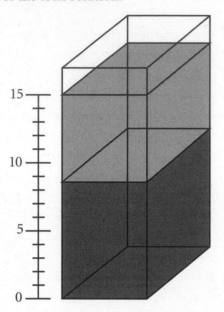

  a. 33%
  b. 40%
  c. 60%
  d. 66%

Section 4: General Science

There are 50 questions in this section. You have 45 minutes to complete this section.

1. Considering the four fundamental forces of physics, this one governs beta decay of radioactive atoms.
  a. strong nuclear force
  b. electromagnetism
  c. gravity
  d. weak nuclear force

2. What important event happened in 1957?
   a. first human to orbit Earth
   b. first landing of a rover on Mars
   c. first human landing on the Moon
   d. first satellite to be put in orbit

3. Common table salt, NaCl, forms from the attraction of positively charged sodium (Na^+) particles and negatively charged chloride (Cl^-) particles. What type of bond is this?
   a. covalent
   b. ionic
   c. metallic
   d. van der Waals

4. The parts of an atom that create the chemical bonds with other atoms are
   a. valence shells.
   b. nuclei.
   c. quark triplets.
   d. isotopes.

5. In this kind of bond between atoms, electrons are shared in pairs.
   a. ionic
   b. hydrogen
   c. van der Waals
   d. covalent

6. Consider the chemical reaction for photosynthesis: $6CO_2 + 6H_2O \rightarrow C_6H_{12}O_6 + \_\_\_\_ O_2$. How many molecules of oxygen (O_2) are made on the right-hand side (that is, what number goes in the blank space)?
   a. 6
   b. 1
   c. 12
   d. 4

7. In photosynthesis, the charge on the carbon in the reactant carbon dioxide is +4, the charge on the carbon in the resulting carbohydrate product is –4. In this reaction, the carbon is said to have been
   a. stripped.
   b. increased.
   c. neutralized.
   d. reduced.

8. Applying an amount of energy less than the heat of fusion to a liquid at the melting point of a particular substance does what?
   a. settles the liquid
   b. warms the liquid
   c. starts to solidify the liquid
   d. evaporates the liquid

9. The basic building blocks of protein are
   a. amino acids.
   b. nucleic acids.
   c. carbohydrates.
   d. lipids.

10. Which is an example of an inorganic material?
   a. blood hemoglobin
   b. quartz
   c. DNA
   d. wood

11. Which biome is characterized by trees that lose their leaves every winter?
   a. boreal forest
   b. tropical rain forest
   c. temperate deciduous forest
   d. tundra

12. Which unit of energy is equivalent to a Newton-meter?
   a. joule
   b. watt
   c. volt
   d. calorie

13. Crude oil originates from
   a. ancient fossilized organic materials.
   b. the natural metabolic processes of plants and organisms.
   c. minerals subjected to high temperatures and pressures.
   d. coal deposits that have liquefied.

14. Albert Einstein developed the
   a. wave theory of light.
   b. general theory of relativity.
   c. three laws of motion.
   d. theory of universal gravitation.

15. Density is the relationship between an object's mass and its volume. It can be measured in grams per cubic centimeter (g/cm^3). A student shakes a jar containing pure water (density = $1.00 \ g/cm^3$), olive oil (density = $0.80 \ g/cm^3$), and saltwater (density = $1.03 \ g/cm^3$) and observes the liquids as they settle out. Starting at the top of the jar and working down, in what order will the liquids settle?
   a. saltwater, olive oil, pure water
   b. olive oil, saltwater, pure water
   c. saltwater, pure water, olive oil
   d. olive oil, pure water, saltwater

16. All forms of energy can be converted at maximum efficiency into
   a. mechanical motion.
   b. electricity.
   c. potential energy.
   d. heat.

17. When entropy decreases, what else must be true?
   a. Entropy must increase on some larger scale.
   b. The decrease must be at the level of the universe.
   c. A mistake was made in the calculation.
   d. Entropy is adjusted to a flow of heat.

18. Which scientist, often called the father of modern science, was tried for heresy by the Roman Inquisition and forced to spend the rest of his life under house arrest?
   a. Isaac Newton
   b. Johannes Kepler
   c. Galileo Galilei
   d. Nikola Tesla

19. When a crane at a building site lifts a beam to its top height, what type of energy is created?
   a. kinetic energy
   b. potential energy
   c. chemical energy
   d. electrical energy

20. Your body operates on
   a. gravitational potential energy.
   b. electrical energy.
   c. chemical potential energy.
   d. nuclear energy.

21. Entomology is the study of
   a. birds.
   b. plants.
   c. insects.
   d. mammals.

22. Bernoulli's Principle states that as the speed of a fluid increases, pressure within the fluid decreases. This explains why it may be helpful to do what to a house during a tornado?
a. open the windows
b. turn off the electricity
c. shut off the main water valve
d. close interior doors

23. Penicillin is a group of antibiotics derived from
a. bacteria.
b. fungi.
c. plants.
d. animals.

24. In the ribosomes, which all cells have, what important cell process occurs?
a. DNA is duplicated.
b. Proteins are assembled.
c. Cell membranes are synthesized.
d. Cell nuclei are degraded.

25. Groups of DNA bases that code for types of amino acids occur as
a. quintuplets.
b. doublets.
c. triplets.
d. quadruplets.

26. In the universal tree of life, derived from comparing the rRNA possessed by all living forms, what does the *r* stand for?
a. rhizocyclic
b. retrospiral
c. recentible
d. ribosomal

27. Liposomes formed from lipids might be naturally occurring structures that formed the precursors for what later structure of cells?
a. immune systems
b. enzymes
c. nuclei
d. membranes

28. In the evolutionary sense, which is most closely related to *Tyrannosaurus rex*?
a. today's rattlesnakes
b. today's pigeons
c. today's lobsters
d. today's frogs

29. If a cell has an organelle called a chloroplast, which type of cell is it?
a. bikaryotic
b. prokaryotic
c. eukaryotic
d. postkaryotic

30. Which of the following places the levels of ecological organization in order from least to most inclusive?
a. population, community, ecosystem, biome
b. biome, ecosystem, community, population
c. ecosystem, population, biome, community
d. community, ecosystem, biome, population

31. Which of the following is true about a hypothesis?
a. It cannot be revised.
b. It can never be proven.
c. It is based on a theory.
d. It is formed before observations are made.

32. What were two evolutionary innovations that led to trees?
a. flowers and cellulose
b. cellulose and xylem
c. xylem and blastula
d. blastula and flowers

33. The bifocal lens was invented by
   a. Thomas Edison.
   b. Benjamin Franklin.
   c. Albert Einstein.
   d. John Isaac Hawkins.

34. What type of organism has an embryonic stage called a *blastula*?
   a. plants
   b. fungi
   c. animals
   d. bacteria

35. What best describes the evolutionary events that were happening around 265 MYA?
   a. radiation of reptiles
   b. origin of life
   c. extinction of the dinosaurs
   d. emergence of australopithecines

36. In plants, which type of vascular tissue takes food made in the leaves all the way down to the roots?
   a. xylem
   b. trachea
   c. capillaries
   d. phloem

37. We know that the Cretaceous-Paleogene (Cretaceous-Tertiary) mass extinction, which killed off the dinosaurs and many other species, was caused from an impact of a giant object from space, because of
   a. a worldwide clay layer that contains lots of the element iridium.
   b. charcoal evidence of worldwide forest fires.
   c. chemical signatures of massive amounts of sulfuric acid aerosols in the atmosphere.
   d. mutations in the surviving organisms caused by UV radiation after the ozone layer was destroyed.

38. A 1,500 kg car traveling at 100 km/h has the same momentum as which of the following cars?
   a. 1,000 kg car traveling at 100 km/h
   b. 1,500 kg car traveling at 50 km/h
   c. 2,000 kg car traveling at 100 km/h
   d. 3,000 kg car traveling at 50 km/h

39. The intensity of an earthquake is measured by what instrument?
   a. altimeter
   b. electrometer
   c. seismometer
   d. spectrometer

40. The first *Homo sapiens* appeared about 150,000 years ago. Approximately how many times longer did dinosaurs roam Earth compared to *Homo sapiens* to this point?
   a. 10
   b. 100
   c. 1,000
   d. 10,000

41. The first American to orbit Earth was
   a. John Glenn.
   b. Neil Armstrong.
   c. Buzz Aldrin.
   d. Mike Adams.

42. If you were a scientist investigating the origin of human social bonding, you would be in the field of
   a. evolutionary psychology.
   b. reversible geology.
   c. physical anthropology.
   d. revolutionary biology.

43. Of the organisms listed, which evolved the most recently?
   a. *Australopithecus*
   b. cyanobacteria
   c. fungi
   d. lichen

44. Considering human ancestry, which of the following is the most distantly related to humans?
   a. bonobo
   b. chimp
   c. gorilla
   d. orangutan

45. If an aqueous solution is alkaline, it is
   a. acidic.
   b. basic.
   c. neutral.
   d. ionic.

46. Alfred Wegener developed the theory of
   a. ice ages.
   b. dinosaur extinction.
   c. polar wander.
   d. continental drift.

47. What is a subduction zone?
   a. places where currents fall toward Earth's core
   b. places where magma oozes downward from a volcano
   c. places where ocean crust plunges toward the mantle
   d. places where currents in the ocean head toward the bottom

48. The Principle of Superposition states that in a sequence of undisturbed rock layers, the oldest rock layer can be found at the bottom of the sequence and the youngest layer on top of the sequence. Why is this principle useful for geologists?
   a. Geologists use this information to reconstruct past tectonic activity.
   b. It provides geologists with exact dates of rock layer formation.
   c. Geologists can use it to determine the type of environment in which the rock layers formed.
   d. It can be used to determine the relative ages of the rock layers.

49. Which geologic timespan accounts for 85% of Earth's history, beginning with Earth's formation and lasting up until about 540 million years ago?
   a. Cenozoic
   b. Precambrian
   c. Paleozoic
   d. Pleistocene

50. Until fairly recently, mammoths roamed Earth during a series of ice ages. This time is called the
   a. Pleistocene.
   b. Anthropocene.
   c. Miocene.
   d. Oligocene.

Section 5: Biology

There are 50 questions in this section. You have 45 minutes to complete this section.

1. Autotrophs are most likely to have which organelle(s)?
   a. Golgi apparatus
   b. chloroplasts
   c. lysosomes
   d. mitochondria

2. In most flowering plants, water moves upward from the roots via which of the following structures?
   a. sieve tubes
   b. phloem
   c. stomata
   d. xylem

3. A third copy of a chromosome is an example of
   a. haploidy.
   b. diplody.
   c. polyploidy.
   d. aneuploidy.

4. The reproductive organ of a plant that is responsible for pollen production is known as the
   a. carpel.
   b. pistil.
   c. stamen.
   d. stigma.

5. Which of the following is a rod-shaped bacteria?
   a. *Lactobacillus*
   b. *Streptococcus*
   c. *Vibrio cholerae*
   d. *Spirillum*

6. Swelling that occurs due to excess fluid accumulating in interstitial spaces is known as
   a. effusion.
   b. erythema.
   c. edema.
   d. progenesis.

7. Pyruvate is converted to carbon dioxide and ethanol during which of the following processes?
   a. photosynthesis
   b. glycolysis
   c. alcoholic fermentation
   d. oxidation

8. Self-fertilization may also be referred to as
   a. syngamy.
   b. autogamy.
   c. allogamy.
   d. incompatibility.

9. The embryological process by which a fertilized ovum divides is known as
   a. the G_2 phase.
   b. the M phase.
   c. cleavage.
   d. cytokinesis.

10. A cell spends most of its time in which stage of the cell cycle?
    a. anaphase
    b. interphase
    c. metaphase
    d. prophase

11. According to Linnaeus's classification system, which of the following groups is the most specific (i.e., has the smallest number of organisms)?
    a. phylum
    b. genus
    c. class
    d. order

12. More than 80% of all the known species of animals belong to the phylum
    a. Mollusca.
    b. Arthropoda.
    c. Echinodermata.
    d. Chordata.

13. Which of the following is the main function of the gallbladder?
    a. to produce enzymes
    b. to digest fats
    c. to produce bile
    d. to store bile

14. Essential amino acids
    a. must be supplied by diet.
    b. are not endogenously synthesized.
    c. include phenylalanine, threonine, and valine.
    d. all of the above

15. The last and longest portion of the small intestine is called the
    a. ascending colon.
    c. jejunum.
    b. duodenum.
    d. ileum.

16. About how much blood does the average person have in his or her body?
    a. 2.5 to 3 liters
    b. 4.5 to 5 liters
    c. 6 to 7 liters
    d. 8 to 9.5 liters

17. Blood from the lungs travels to the left atrium of the heart through the
    a. aorta.
    b. superior vena cava.
    c. pulmonary artery.
    d. pulmonary veins.

18. A person with phenylketoneuria should limit intake of what amino acid?
    a. tyrosine
    b. phenylalanine
    c. histidine
    d. asparagine

19. Transfusion of incorrect blood types results in
    a. excess production.
    b. chemical reduction of hemoglobin.
    c. agglutination of erythrocytes.
    d. lymphocytosis.

20. Plants differ from animals because plants
    a. cannot live in water.
    b. have cell walls.
    c. are prokaryotes.
    d. do not have specialized tissues.

21. The hypothalamus stimulates the pituitary gland to secrete vasopressin when
    a. the amount of water in the blood is too low.
    b. a woman's estrogen level increases.
    c. the thyroid is not functioning properly.
    d. insulin production is too high.

22. A bacteriophage can be described as
    a. a bacterium that causes illness.
    b. a virus that infects bacteria.
    c. a bacteria-fighting organelle.
    d. an inner membrane of bacteria.

23. Which of the following is characteristic of smooth, or nonstriated, muscles?
   a. They are voluntary muscles, controlled at will.
   b. When viewed under a microscope, they have a striped appearance.
   c. They make up the walls of the hollow organs of the body.
   d. They are not stimulated by nerves.

24. Contraction of the biceps muscle causes the
   a. elbow joint to bend.
   b. arm to straighten.
   c. triceps muscle to contract simultaneously.
   d. shoulder to relax.

25. Which of the following is true of a resting neuron?
   a. There is an equal concentration of both sodium and potassium within the cell.
   b. The cell membrane becomes more permeable, and a flow of sodium and potassium ions causes a depolarization.
   c. The concentration of sodium outside the cell is higher than it is inside; the concentration of potassium inside the cell is lower than it is outside.
   d. The concentration of sodium outside the cell is higher than it is inside; the concentration of potassium inside the cell is higher than it is outside.

26. What is the main function of the cerebellum?
   a. to control respiration and heartbeat
   b. to coordinate skeletal movements
   c. to determine personality
   d. to act as a relay center between the cerebrum and the medulla

27. Which organelle has the main function of providing the cell with energy?
   a. nucleus
   b. ribosomes
   c. mitochondria
   d. endoplasmic reticulum

28. Which of the following is an example of an exocrine gland?
   a. pineal
   b. pituitary
   c. salivary
   d. adrenal

29. Urine produced by the kidneys first flows into which structure?
   a. bladder
   b. ureter
   c. urethra
   d. adrenal gland

30. In plants, the reverse reaction of photosynthesis is
   a. anabolism.
   b. fermentation.
   c. oxidation.
   d. respiration.

31. The ventricles are actively filled during which phase of the cardiac cycle?
   a. atrial systole
   b. atrial diastole
   c. ventricular systole
   d. valvular stenosis

32. In pea plants, purple flower color (P) is dominant to white flower color (p). If two pea plants with genotypes Pp are crossed, what percentage of the offspring would be expected to have purple flowers?
   a. 25%
   b. 50%
   c. 75%
   d. 100%

33. Which of the following is the site of protein synthesis within a eukaryotic cell?
  a. the ribosomes
  b. the nucleus
  c. the mitochondria
  d. the Golgi apparatus

34. Hypertension is commonly known as
  a. high blood pressure.
  b. diabetes.
  c. high cholesterol.
  d. arthritis.

35. Nutrients, wastes, and gases are exchanged between maternal and fetal blood via the
  a. placenta.
  b. amnion.
  c. yolk sac.
  d. fallopian tube.

36. The gene for blue eyes is recessive. If your mother has blue eyes and your brown-eyed father has one gene for blue eyes and one for brown eyes, what are your chances of having blue eyes?
  a. 100%
  b. 75%
  c. 50%
  d. 25%

37. On some invertebrates, which of the following are the bristle-like, hollow, or chitinous outgrowths of the epidermis?
  a. the setae
  b. the cilia
  c. the hair
  d. the whiskers

38. A low hematocrit is a symptom of
  a. anemia.
  b. atherosclerosis.
  c. type I diabetes.
  d. arthritis.

39. What are the tiny air sacs where exchange of respiratory gases occurs in mammals and reptiles?
  a. the bronchioles
  b. the bronchi
  c. the sinuses
  d. the alveoli

40. During anaphase of mitosis, chromosomes separate into two sister
  a. alleles.
  b. centrosomes.
  c. chromatids.
  d. homologues.

41. Which of the following is the bony material perforated by tiny canals containing nerve cells in human teeth?
  a. gingiva
  b. pulp
  c. enamel
  d. dentin

42. Macular degeneration is a condition affecting what organ?
  a. the kidney
  b. the liver
  c. the eye
  d. the brain

43. A symbiotic relationship where one member benefits and the other is unaffected is known as
  a. mutualism.
  b. commensalism.
  c. parasitism.
  d. predation.

44. Which of the following is considered an accessory organ in the digestive system?
  a. the anus
  b. the liver
  c. the esophagus
  d. the pharynx

45. Which of the following would be considered an acquired characteristic?
  a. the large muscles of a weight lifter
  b. the appendix of a human being
  c. the nocturnal vision of an owl
  d. the large ears of a rabbit

46. What is the fluid found in animals with open circulatory systems?
  a. blood
  b. adrenaline
  c. hemolymph
  d. protoplasm

47. The human pelvic girdle consists of the ischium, pubis, and
  a. scapulae.
  b. clavicles.
  c. sternum.
  d. ilium.

48. The volume of air that remains in the lungs after strenuous exhalation is the
  a. volume capacity.
  b. residual volume.
  c. tidal volume.
  d. vital capacity.

49. Groups of three nucleotides that specify a particular amino acid to be added in a protein sequence are known as
  a. base pairs.
  b. chromosomes.
  c. genes.
  d. codons.

50. The formation of rhizomes is an example of which type of asexual reproduction?
  a. fragmentation
  b. binary fission
  c. budding
  d. vegetative reproduction

1 IA																	18 VIIIA
1 **H** 1.00794	2 IIA											13 IIIA	14 IVA	15 VA	16 VIA	17 VIIA	2 **He** 4.002602
3 **Li** 6.941	4 **Be** 9.012182											5 **B** 10.811	6 **C** 12.0107	7 **N** 14.00674	8 **O** 15.9994	9 **F** 8.9984032	10 **Ne** 20.1797
11 **Na** 22.989770	12 **Mg** 24.3050	3 IIIB	4 IVB	5 VB	6 VIB	7 VIIB	8	9 VIIIB	10	11 IB	12 IIB	13 **Al** 26.981538	14 **Si** 28.0855	15 **P** 30.973761	16 **S** 32.066	17 **Cl** 35.4527	18 **Ar** 39.948
19 **K** 39.0983	20 **Ca** 40.078	21 **Sc** 44.955910	22 **Ti** 47.867	23 **V** 50.9415	24 **Cr** 51.9961	25 **Mn** 54.938049	26 **Fe** 55.845	27 **Co** 58.933200	28 **Ni** 58.6934	29 **Cu** 63.546	30 **Zn** 65.39	31 **Ga** 69.723	32 **Ge** 72.61	33 **As** 74.92160	34 **Se** 78.96	35 **Br** 79.904	36 **Kr** 83.80
37 **Rb** 85.4678	38 **Sr** 87.62	39 **Y** 88.90585	40 **Zr** 91.224	41 **Nb** 92.90638	42 **Mo** 95.94	43 **Tc** (98)	44 **Ru** 101.07	45 **Rh** 102.90550	46 **Pd** 106.42	47 **Ag** 107.8682	48 **Cd** 112.411	49 **In** 114.818	50 **Sn** 118.710	51 **Sb** 121.760	52 **Te** 127.60	53 **I** 126.90447	54 **Xe** 131.29
55 **Cs** 132.90545	56 **Ba** 137.327	57 **La*** 138.9055	72 **Hf** 178.49	73 **Ta** 180.9479	74 **W** 183.84	75 **Re** 186.207	76 **Os** 190.23	77 **Ir** 192.217	78 **Pt** 195.078	79 **Au** 196.96655	80 **Hg** 200.59	81 **Tl** 204.3833	82 **Pb** 207.2	83 **Bi** 208.98038	84 **Po** (209)	85 **At** (210)	86 **Rn** (222)
87 **Fr** (223)	88 **Ra** (226)	89 **Ac**** (227)	104 **Rf** (265)	105 **Db** (268)	106 **Sg** (271)	107 **Bh** (270)	108 **Hs** (277)	109 **Mt** (276)	110 **Ds** (281)	111 **Rg** (280)	112 **Cn** (285)	113 **Nh** (286)	114 **Fl** (289)	115 **Mc** (289)	116 **Lv** (293)	117 **Ts** (294)	118 **Og** (294)

* Lanthanide series	58 **Ce** 140.116	59 **Pr** 140.90765	60 **Nd** 144.24	61 **Pm** (145)	62 **Sm** 150.36	63 **Eu** 151.964	64 **Gd** 157.25	65 **Tb** 158.92534	66 **Dy** 162.50	67 **Ho** 164.93032	68 **Er** 167.26	69 **Tm** 168.93421	70 **Yb** 173.04	71 **Lu** 174.967
** Actinide series	90 **Th** 232.0381	91 **Pa** 231.03588	92 **U** 238.0289	93 **Np** (237)	94 **Pu** (244)	95 **Am** (243)	96 **Cm** (247)	97 **Bk** (247)	98 **Cf** (251)	99 **Es** (252)	100 **Fm** (257)	101 **Md** (258)	102 **No** (259)	103 **Lr** (262)

Section 6: Chemistry

There are 50 questions in this section. You have 45 minutes to complete this section. Use the periodic table on page 310 to help you answer the questions when necessary.

1. Which of the following has the greatest mass?
   a. one water molecule
   b. one mole of electrons
   c. one mole of protons
   d. five molecules of benzene

2. Which of the following is immiscible with water?
   a. HCl
   b. CCl_4
   c. methanol
   d. KOH

3. How many moles of hydrogen are in 18.0 g H_2O?
   a. one
   b. two
   c. nine
   d. 18

4. The reaction $Fe_2O_3 + 2Al \rightarrow 2Fe + Al_2O_3$ is best classified as what type of reaction?
   a. double displacement reaction
   b. oxidation-reduction reaction
   c. acid–base reaction
   d. decomposition reaction

5. Which of the following elements is in period V of the periodic table?
   a. B
   b. N
   c. Nb
   d. Rb

6. Which of the following is a noble gas?
   a. xenon
   b. potassium
   c. iodine
   d. barium

7. What is the formula for cobalt (II) phosphate?
   a. $CoPO_4$
   b. Co_2PO_4
   c. $Co_3(PO_4)_2$
   d. $Co_2(PO_4)_3$

8. Which of the following choices best describes the structure of the class of molecules that is the major constituent of cell membranes?
   a. a carboxylic acid bonded to an amino group
   b. one molecule of glycerol bonded to three fatty acids
   c. one molecule of glycerol bonded to two fatty acids and one phosphate group
   d. one molecule of glycerol bonded to one fatty acid and two hydroxyl groups

9. Osmotic pressure is defined as
   a. the change in pressure of a liquid undergoing osmosis.
   b. pressure that must be applied to prevent net diffusion of pure solvent through a semipermeable membrane into solution.
   c. the combined pressure of gases in the external atmosphere of a system undergoing osmosis.
   d. pressure that is proportional to osmotic potential.

10. Which of the following is classified as an aldehyde?
    a. CH_4
    b. CH_2Cl_2
    c. $CH_3C(O)CH_3$
    d. $CH_3CH_2C(O)H$

11. The nuclear process $^{238}_{92}U \rightarrow\, ^{234}_{90}Th + ^4_2He$ is an example of
    a. α decay.
    b. β decay.
    c. γ emission.
    d. nuclear fusion.

12. What is the formula for bismuth (III) hydroxide?
    a. Bi_3OH
    b. $Bi(OH)_3$
    c. $Bi(OH)_2$
    d. $BiOH$

13. What are the products of the reaction between sodium metal and water?
    a. $NaH^+_{(aq)} + OH^-_{(aq)}$
    b. $NaOH_{(aq)} + H_{2(g)}$
    c. $Na_{(s)} + H_{2(g)} + O_{2(g)}$
    d. $NaOH_{(aq)} + H_{2(g)} + O_{2(g)}$

14. Which best describes the following redox reaction:
    $Br^-_{(aq)} + MnO^-_{4(aq)} \rightarrow Br_{2(l)} + Mn^{+2}_{(aq)}$?
    a. Br and Mn are both reduced.
    b. Br is oxidized and Mn is reduced.
    c. Br is oxidized and O is reduced.
    d. Br is reduced and Mn is oxidized.

15. Which type of bonding occurs in ammonia (NH_3)?
    a. covalent
    b. ionic
    c. metallic
    d. covalent network

16. Which of the following is a weak acid?
    a. HCl
    b. HNO_3
    c. H_2SO_4
    d. H_2CO_3

17. What is the molecular formula of a compound with empirical formula CH_2O and molar mass 90 g?
    a. CH_2O
    b. $C_3H_3O_3$
    c. $C_3H_6O_3$
    d. $C_6H_{14}O$

18. Which of the following has the largest radius?
    a. K
    b. Rb
    c. Ca
    d. Sr

19. Avogadro's number, 6.02×10^{23}, is equal to
    a. the number of atoms or molecules in one mole of any substance.
    b. the number of atoms or molecules in 1.0 gram of any substance.
    c. the number of carbon atoms in 1.0 gram of carbon.
    d. the number of atoms in 12.0 grams of any element.

20. Which of the following species is being oxidized in this redox reaction?
    $Zn_{(s)} + Cu^{2+}_{(aq)} \rightarrow Zn^{2+}_{(aq)} + Cu_{(s)}$
    a. $Zn_{(s)}$
    b. $Cu^{2+}_{(aq)}$
    c. $Zn^{2+}_{(aq)}$
    d. $Cu_{(s)}$

21. What is the oxidation number of nickel in nickel oxide (NiO_2)?
    a. +2
    b. +4
    c. −2
    d. −4

22. Which of the following is a key characteristic of the alkali metals?
a. highly stable
b. poor coductivity
c. highly reactive with water
d. gases at room temperature

23. β decay results in the emission of _____ from a heavy atom.
a. a helium nucleus
b. an electron
c. a proton
d. a high-energy photon

24. A "trans" fat describes fatty acids that contain
a. no C–C double bonds.
b. multiple C–C double bonds and some C–C single bonds.
c. at least one C–C double bond with a trans geometry.
d. only C–C double bonds.

25. Which of the following are the general products of a hydrocarbon combustion reaction?
a. $C_{(s)}$, O_2, and H_2
b. $C_{(s)}$, H_2O, and O_2
c. CO_2 and H_2
d. CO_2 and H_2O

26. The normal boiling point of water is 100°C. Suppose 256 grams of a compound with the formula $C_{10}H_8$ is dissolved in 5.15 kg of water. K_b of water is 0.52°C kg/mol. What is the change in the boiling point?
a. 0.2°
b. 0.05°
c. 0.4°
d. 2.0°

27. Which of the following has the greatest number of atoms?
a. 1.0 mol N
b. 1.0 g N
c. 1.0 mol NO_2
d. 0.5 mol NH_3

28. Which of the following equations describes the reaction between $Al_{(s)}$ and H_2SO_4?
a. $2Al_{(s)} + 3H_2SO_{4(aq)} \rightarrow Al_2(SO_4)_3 + 3H_{2(g)}$
b. $Al_{(s)} + H_2SO_{4(aq)} \rightarrow Al(SO_4) + H_{2(g)}$
c. $2Al_{(s)} + 3H_2SO_{4(aq)} \rightarrow Al_2(SO_3)_3 + 3H_2O_{(l)}$
d. No reaction occurs.

29. Which of the following is a transition metal?
a. lithium
b. iron
c. aluminum
d. tin

30. Which of the following is the probable charge for an ion formed from Ca?
a. +1
b. +2
c. −1
d. −2

31. Which of the following is the electron configuration of a neutral atom of Ca?
a. $[Ar]\, 3s^2$
b. $[Ar]\, 3d^2$
c. $[Ar]\, 4p^2$
d. $[Ar]\, 4s^2$

32. The phosphate buffer system helps maintain a relatively constant pH within living cells:

$$H_2PO_{4(aq)}^- \rightleftarrows H_{(aq)}^+ + HPO_{4(aq)}^{2-}$$

What happens to this equilibrium reaction if the interior of the cell becomes more acidic?
a. less HPO_4^{2-} is consumed
b. less $H_2PO_4^{2-}$ is produced
c. more H^+ is produced
d. more HPO_4^{2-} is consumed

33. What is the equilibrium constant, K_c, of the following reaction?

$$Xe_{(g)} + 2F_{2(g)} \rightleftarrows XeF_{4(g)}$$

a. $K_c = \dfrac{[XeF_4]}{[Xe][F_2]}$

b. $K_c = \dfrac{[Xe][F_2]}{[XeF_4]}$

c. $K_c = \dfrac{[XeF_4]}{[Xe][F_2]^2}$

d. $K_c = \dfrac{[Xe][F_2]^2}{[XeF_4]}$

34. What is the oxidation number of sodium in the following reaction? $Pb(NO_3)_{2(aq)} + 2NaI_{(aq)} \rightarrow PbI_{2(s)} + 2NaNO_{3(aq)}$

a. +1

b. +2

c. −1

d. −2

35. Carbon dating takes advantage of the beta decay of a carbon-14 isotope. Which of the following equations describes this decay?

a. $^{14}_{6}C \rightarrow {}^{13}_{5}B + {}^{1}_{1}H$

b. $^{14}_{6}C \rightarrow {}^{14}_{7}N + {}^{0}_{-1}\beta$

c. $^{14}_{6}C \rightarrow {}^{13}_{5}B + {}^{1}_{0}n$

d. $^{14}_{7}N + {}^{1}_{0}n \rightarrow {}^{14}_{6}C + {}^{1}_{1}H$

36. A dating technique involves electron capture by the potassium-40 isotope according to the following equation: $^{40}_{19}K + {}^{0}_{-1}e \rightarrow {}^{40}_{18}Ar$. If the half-life is 1.2×10^9 years, how long does it take for only 10 g to remain of the original 40 g of potassium-40 in a rock sample?

a. 1.2×10^9 years

b. 0.6×10^9 years

c. 2.4×10^9 years

d. 1.8×10^9 years

37. Which of the following elements is a member of the actinide series?

a. uranium

b. terbium

c. tellurium

d. radon

38. Which of the following is the symbol for the isotope with 18 protons and 22 neutrons?

a. $^{40}_{18}Ar$

b. $^{22}_{18}Ar$

c. $^{40}_{22}Ti$

d. $^{90}_{40}Zr$

39. Vanillin, the molecule shown here that is responsible for vanilla's taste and smell, possesses all of the following functional groups EXCEPT

a. aldehyde.

b. ketone.

c. alcohol.

d. ether.

40. What is the effect of the addition of a catalyst to a reaction in equilibrium?

a. The reaction favors the formation of the products.

b. The reaction favors the formation of the reactants.

c. There is no change in composition of the reaction.

d. The rate of the reaction slows.

41. Which of the following pairs are allotropes?
   a. O_2 and O_3
   b. Fe^{2+} and Fe^{3+}
   c. OH^- and H_3O^+
   d. H_2O_2 and H_2O

42. A gas is held in a rigid 4 L container at 1 atm and 27°C. If the temperature is raised to 117°C, what will the pressure in the container be?
   a. 4.3 atm
   b. 0.77 atm
   c. 1.3 atm
   d. 0.23 atm

43. The combustion of methane with oxygen produces carbon dioxide and water:

$$CH_{4(g)} + 2O_{2(g)} \rightarrow CO_{2(g)} + 2H_2O_{(g)}$$

If 4.00 g of CH_4 and 4.00 g of O_2 are combusted in a closed container, what is the maximum amount of CO_2 that can be produced?
   a. 2.25 g
   b. 2.75 g
   c. 5.50 g
   d. 11.0 g

44. Which fuctional group characterizes carboxylic acid?
   a. COOH
   b. C=O
   c. OH
   d. C=C

45. Which of the following does NOT have the electron configuration [Ne] $3s^2 3p^6$?
   a. Cl
   b. S^{2-}
   c. K^+
   d. Ca^{2+}

46. Which of the following classes of molecules does NOT have a carbonyl group?
   a. ester
   b. amide
   c. aldehyde
   d. amine

47. If temperature and pressure are held constant for a sample of gas, and the number of moles is doubled, in what manner will the volume change?
   a. It will double.
   b. It will quadruple.
   c. It will be halved.
   d. There will be no change.

48. What will happen if a semipermeable membrane is placed between two different concentrations of a NaCl solution?
   a. The solute will move toward the higher concentration of NaCl.
   b. The solute will move toward the lower concentration of NaCl.
   c. The solvent will move toward the higher concentration of NaCl.
   d. The solvent will move toward the lower concentration of NaCl.

49. Ethyl acetate has the molecular formula $C_4H_8O_2$. What is the empirical formula of ethyl acetate?
   a. CHO
   b. C_2H_4O
   c. CH_2O
   d. C_2H_6O

50. Proteins are polymers of which of the following organic compounds?
   a. amino acids
   b. alkynes
   c. alcohols
   d. fatty acids

Answers

Section 1: Verbal Ability

1. a. commitment
2. c. ridiculous
3. b. respiratory
4. c. precise
5. b. assurance
6. a. frequently
7. c. development
8. a. concede
9. b. encouraging
10. c. phenomena
11. c. compatible
12. a. clinician
13. b. commencement
14. b. supervisor
15. b. pneumonia
16. c. annoyed
17. c. apparatus
18. c. codeine
19. a. accompany
20. b. incessant
21. b. dilemma
22. c. efficient
23. b. therapy
24. a. viewpoint
25. c. aggravated
26. c. arteries
27. a. alumni
28. a. announcement
29. c. aisle
30. b. sensible
31. a. heifer
32. a. association
33. b. rehearsal
34. c. fascinated
35. a. destructive
36. c. dissolve
37. a. illuminate
38. c. knowledge
39. b. meteorology
40. a. adjournment
41. c. vengeance
42. c. tremendous
43. b. immortality
44. c. capitalization
45. a. brilliant
46. b. parenthesis
47. c. weird
48. c. sonnet
49. a. depot
50. c. presume

Section 2: Reading Comprehension

1. b. See the third paragraph: *One in ten* (10% of) cases of anorexia end in death.

2. a. See the second and third paragraphs for reference to heart problems with anorexia, the fourth and fifth paragraphs for discussion of heart problems with bulimia, and the last paragraph, where heart disease is mentioned as a risk in obese people who suffer from binge-eating disorder.

3. c. Each answer choice can be a synonym of *withdrawn*, but in this context, only *introverted* describes the condition of being emotionally removed, which is how the word is used to describe people who suffer from anorexia in paragraph 3.

4. b. According to the second paragraph, the disorder *usually begins around the time of puberty*, which occurs during adolescence.

5. b. The first sentence of the fifth paragraph tells us that bulimia sufferers are often able to keep their problem a secret, partly because they maintain a normal or above-normal weight.

6. b. In the second paragraph, the thyroid gland function is mentioned as slowing down— one effort on the part of the body to protect itself.

7. a. According to the last paragraph, about 30% of people participating in medically supervised weight-control programs have binge-eating disorder.

8. **b.** As stated in the opening sentence of the fourth paragraph, bulimia patients may exercise obsessively.

9. **d.** The main idea of the passage is stated in the first paragraph: *all eating disorders share some common manifestations,* but *each has distinctive symptoms and risks.* Disorders and diseases are not the same things, and choice **b** is incorrect.

10. **b.** The author uses the phrase *going gray* as a metaphor for growing older. It describes the phenomenon of a large segment of a population growing older.

11. **d.** The passage emphasizes the need for age-specific care.

12. **c.** According to the fifth paragraph of the passage, depression is *a treatable condition that affects nearly five million seniors.*

13. **c.** The sixth paragraph is mainly about how the diverse ethnicities and races of patients raise new challenges for healthcare providers. Choice **c** is correct because it takes both race and ethnicity into account.

14. **b.** What the average life expectancy will be in 2080 can only be determined with speculation since no one can read the future.

15. **c.** See the second paragraph of the passage. It explains that as radon decays further it releases radiation and transforms into radon daughters.

16. **b.** That inert gases are chemically inactive can be inferred from the second paragraph, which says that radon is unlike its *chemically active* daughters.

17. **d.** The fifth paragraph says that the unattached daughters pose danger to the lungs because they can travel directly to those organs.

18. **a.** The fourth paragraph says that *plating out* is the process by which radon daughters attach to matter.

19. **a.** The sixth paragraph states that a study found an equal chance of getting cancer from exposure to the same amount of radon, X-rays, and atomic bombs.

20. **b.** The beginning of the second paragraph says that radon is formed as uranium and radium decay.

21. **d.** The answer to this question can be found in the first sentence of the third paragraph, which states that *radon gas released directly into the atmosphere poses slight health risks.*

22. **b.** The fifth paragraph describes torticollis and states that 10% to 20% of patients experience spontaneous remission, but it may not last long. Details also reveal it is the most common of focal dystonias, affects people at any age, and affects the neck muscles.

23. **d.** Emotional imbalance is not usually a feature of the dystonias, as stated in the last sentence of the first paragraph.

24. **a.** According to the fourth paragraph, torsion dystonia may be inherited.

25. **c.** Meige's syndrome combines symptoms of blepharospasm (affecting the eyes) and oromandibular dystonia (affecting the lips and tongue).

26. **a.** Both torticollis and cranial dystonia affect the neck and head, as indicated in the fifth and seventh paragraphs.

27. **d.** The first sentence of the last paragraph states that DRD patients can be successfully treated with drugs.

28. **a.** The second sentence states that dystonia-related movements are involuntary.

29. **c.** Cranial dystonia affects muscles in the head, face, and neck. Since it affects two or more adjacent body parts, cranial dystonia is a segmental dystonia.

30. d. Each answer choice can be used as a synonym of *progressive*, but the context of this particular passage must be used to determine the correct answer. It is used in the final paragraph of this passage to describe the increased difficulty in walking of children and adolescents who suffer from DRD.

31. d. See the second paragraph of the passage.

32. c. See the last paragraph of the passage.

33. d. The third paragraph deals with the nymph stage as a whole, including how larvae become nymphs by molting, how they affect human hosts, and when they mate.

34. a. See the first sentence of the passage.

35. b. The end of the second paragraph says that larval infection is a *rare occurrence*.

36. c. After the rash, which may or may not appear, the next symptoms are the flu-like symptoms listed in the fifth paragraph.

37. d. The second paragraph chiefly describes how diabetes makes it difficult for the body to use glucose, which is another name for sugar.

38. b. According to the end of the first paragraph, only the long-term health problems are the same for these two different disorders.

39. d. This answer choice can be found in the final paragraph of the passage, which states that *foods that are rich in carbohydrates, like breads, cereals, fruits, and vegetables, break down into glucose during digestion, causing blood glucose to rise.*

40. c. According to the last paragraph, non-insulin-dependent diabetics should stick to a diet consisting of 50% to 60% carbohydrates. The paragraph also notes that raw foods do not cause as high a blood sugar level as cooked foods.

41. a. The second and fourth paragraphs mention that the main role of insulin is to signal the burning of glucose/sugar for energy. Most hormones function as stimuli for other processes.

42. b. Type II, or non-insulin-dependent, diabetes is the main subject of the passage, which distinguishes Type II from Type I and goes on to stress the importance of diet.

43. d. The fourth paragraph of the passage says that possible problems with insulin receptors include a paucity of receptors or a defect causing improper binding of the insulin to the receptors.

44. c. The first paragraph of the passage indicates that *13 to 14 million people in the United States* have diabetes, and 2004 is the only year in the list indicating such an average. Although it is possible that this number has dropped since 2004, there is no way of knowing it from the passage and table, so choice **c** remains the likeliest answer.

45. c. Type I diabetes is the insulin-dependent form of this condition. The minority of diabetics are afflicted with this form. They are diagnosed as children and must take daily injections of insulin to make up for what their pancreases do not produce.

Section 3: Math

1. c. $4\frac{2}{5} + 3\frac{1}{2} + \frac{3}{8}$ can be rewritten: $4 + 3 + \frac{2}{5} + \frac{1}{2} + \frac{3}{8}$. To add the fractions, find the least common multiple of 5, 2, and 8, which is 40. Next, rewrite the problem: $7 + \frac{16}{40} + \frac{20}{40} + \frac{15}{40} = 7\frac{51}{40} = 8\frac{11}{40}$.

2. b. Multiply 9 by 60 to get 540 minutes in 9 hours. Then divide 540 by 32. The quotient is 16.875, or rounded to the nearest minute, 17 minutes.

3. b. Add all four weights for a total of 703; 703 rounded to the nearest tenth is 700.

4. b. Substitute the values into the given expression: $\frac{6(3)-6(-2)}{9}$ then becomes $\frac{18-(-12)}{9} = \frac{30}{9}$, or $3\frac{1}{3}$.

5. a. The formula to use here is $A = \frac{1}{2}bh$ or $A = \frac{1}{2}(10)(2) = 10$ square inches.

6. d. This problem is solved by dividing 60 by 0.75 to get 80.

7. d. First, find the least common denominator, which is 6. The equation then becomes $\frac{3x}{6} + \frac{x}{6} = 4$, or $\frac{4x}{6} = 4$. Multiply both sides by 6 to get $4x = 24$. Divide through by 4 to get $x = 6$.

8. b. To divide exponential expressions containing the same base, subtract the exponents.

9. d. This is a simple division problem as long as you keep the decimal values straight.

10. b. First, convert the mixed number in the numerator to a fraction: $\frac{21}{8}$. Then, invert the denominator and multiply: $(\frac{21}{8})(\frac{3}{1}) = \frac{63}{8}$, or $7\frac{7}{8}$.

11. b. To solve this problem, find the area of two rectangles and then add the results. Use an imaginary line to block off the first rectangle at the top of the figure. This rectangle measures 5 feet by 2 feet. Using the formula $A = lw$, this comes to 10 square feet. The second rectangle is also 5 feet by 2 feet. Add the two together for a total of 20 square feet.

12. c. Change the percent to a decimal and then multiply: $0.072 \times 465 = 33.48$, which, rounded to the nearest tenth, is 33.5.

13. c. Solve the problem: 855 is 57% of what number? Then solve $855 = 0.57x$. $x = \frac{855}{0.57} = 1,500$. There are 1,500 nurses.

14. a. The halfway point on the number line is between 0 and $-\frac{1}{2}$, which is $-\frac{1}{4}$.

15. d. A heptagon has seven sides.

16. a. To square y, multiply y times y.

17. c. This is a simple multiplication problem as long as you keep the decimal values straight.

18. c. Do the operations in order from left to right: $-10 + (-4) = -14$. Next, $-14 + \frac{1}{2} = -13\frac{1}{2}$. Then, $-13\frac{1}{2} - (-\frac{1}{4}) = -13\frac{1}{2} + \frac{1}{4} = -13\frac{1}{4}$.

19. a. $2(x - 14) = -6(-3x - 4)$. Multiply 2 by the terms in parentheses on the left side of the equation and multiply -6 by the terms in the parentheses on the right hand side: $2x - 28 = 18x + 24$. Then add 28 to both sides: $2x = 18x + 52$. Subtract $18x$ from both sides: $-16x = 52$. Divide both sides by -16 and reduce the fraction: $x = -\frac{52}{16} = -\frac{13}{4}$.

20. c. $(\frac{1}{3})(5)(3)(8) = 40$

21. b. $(7.25)(10)(10)(10) = 7,250$

22. a. Subtract 25 from both sides to get $8n = 40$, and divide both sides by 8 to get $n = 5$.

23. a. Convert the mixed number $3\frac{7}{8}$ to the improper fraction $\frac{31}{8}$ and then invert.

24. d. $z(x^2 - y) = -5(3^2 - 2) = -5(9 - 2) = -5(7) = -35$

25. b. $\sqrt{400} + \sqrt{625} = 20 + 25 = 45$

26. c. From 10:42 to 12:42, 2 hours have elapsed. From 12:42 to 1:00, another 18 minutes have elapsed ($60 - 42 = 18$). Next, between 1:00 and 1:19, there are another 19 minutes, for a total of 2 hours 37 minutes.

27. a. The salary increase $72,450 - $69,000 = $3,450. To calculate percentage increase, divide this increase of $3,450 by the original salary of $69,000 to get 0.05, which equals 5%.

28. d. First, you have to determine the perimeters of all four rooms. This is done by using the formula for a square ($P = 4s$), or for a rectangle ($P = 2l + 2w$), as follows: $(2 \times 12) + (2 \times 8) = 40$ for choice **a**; $(2 \times 14) + (2 \times 7) = 42$ for choice **b**; $4 \times 10 = 40$ for choice **c**; $4 \times 11 = 44$ for the correct answer, choice **d**.

29. b. Convert Fahrenheit to Centigrade using the formula given: $C = \frac{5}{9}(122 - 32)$; that is, $C = \frac{5}{9} \times 90$; so $C = 50°$.

30. b. You cannot just take 25% off the original price, because the 10% discount after three years of service is taken off the price that has already been reduced by 15%. Figure the problem in two steps: After the 15% discount, the price is $71.83. Ninety percent of that—subtracting 10%—is $64.65.

31. a. Add the number of men and number of women to get the total number of staff: 200. The number of women, 24, is 12% of 200.

32. b. Substituting known quantities into the formula yields $20 = \frac{64.8}{x^2}$. Next, multiply both sides by x^2 to get $20x^2 = 64.8$, and then divide through by 20 to get $x^2 = 3.24$. Now take the square root of both sides to get $x = 1.8$.

33. a. The sum of $4,000 and y is written as $4,000 + y$. Three times the sum of $4,000 and y is $3(4,000 + y)$. The correct translation of the sentence is $x = 3(4,000 + y)$.

34. c. You must break the 92,000 into the amounts mentioned in the policy: $92,000 = 20,000 + 40,000 + 32,000$. The amount the policy will pay is $(0.8)(20,000) + (0.6)(40,000) + (0.4)(32,000) = 16,000 + 24,000 + 12,800 = 52,800$.

35. a. Each Alzheimer's patient takes $\frac{1}{4}$ hour. Each stroke patient thus takes $\frac{3}{4}$ hour. The doctor has already spent $10(\frac{1}{4}) + 3(\frac{3}{4}) = \frac{10}{4} + \frac{9}{4} = \frac{19}{4} = 4\frac{3}{4}$ hours with patients today. Her 6-hour schedule minus $4\frac{3}{4}$ hours leaves $1\frac{1}{4}$ hours left to see patients. Since each stroke patient takes $\frac{3}{4}$ hour, the doctor has time to treat only one more stroke patient in the $1\frac{1}{4}$ hours remaining.

36. b. Solving this problem requires converting 15 minutes to 0.025 hour, which is the time, then using the formula *distance = rate × time*: 62 mph × 0.25 hour = 15.5 miles.

37. b. Use the Pythagorean theorem: $1^2 + x^2 = (\sqrt{10})^2$; $1 + x^2 = 10$, so $x^2 = 9$. Thus, $x = 3$.

38. d. The radius of the circle is $r = 6$. The formula for the area of a circle is given by $A = \pi r^2$. The area of the circle is $A = \pi 6^2 = (3.14)(36) = 113.04$ square feet.

39. c. Let T = Ted's age; S = Sam's age $= 3T$; R = Ron's age $= \frac{S}{2} = \frac{3T}{2}$. The sum of the ages is $\frac{3T}{2} + 3T + T = \frac{3T}{2} + \frac{6T}{2} + \frac{2T}{2} = \frac{11T}{2}$, which is equal to 55. Now multiply both sides of the resulting equation, $55 = \frac{11T}{2}$, by 2 to get $110 = 11T$. Divide through by 11 to get $10 = T$. That is Ted's age, so Sam is $3T = 3(10) = 30$ years old, and Ron is $\frac{S}{2} = \frac{30}{2} = 15$ years old.

40. c. The formula for the area of a triangle is $A = (\frac{1}{2})bh$. The value of b is 5, so $45 = (\frac{1}{2})(5)h$. Multiply both sides of the equation by 2 to get rid of the $(\frac{1}{2})$: $90 = 5h$. Divide both sides by 5: $18 = h$. The height is 18 feet.

41. d. Four inches is equal to 16 quarter inches. Since each quarter inch is 2 feet, multiply 16 by 2 to get 32 feet.

42. d. 160% is equal to $\frac{160}{100}$. Reduce this fraction by dividing both top and bottom by 20 to get $\frac{8}{5}$.

43. c. The surface area of a cylinder is equal to the area of the two circles on the top and bottom plus the area of a rectangle that is as tall as the cylinder and as wide as the circumference of the circles. The area of the two circles $= 2\pi r^2 = 2\pi(0.4)2 = 2\pi(0.16) = 0.32\pi$. The area of the rectangle is its height multiplied by the circumference of the circle $= 2(2\pi r) = 2(2\pi)(0.4) = 1.6\pi$. Now add: $0.32\pi + 1.6\pi = 1.92\pi$.

44. a. Use the Pythagorean formula to find the height of the smaller triangle:

$a^2 + b^2 = c^2$

$90^2 + b^2 = 150^2$

$8,100 + b^2 = 22,500$

$b^2 = 14,400$

$b = 120$, which is the height of both the smaller triangle and the larger triangle. Use the Pythagorean formula again to find the length of x:

$a^2 + b^2 = x^2$

$160^2 + 120^2 = x^2$

$40,000 = x^2$

$200 = x$

45. d. If the figure is a regular decagon, it can be divided into 10 equal sections by lines passing through the center. Two such lines form the indicated angle, which includes three of the 10 sections; $\frac{3}{10}$ of 360° = 108°.

46. c. 7.91 is read as *seven and ninety-one hundredths*. 791.91 is read as *seven hundred ninety-one and ninety-one hundredths*. 7.0091 is read as *seven and ninety-one hundred thousandths*.

47. a. At the end of three hours, the organ still has 100% function. After four hours, it has 80% of that 100%, or 0.8. After five hours, it has 80% of the 80% it had at the end of four hours: (0.8)(0.8) = 64%. After six hours, it has 80% of the 64% it had after five hours: (0.8)(0.64) = 0.512, or about 50%.

48. d. Let E = the estimate. One-fifth more than the estimate means $\frac{6}{5}$ or 120% of E, so 600,000 = 1.2(E). Divide both sides by 1.2 to get E = 500,000.

49. b. The difference between 105° and 99° is 6°. Application of the ice pack plus a resting period of 5 minutes before reapplication means that the temperature is lowered by half a degree every 6 minutes, or 1° every 12 minutes. Six degrees times 12 minutes per degree is 72 minutes, or 1 hour 12 minutes.

50. b. The lighter liquid is $\frac{6}{15}$, or $\frac{2}{5}$, of the total solution; $\frac{2}{5}$ = 0.4, or 40%.

Section 4: General Science

1. d. The weak nuclear force determines beta decay, which occurs when a neutron converts to a proton, with the ejection of an electron.

2. d. Sputnik 1 was the first satellite to be put into Earth's orbit in 1957 by the Soviet Union.

3. b. Ionic bonds form when oppositely charged ions attract in order to become neutral and stable. Sodium gives up its one outer shell electron leaving it with a +1 positive charge, and chlorine gains this electron, giving it a −1 charge. Together, they form the chemically neutral salt molecule NaCl.

4. a. The valence shell either gains or loses electrons to create bonds with other atoms. Valence means *strength* (think *valiant*).

5. d. The covalent bond is a shared pair of electrons, which "spend time" in both atoms, though often in one more than the other.

6. a. The number 6 brings the total number of oxygen atoms on the right-hand side to 18, the same as the total on the left-hand side, thereby balancing the reaction.

7. d. Reduction of an element in a chemical reaction occurs when its charge is numerically lowered (in this case, from +4 to −4).

8. b. The liquid is warmed. The heat of fusion is the amount of energy is takes to melt a solid, to turn it into liquid at the same temperature. Because our example is already liquid, applying any heat at all only warms it up. This may or may not also evaporate the liquid, we don't know without more information.

9. a. Amino acids combine to form proteins. Nucleic acids combine to form DNA and RNA.

10. b. Only quartz contains no carbon, a necessary condition for an organic molecule. Therefore, quartz is an inorganic molecule.

11. c. Temperature deciduous forests have hot summers and cold winters. During the winter, there is not enough sunlight to support tree growth, so trees lose their leaves every winter. In tropical rain forests, there is enough sunlight and rain to support greenery year-round.

12. a. The joule is 1 N-m. The calorie is also a unit of energy but is not equal to an N-m. The watt is a unit of energy flow rate, or power, not energy itself.

13. a. The breakdown of plant and animal matter over long periods of time under special conditions leads to the formation of oil.

14. b. Albert Einstein published the general theory of relativity in 1916. It describes gravity as a geometric property of space and time.

15. d. Less dense liquids will float on top of more dense liquids. In this case, the olive oil has the lowest density, then the pure water, and finally the saltwater. This also explains why oil floats on ocean water when oil spills occur.

16. d. Though all forms of energy can be converted into all other forms, the efficiency varies and is sometimes very low. Heat, the most degraded form of energy, according to the law of entropy, can be made from the other forms with a conversion rate that is theoretically 100%.

17. a. Entropy can decrease only if the decrease is strictly local and is more than balanced by an increase on some larger scale.

18. c. Galileo Galilei was called the father of modern science. The Roman Inquisition investigated him and believed that his work challenged the Catholic Church. He was found guilty of heresy and ordered to live under house arrest.

19. b. Potential energy is created at the top, when the crane stops. Kinetic energy would occur were the beam dropped.

20. c. Chemical potential energy is released from the food we eat, when combined with oxygen in the air.

21. c. Entomology is the scientific study of insects. The word comes from the Greek *entomos*, which means "that which is cut into pieces or segmented" (meaning insects).

22. a. The fast blowing wind around the house creates an area of low pressure. If the house is tightly sealed, its pressure will remain higher inside. The higher pressure area within the house will try to stabilize by potentially "blowing" the windows and roof out into the lower pressure area surrounding the house. Thus, opening the windows may help to stabilize the pressure.

23. b. Penicillin is derived from the fungi *Penicillium*. Penicillin antibiotics were the first drugs to cure serious bacterial infections, and are still widely used today.

24. b. Proteins are assembled at ribosomes, from amino acids brought to the ribosomes by transfer RNA molecules, according to the genetic code.

25. c. Triplets of bases—for example, AAT, CGT, or GAC—code for amino acids. This was discovered by, among others, English biologist Francis Crick, who first discovered the double helix structure of DNA many years earlier.

26. d. The *r* in rRNA stands for *ribosomal*. The ribosomes are used to construct the universal tree of life because all organisms possess ribosomes.

27. d. Liposomes are hollow spheres of lipid molecules, which are similar to (though simpler than) membranes of cells. Liposomes might have played a role in the origin of life and the evolution of cells.

28. b. Today's pigeons descended from ancestral birds, which descended directly from bipedal dinosaurs.

29. c. Eukaryotic cells have organelles while prokaryotic cells do not.

30. a. A population is all the individuals of the same species living in the same place at the same time. A community is all the populations in that place and time. An ecosystem includes the community and nonliving (abiotic) factors in that place and time. A biome is a set of ecosystems with similar environmental conditions.

31. b. A hypothesis can never be absolutely proven, only disproven. There can be so much data that supports it that it becomes a theory or law, but new data can always refute or revise it. A hypothesis is formed after observations are made.

32. b. The cellulose molecule and the xylem tube system inside plants enabled tallness to evolve, and thus paved the way for trees. The blastula is a feature of the animal embryo, and flowers only came millions of years after the evolution of trees.

33. b. Benjamin Franklin is credited for inventing bifocal lenses, and was one of the first to use them. The term *bifocal* was introduced in 1824 by John Isaac Hawkins, the creator of trifocals, but the invention was credited to Franklin by Hawkins.

34. c. Animals have the blastula stage of embryonic development, which is a tiny hollow sphere of cells.

35. a. It's the radiation of reptiles. The other answers are either much earlier (the origin of life) or substantially later.

36. d. Phloem is the special tube-like tissue in plants that transports food downward. Xylem conducts water and minerals up from the soil. The other choices are found in animals.

37. a. The evidence of a worldwide clay layer that contains lots of the element iridium was found first in Italy, and then in many parts of the world. Iridium at those concentrations must have come from an impactor from space.

38. d. Momentum equals mass times velocity, so the momentum of the first car is $(1{,}500 \text{ kg})(100 \text{ km/h}) = 150{,}000 \text{ kg·km/h}$. The only other car with the same value for mass times velocity is the heaviest car: $(3{,}000 \text{ kg})(50 \text{ km/h}) = 150{,}000 \text{ kg·km/h}$.

39. c. A seismometer (or seismograph) measures motions of the ground, including those caused by earthquakes and volcanoes. The term comes from the Greek *seismos*, meaning "shaking or quaking," and *metron*, meaning "measure."

40. c. Dinosaurs roamed Earth for about 150 million years. 150,000,000 divided by 150,000 is about 1,000 times longer that the dinosaurs dominated Earth than *Homo sapiens* have.

41. a. John Glenn orbited Earth in 1962 in *Friendship 7*. He was the first American to do so.

42. a. The field that studies the evolution of human behavior and the evolution of the human mind is called evolutionary psychology.

43. a. *Australopithecus*, a human ancestor (a hominid), is the most recent by far.

44. d. The orangutan is most distantly related to us. Its lineage diverged from the lineage that led to humans the longest time ago.

45. b. Alkaline is another term for basic, which is defined by a pH > 7.

46. d. Wegener called his idea "continental drift," because it looked like South America and Africa were once together and then drifted apart.

47. c. Places where ocean crust plunges toward the mantle are called subduction zones, because the crust is subducted down into the deeper layers of rock.

48. d. Superposition is one of several relative dating techniques geologists use to identify the age of rocks in comparison to other rock layers surrounding them. Although this is useful for determining the sequence of rock formation, it does not directly provide the exact dates of rock formation— other techniques, such as radiometric dating, would be required.

49. b. The Precambrian or "time of hidden life" encompassed about the first four billion years of Earth's history. The Precambrian can further be subdivided into the Hadean, Archean, and Proterozoic Eons.

50. a. The time of recent ice ages was the Pleistocene, near the end of which (defined by the last melting of the ice sheets), humans reached a high level of culture, as shown by cave art. They also hunted mammoths.

Section 5: Biology

1. b. Autotrophs generate energy from sunlight rather than consuming other sources of energy. Chloroplasts contain the photosynthetic machinery necessary for harvesting solar energy.

2. d. Xylem tissue conducts water and minerals from the roots to the rest of the plant, while phloem tissue carries sugars from the leaves to other parts of the plant. Sieve tubes are phloem components. Stomata are minute openings in leaves that allow air to enter.

3. d. Aneuploidy describes extra individual chromosomes, while polyploidy describes extra sets of homologous chromosomes.

4. c. Pollen released by the stamen is captured by the stigma and reaches the carpels, where the ovum cells are located.

5. a. The shapes of bacteria can be determined from their names, where "coccus" describes a spherical shape, "bacillus" describes a rod-like shape, and "vibrios" and "spirilla" describe spiral shapes.

6. c. Edema, also known as *dropsy*, is the interstitial collection of watery fluid.

7. c. Alcoholic fermentation occurs during anaerobic respiration, producing ethanol and carbon dioxide.

8. b. Remember that the prefix *auto* means *self*. Autogamy is a common method of fertilization used in plants. Syngamy is the union of male and female gametes also known as fertilization, and allogamy is cross-fertilization.

9. c. A single fertilized egg cell divides and becomes multicellular during cleavage. The other answers are all stages that a cell passes through during the four-stage cell cycle: G_2 phase, M phase (mitosis and cytokinesis), G_1 phase, and S phase.

10. b. A cell spends most of its time in interphase, which includes all phases of the cell cycle except for mitosis (M phase). The remaining choices are all phases of mitosis.

11. b. In the complete Linnaean classification of an organism, the groups from most inclusive to most exclusive are kingdom, phylum, class, order, family, genus, and species.

12. b. The largest phylum is Arthropoda, the arthropods, which include insects. Insects make up approximately 80% of all known animal species.

13. d. Bile is produced in the liver and stored in the gallbladder.

14. d. Essential amino acids cannot be synthesized by the body and must be ingested. In addition to phenylalanine, threonine, and valine, the complete list of essential amino acids contains tryptophan, isoleucine, methionine, leucine, lysine, and histidine.

15. d. The first part of the small intestine is the duodenum; the second part is the jejunum; the third, last, and longest part is the ileum.

16. b. Every person's body contains an average of 4.5 to 5 liters of blood.

17. d. Oxygen-rich blood collects into venules and finally into a pulmonary vein from each lung. Veins return blood to the heart, while arteries carry blood away from the heart.

18. b. Phenylketoneuria (PKU) is a hereditary disease that results in loss of function of the enzyme that converts phenylalanine to tyrosine. Buildup of phenylalanine can cause many deleterious effects, so only limited amounts may be safely consumed by those with PKU.

19. c. If incorrect blood types are transfused (for example, if type B blood is injected into a person with type A blood), red cells will clump together. This process is called agglutination.

20. b. Unlike animals, plants have cell walls made out of cellulose. Plants can live in water and do have specialized tissues, like animals. Plants and animals are both eukaryotes, not prokaryotes.

21. a. Water balance in the blood is controlled by the hormone vasopressin, which is secreted by the pituitary gland.

22. b. Bacteriophages are viruses that infect bacteria.

23. c. Smooth muscles are called involuntary muscles. They make up the walls of the hollow organs of the body, such as those of the alimentary canal.

24. a. Muscles work in pairs. Contraction of the biceps muscle bends the elbow; contraction of the triceps muscle straightens the arm.

25. d. Because a resting neuron's cell membrane is relatively impermeable to both sodium and potassium, and because active transport systems work to move sodium to the extracellular fluid and potassium to the intracellular fluid, the concentration of sodium ions is about 14 times higher outside the cell than inside, and the concentration of potassium ions is 20 to 30 times higher inside the cell than outside.

26. b. The cerebellum coordinates impulses sent out from the cerebrum. Its main function is to coordinate skeletal movements.

27. c. Mitochondria are organelles present in both plant and animal cells. The main function of mitochondria is to provide the cell with energy.

28. c. The salivary glands have ducts and are called exocrine glands. The others are endocrine glands, which are ductless and release their secretions directly into the blood.

29. b. The urine produced by the kidneys first drains into the ureters, which carry the urine to the bladder, where it is stored. It then flows out of the body via the urethra. The adrenal glands sit on top of the kidneys and are part of the endocrine system, not the renal system.

30. d. The overall reaction for photosynthesis is $6CO_2 + 6H_2O \rightarrow C_6H_{12}O_6 + 6O_2$ so the reverse reaction is $C_6H_{12}O_6 + 6O_2 \rightarrow 6CO_2 + 6H_2O$. This reverse reaction is the overall reaction for respiration, the breakdown of sugar into carbon dioxide and water, which releases energy for the cell to use. Fermentation does break down sugar, but into ethanol or lactic acid, not carbon dioxide and water.

31. b. The diastole phase of a heartbeat occurs between two contractions of the heart during which the heart muscles relax and the ventricles fill up with blood.

32. c. A Punnett square of Pp and Pp shows that offspring would have three potential genotypes: PP, Pp, and pp. Half of the offspring would be Pp, one-fourth PP, and one-fourth pp. Since P is dominant, it would be expressed for two of the genotypes, PP and Pp, and therefore three-fourths of the offspring. Therefore, 75% of the offspring would be expected to have purple flowers.

33. a. Ribosomes, located on the endoplasmic reticulum (ER) and the cytoplasm, are where protein synthesis occurs.

34. a. Hypertension is the medical term for increased blood pressure.

35. a. The placenta is the organ in viviparous animals that connects the embryo to its mother's uterus.

36. c. Draw a Punnett square diagram. Blue eye color (b) is a recessive trait and brown (B) is dominant. Your mother must be homozygous recessive to have blue eyes (bb) and your father is heterozygous (Bb). Therefore, your chances of having blue eyes is 50%.

37. a. Setae (singular *seta*) are the bristle-like projections on some invertebrates. Hair only occurs on mammals, and whiskers are a type of hair.

38. a. Hematocrit describes the percentage of blood volume occupied by red blood cells. Anemia is a condition characterized by too few healthy red blood cells.

39. d. The alveoli, where carbon dioxide and oxygen are exchanged, are located at the ends of tubes called bronchioles.

40. c. During anaphase, the centrosome holding the two identical halves of each chromosome disintegrates and the chromosome separates into sister chromatids. It is during anaphase I of meiosis, not mitosis, that homologous chromosomes separate.

41. d. Dentin is the thick, bony layer underneath the calcium phosphate deposit that makes up the enamel of teeth.

42. c. The macula is a spot near the center of the retina in the eye. Macular degeneration results in loss of central vision.

43. b. Symbiotic relationships can be divided into three categories: mutualism, commensalism, and parasitism. Commensalism occurs where one member of the pair benefits from the other without either harming or helping the other.

44. b. Digestive organs called accessory organs contribute to the digestive process, but food does not pass through them. Choice **b**, the liver, is an example. The other choices are part of the alimentary canal or gastrointestinal tract, which is the tube through which food passes as it is digested.

45. a. Acquired characteristics are features that develop within the lifetime of an individual organism, as do large muscles in a weight lifter. The large ears of rabbits and nocturnal vision of owls have developed over generations to help these animals survive. The human appendix is a vestigial organ.

46. c. In arthropods, hemolymph carries nutrients and oxygen to cells.

47. d. The ilium is the third component of the human pelvic girdle. The human pectoral girdle consists of the scapulae and clavicles.

48. b. After exhalation, a volume of air still remains in the lungs. Residual volume is a measure of lung capacity that measures the amount of air remaining in the lungs after strenuous exhalation.

49. d. Codons are three-letter codes of either DNA or mRNA that code for a specific amino acid that is added during translation.

50. d. Vegetative reproduction refers to types of asexual reproduction where parts of a parent plant form new individual plants. Rhizomes are stems that form near a parent plant and grow into new individual plants.

Section 6: Chemistry

1. c. A proton weighs considerably more than an electron, so one mole of protons weighs more than one mole of electrons. A water molecule weighs approximately the same as 18 protons, and 5 molecules of benzene weighs approximately the same as 390 protons, both considerably less than the 6.02×10^{23} protons in a mole.

2. b. Water is a polar molecule, so other polar molecules will be soluble in it but nonpolar molecules will not. Like dissolves like. CCl_4 is the only choice that is nonpolar.

3. b. There is one mole of H_2O in 18.0 g water. Each mole of water contains two moles of hydrogen.

4. b. In this reaction, the iron is reduced from Fe (III) to Fe (0) and the aluminum is oxidized from Al (0) to Al (III).

5. d. Periods are the horizontal rows on the periodic table. Period V is the fifth row down from the top, which begins with Rb (rubidium) and ends with Xe (xenon). N (nitrogen) and Nb (niobium) are in groups VA (15) and VB (5), respectively, which are the vertical columns on the table. B (boron) has an atomic number of 5 but is not in period 5.

6. a. Noble gases are the elements in group VIIIA (group 18) of the periodic table. The noble gases are helium, neon, argon, krypton, xenon, and radon.

7. c. Phosphate has a charge of −3, and cobalt (II) has a charge of +2. To balance the charges, they must be combined in the ratio $Co_3(PO_4)_2$.

8. c. Phospholipids, the major components of cell membranes, are made up of one molecule of glycerol bonded to two fatty acids and one phosphate group. Choice **a** describes a peptide bond, and choice **b** describes a triglyceride.

9. b. Choice **b** is the definition of osmotic pressure. Osmotic potential, mentioned in choice **d**, is inversely proportional to osmotic pressure and is the Gibbs free energy value for the osmosis reaction.

10. d. An aldehyde is a molecule containing a carbonyl group (C=O), a hydrogen atom, and an alkyl group. The only choice that fits this definition is choice **d**.

11. a. α decay is a decay process where a helium nucleus is released.

12. b. Bismuth (III) has an oxidation number of +3, and the hydroxide ion has an oxidation number of −1. Therefore, three hydroxide ions must bond to each bismuth atom to form an uncharged compound.

13. b. When an alkali metal such as sodium reacts with water, an explosive reaction takes place, and the result is a metal hydroxide and hydrogen gas.

14. b. When an atom loses electrons, it is said to be oxidized; and when an atom gains electrons, it is said to be reduced. In this reaction, Br goes from negatively charged to neutral, thus losing an electron and being oxidized. Mn goes from a charge of +7 to a charge of +2, gaining electrons in the process and becoming reduced.

15. a. Covalent bonding occurs when two atoms share electrons. In ammonia, each hydrogen atom shares an electron with the nitrogen atom.

16. d. Carbonic acid, H_2CO_3, has a pK$_a$ of 6.35. The other choices are all strong acids.

17. c. The mass of the empirical compound $CH_2O = (1C \times 12\ g) + (2H \times 1\ g) + (1O \times 16\ g) = 30\ g$. Since the molar mass of the compound is 90 g, the multiplier is $\frac{90}{30} = 3$, yielding a molecular formula of $C_3H_6O_3$.

18. b. As a general rule, radius increases as you go down and to the left in the periodic table. Rb is the farthest down and to the left.

19. a. The number of atoms or molecules in one mole of a substance is 6.02×10^{23}. This number is known as Avogadro's number and is derived from the number of carbon-12 atoms in 12.0 grams of carbon.

20. a. In redox reactions, atoms that lose electrons are being oxidized. The half reaction $Zn_{(s)} \rightarrow Zn^{2+}_{(aq)} + 2e^-$ shows that $Zn_{(s)}$ is losing two electrons in this reaction.

21. b. The oxidation number of an atom in a compound is equal to the charge carried by the ion. In the compound NiO_2, the nickel ion has a charge of +4.

22. c. The alkali metals are found in group IA (group 1) of the periodic table. They share the characteristic of being highly reactive with water. When in contact with water, a rapid reaction occurs that produces metal hydroxide and hydrogen gas.

23. b. β decay results in the conversion of a neutron into a proton and an electron and the expulsion of the electron from the nucleus.

24. c. Trans fats are fatty acids with at least one trans C–C double bond. These fats are found in partially hydrogenated oils and have been associated with many negative health effects.

25. d. Combustion of hydrocarbons produces CO_2 and H_2O.

26. a. Use the equation $\Delta T = \frac{K_b(\text{moles solute})}{\text{mass of solvent}}$. This gives $\frac{0.52(\frac{256}{128})}{5.15}$; $\frac{0.52}{5.15}$ is approximately $\frac{1}{10}$, and $\frac{256}{128} = 2$, so the answer is 0.2.

27. c. Because the molar mass of N is greater than 1, there are more atoms in 1 mole of N than in 1 gram. There are obviously more atoms in 1 mole of NO_2 than in 1 mole of N, since NO_2 has 3 atoms compared with 1 atom in N. While there are 4 atoms in each molecule of NH_3, there are half as many molecules in the NH_3 as in the NO_2 (0.5 mol compared to 1 mol).

28. a. Because H_2SO_4 is a strong acid, it will react with Al. Choice **a** is the only option that is balanced.

29. b. Transition metals are those with partially filled d orbitals. Iron is the only element of the list that fits that criterion.

30. b. Use the periodic table to answer this question. Elements in group IIA (group 2) tend to go to a +2 ion.

31. d. Ca has two valence shells, which occur in the 4s shell.

32. d. If the cell becomes more acidic, this means that more H$^+$ ions are introduced into the system. This will cause more HPO_4^{2-} to be consumed as it reacts with this additional H$^+$, regenerating more $H_2PO_4^{2-}$ (the equilibrium shifts to the left). More H$^+$ ions would not be produced since this would make the cell even more acidic and would not counteract the change in pH.

33. c. For a given reaction, $wA + xB \rightleftarrows yC + zD$, $K_c = \frac{[C]^y[D]^z}{[A]^w[W]^x}$. There are 2 moles of F_2 reacting for every mole of Xe, so be sure to square the concentration of F_2 in the equilibrium constant.

34. a. The oxidation numbers of NO_3^- and I$^-$ are generally both −1; to make the net charge zero, the oxidation number for Na must be +1.

35. b. Choice **b** is the only one involving a beta particle.

36. c. It will take one half-life to go from 40 g to 20 g; it will take another half-life to go from 20 g to 10 g. This gives a total of 2.4×10^9 years.

37. a. Uranium is an actinide. Actinides are elements with partially filled $5f$ orbitals (elements 89 to 103).

38. a. The number of protons is the atomic number, or the lower number; the upper number is the sum of the protons and neutrons.

39. b. A ketone features a carbonyl group (C=O) with two carbons bound to either side of it.

40. c. The only effect of the addition of a catalyst is to increase the rate of reaction. There is no change in the composition.

41. a. Allotropes are two different formats of an element. Ozone and O_2 are two different formats for the element oxygen.

42. c. For an ideal gas in a fixed volume, temperature and pressure are directly proportional. The temperature must be converted to Kelvin (27°C = 300 K and 117°C = 390 K). The temperature is increased by $\frac{390}{300} = 1.3$, so the new pressure must be 1 atm × 1.3 = 1.3 atm.

43. b. $\frac{4.00\text{ g}}{16\text{ g/mol}} = 0.25$ mol CH_4; $\frac{4.00\text{ g}}{32\text{ g/mol}}$

$= 0.125$ mol O_2

The limiting reactant in this reaction is oxygen.

$\frac{1\text{ mol }CO_2}{1\text{ mol }O_2} \times 0.125$ mol $O_2 \times 44$ g/mol CO_2

$= 2.75$ g CO_2

44. a. Carboxylic acids are organic compounds characterized by the presence of a carboxyl group, COOH. The carboxyl group is a carbon atom with a double-bonded oxygen atom and a hydroxyl group.

45. a. The electron configuration for Cl is [Ne] $3s^2 3p^5$.

46. d. Amines are organic molecules with an NR_3 (R = alkyl or hydrogen) group.

47. a. This problem follows Avogadro's law, which states that volume is proportional to the number of moles if temperature and pressure are constant.

48. c. This is an example of osmosis. If the concentration of solute is unequal on either side, the solvent will move toward the higher concentration of solute.

49. b. The molecular formula describes the actual atoms of the molecule. The empirical formula reduces the empirical formula to the simplest ratio of molecules. $C_4H_8O_2$ is reduced to C_2H_4O.

50. a. Proteins are macromolecules consisting of amino acids.

Scoring

After you take your actual exam, a complicated formula will be used to convert your raw score on each section of the test into a percentile. The raw score is simply the number you get right on each section; wrong answers don't count against you. A percentile is a way of comparing your score with that of other test takers; this number indicates what percent of other test takers scored lower than you did on this section.

First, count the number of questions you got right in each section, and record them in the blanks:

Section 1: _____ of 50 questions right
Section 2: _____ of 45 questions right
Section 3: _____ of 50 questions right
Section 4: _____ of 50 questions right
Section 5: _____ of 50 questions right
Section 6: _____ of 50 questions right

Next, convert your raw score into a *percentage* for each section of the exam. (Remember that this percentage is not the same as a *percentile*.) By now, your quantitative ability should be good enough to tell you how to arrive at a percentage, but if you've forgotten, refer back to the scoring instructions in Chapter 3.

Now you can compare your scores on this test with those on the first practice exam. Chances are, your scores went up. If they didn't, it's probably because you took the first practice exam without having to worry about time, whereas in this exam, you had some fairly tight time limits to meet.

So if your scores went *down* between the first practice exam and this one, the problem is not so much the limits of your knowledge as your ability to work quickly without sacrificing accuracy. In that case, reread Chapter 2, "LearningExpress Test Preparation System," for tips on how to improve your time management during the exam. Then, practice your time management skills on the sample exam in the next chapter. Before you begin each section, figure out the average amount of time allotted for each question by dividing the number of minutes allowed by the number of questions. Then, as you work through the section, keep yourself moving according to the schedule you've worked out. Remember to rack up the easy points by answering the easiest questions first, leaving the harder questions for last.

On the other hand, if your scores went up, you're probably wondering if they went up enough and, if not, what you should do about it. First of all, remember that no one is expected to score 100% on a section, so don't be too hard on yourself. Here's what you should do, based on your percentage scores on this practice exam:

- **For sections on which you scored less than 50%,** you need some concentrated work in those areas. (If you scored under 50% on all five sections, you might have to postpone taking the exam while you work on your skills.) If biology and chemistry were your problem areas, more work with your textbooks and other materials might be enough, especially if you weren't very conscientious about reviewing before you took this practice exam. For other areas, and for biology and chemistry if you did review your textbooks, an extra college course

is your best bet. If you don't have time or money for a complete course, find a tutor who will work with you individually. Most colleges have free or low-cost peer tutorial programs, or you may be able to get help from a professional teacher for a reasonable hourly fee.

- **For sections on which you scored 50–70%,** more review and practice is in order. Find a tutor, or form a study group with other students who are preparing for the exam. Go to the library or bookstore for other books that review the relevant areas; if those books also contain practice test questions, all the better. When you've done a fair amount of review, go back to the appropriate chapters of this book to review the practice questions and strategies.

- **For sections on which you scored 70–80%,** you're on your way to a score that will look good to the admissions department of your chosen program, but a little more work wouldn't hurt. Start by reviewing the appropriate chapters in this book. If you feel at all shaky about the material, use other resources: additional books, a friend who's good at the appropriate subject, a study group, or a peer tutor.

- **For sections on which you scored more than 80%,** you're in pretty good shape. But you should keep studying and practicing up to the day before the test, so you'll know that you're as prepared as possible to score as well as you can. Keep reviewing Chapters 4–9 of this book right up until test day, and use additional resources whenever you can.

One of the biggest keys to your success on the exam is your self-confidence. The more comfortable you are with your ability to perform, the more likely you are to do well. You know what to expect, you know your strengths and weaknesses, and you can work to turn those weaknesses into strengths before the actual exam. Your preparedness should give you the confidence that you'll need to do well on exam day.

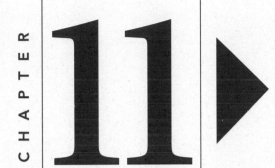

PRACTICE EXAM III

CHAPTER SUMMARY

How ready are you? This is the last of the three practice exams presented in this book. Use this test for extra practice and to determine the areas in which you should concentrate your attention in the time leading up to exam day.

This practice test will give you additional preparation and help you focus your study in the final days before the exam. As with the two earlier practice exams, this multiple-choice test is designed to reflect the topics and format of the entrance exams used by health training programs. The six test sections include Verbal Ability, Reading Comprehension, Math, General Science, Biology, and Chemistry. Although this practice test is general enough to prepare you for any health occupations entrance exam, be sure to investigate the specifics of the test you will be taking. The more you know, the better prepared you will be.

Before you take this third exam, find a quiet place where you can work undisturbed for four hours. Set a timer, stopwatch, or alarm clock to time yourself according to the directions in each section. Work as quickly as you can to meet the time limits, but do not sacrifice accuracy. Stop working when you run out of time even if you have not answered all of the questions. Allow yourself a five-minute break between each section and a 15-minute break after Section 3.

Using a number 2 pencil, mark your answers on the answer sheet on the following pages. The answer key is located on page 372—refer to this only once you have completed the test. A section about how to score your exam follows the answer key.

Section 1: Verbal Ability

1. (a) (b) (c) (d)
2. (a) (b) (c) (d)
3. (a) (b) (c) (d)
4. (a) (b) (c) (d)
5. (a) (b) (c) (d)
6. (a) (b) (c) (d)
7. (a) (b) (c) (d)
8. (a) (b) (c) (d)
9. (a) (b) (c) (d)
10. (a) (b) (c) (d)
11. (a) (b) (c) (d)
12. (a) (b) (c) (d)
13. (a) (b) (c) (d)
14. (a) (b) (c) (d)
15. (a) (b) (c) (d)
16. (a) (b) (c) (d)
17. (a) (b) (c) (d)

18. (a) (b) (c) (d)
19. (a) (b) (c) (d)
20. (a) (b) (c) (d)
21. (a) (b) (c) (d)
22. (a) (b) (c) (d)
23. (a) (b) (c) (d)
24. (a) (b) (c) (d)
25. (a) (b) (c) (d)
26. (a) (b) (c) (d)
27. (a) (b) (c) (d)
28. (a) (b) (c) (d)
29. (a) (b) (c) (d)
30. (a) (b) (c) (d)
31. (a) (b) (c) (d)
32. (a) (b) (c) (d)
33. (a) (b) (c) (d)
34. (a) (b) (c) (d)

35. (a) (b) (c) (d)
36. (a) (b) (c) (d)
37. (a) (b) (c) (d)
38. (a) (b) (c) (d)
39. (a) (b) (c) (d)
40. (a) (b) (c) (d)
41. (a) (b) (c) (d)
42. (a) (b) (c) (d)
43. (a) (b) (c) (d)
44. (a) (b) (c) (d)
45. (a) (b) (c) (d)
46. (a) (b) (c) (d)
47. (a) (b) (c) (d)
48. (a) (b) (c) (d)
49. (a) (b) (c) (d)
50. (a) (b) (c) (d)

Section 2: Reading Comprehension

1. (a) (b) (c) (d)
2. (a) (b) (c) (d)
3. (a) (b) (c) (d)
4. (a) (b) (c) (d)
5. (a) (b) (c) (d)
6. (a) (b) (c) (d)
7. (a) (b) (c) (d)
8. (a) (b) (c) (d)
9. (a) (b) (c) (d)
10. (a) (b) (c) (d)
11. (a) (b) (c) (d)
12. (a) (b) (c) (d)
13. (a) (b) (c) (d)
14. (a) (b) (c) (d)
15. (a) (b) (c) (d)
16. (a) (b) (c) (d)
17. (a) (b) (c) (d)

18. (a) (b) (c) (d)
19. (a) (b) (c) (d)
20. (a) (b) (c) (d)
21. (a) (b) (c) (d)
22. (a) (b) (c) (d)
23. (a) (b) (c) (d)
24. (a) (b) (c) (d)
25. (a) (b) (c) (d)
26. (a) (b) (c) (d)
27. (a) (b) (c) (d)
28. (a) (b) (c) (d)
29. (a) (b) (c) (d)
30. (a) (b) (c) (d)
31. (a) (b) (c) (d)
32. (a) (b) (c) (d)
33. (a) (b) (c) (d)
34. (a) (b) (c) (d)

35. (a) (b) (c) (d)
36. (a) (b) (c) (d)
37. (a) (b) (c) (d)
38. (a) (b) (c) (d)
39. (a) (b) (c) (d)
40. (a) (b) (c) (d)
41. (a) (b) (c) (d)
42. (a) (b) (c) (d)
43. (a) (b) (c) (d)
44. (a) (b) (c) (d)
45. (a) (b) (c) (d)

Section 3: Math

1.	ⓐ	ⓑ	ⓒ	ⓓ	18.	ⓐ	ⓑ	ⓒ	ⓓ	35.	ⓐ	ⓑ	ⓒ	ⓓ
2.	ⓐ	ⓑ	ⓒ	ⓓ	19.	ⓐ	ⓑ	ⓒ	ⓓ	36.	ⓐ	ⓑ	ⓒ	ⓓ
3.	ⓐ	ⓑ	ⓒ	ⓓ	20.	ⓐ	ⓑ	ⓒ	ⓓ	37.	ⓐ	ⓑ	ⓒ	ⓓ
4.	ⓐ	ⓑ	ⓒ	ⓓ	21.	ⓐ	ⓑ	ⓒ	ⓓ	38.	ⓐ	ⓑ	ⓒ	ⓓ
5.	ⓐ	ⓑ	ⓒ	ⓓ	22.	ⓐ	ⓑ	ⓒ	ⓓ	39.	ⓐ	ⓑ	ⓒ	ⓓ
6.	ⓐ	ⓑ	ⓒ	ⓓ	23.	ⓐ	ⓑ	ⓒ	ⓓ	40.	ⓐ	ⓑ	ⓒ	ⓓ
7.	ⓐ	ⓑ	ⓒ	ⓓ	24.	ⓐ	ⓑ	ⓒ	ⓓ	41.	ⓐ	ⓑ	ⓒ	ⓓ
8.	ⓐ	ⓑ	ⓒ	ⓓ	25.	ⓐ	ⓑ	ⓒ	ⓓ	42.	ⓐ	ⓑ	ⓒ	ⓓ
9.	ⓐ	ⓑ	ⓒ	ⓓ	26.	ⓐ	ⓑ	ⓒ	ⓓ	43.	ⓐ	ⓑ	ⓒ	ⓓ
10.	ⓐ	ⓑ	ⓒ	ⓓ	27.	ⓐ	ⓑ	ⓒ	ⓓ	44.	ⓐ	ⓑ	ⓒ	ⓓ
11.	ⓐ	ⓑ	ⓒ	ⓓ	28.	ⓐ	ⓑ	ⓒ	ⓓ	45.	ⓐ	ⓑ	ⓒ	ⓓ
12.	ⓐ	ⓑ	ⓒ	ⓓ	29.	ⓐ	ⓑ	ⓒ	ⓓ	46.	ⓐ	ⓑ	ⓒ	ⓓ
13.	ⓐ	ⓑ	ⓒ	ⓓ	30.	ⓐ	ⓑ	ⓒ	ⓓ	47.	ⓐ	ⓑ	ⓒ	ⓓ
14.	ⓐ	ⓑ	ⓒ	ⓓ	31.	ⓐ	ⓑ	ⓒ	ⓓ	48.	ⓐ	ⓑ	ⓒ	ⓓ
15.	ⓐ	ⓑ	ⓒ	ⓓ	32.	ⓐ	ⓑ	ⓒ	ⓓ	49.	ⓐ	ⓑ	ⓒ	ⓓ
16.	ⓐ	ⓑ	ⓒ	ⓓ	33.	ⓐ	ⓑ	ⓒ	ⓓ	50.	ⓐ	ⓑ	ⓒ	ⓓ
17.	ⓐ	ⓑ	ⓒ	ⓓ	34.	ⓐ	ⓑ	ⓒ	ⓓ					

Section 4: General Science

1.	ⓐ	ⓑ	ⓒ	ⓓ	18.	ⓐ	ⓑ	ⓒ	ⓓ	35.	ⓐ	ⓑ	ⓒ	ⓓ
2.	ⓐ	ⓑ	ⓒ	ⓓ	19.	ⓐ	ⓑ	ⓒ	ⓓ	36.	ⓐ	ⓑ	ⓒ	ⓓ
3.	ⓐ	ⓑ	ⓒ	ⓓ	20.	ⓐ	ⓑ	ⓒ	ⓓ	37.	ⓐ	ⓑ	ⓒ	ⓓ
4.	ⓐ	ⓑ	ⓒ	ⓓ	21.	ⓐ	ⓑ	ⓒ	ⓓ	38.	ⓐ	ⓑ	ⓒ	ⓓ
5.	ⓐ	ⓑ	ⓒ	ⓓ	22.	ⓐ	ⓑ	ⓒ	ⓓ	39.	ⓐ	ⓑ	ⓒ	ⓓ
6.	ⓐ	ⓑ	ⓒ	ⓓ	23.	ⓐ	ⓑ	ⓒ	ⓓ	40.	ⓐ	ⓑ	ⓒ	ⓓ
7.	ⓐ	ⓑ	ⓒ	ⓓ	24.	ⓐ	ⓑ	ⓒ	ⓓ	41.	ⓐ	ⓑ	ⓒ	ⓓ
8.	ⓐ	ⓑ	ⓒ	ⓓ	25.	ⓐ	ⓑ	ⓒ	ⓓ	42.	ⓐ	ⓑ	ⓒ	ⓓ
9.	ⓐ	ⓑ	ⓒ	ⓓ	26.	ⓐ	ⓑ	ⓒ	ⓓ	43.	ⓐ	ⓑ	ⓒ	ⓓ
10.	ⓐ	ⓑ	ⓒ	ⓓ	27.	ⓐ	ⓑ	ⓒ	ⓓ	44.	ⓐ	ⓑ	ⓒ	ⓓ
11.	ⓐ	ⓑ	ⓒ	ⓓ	28.	ⓐ	ⓑ	ⓒ	ⓓ	45.	ⓐ	ⓑ	ⓒ	ⓓ
12.	ⓐ	ⓑ	ⓒ	ⓓ	29.	ⓐ	ⓑ	ⓒ	ⓓ	46.	ⓐ	ⓑ	ⓒ	ⓓ
13.	ⓐ	ⓑ	ⓒ	ⓓ	30.	ⓐ	ⓑ	ⓒ	ⓓ	47.	ⓐ	ⓑ	ⓒ	ⓓ
14.	ⓐ	ⓑ	ⓒ	ⓓ	31.	ⓐ	ⓑ	ⓒ	ⓓ	48.	ⓐ	ⓑ	ⓒ	ⓓ
15.	ⓐ	ⓑ	ⓒ	ⓓ	32.	ⓐ	ⓑ	ⓒ	ⓓ	49.	ⓐ	ⓑ	ⓒ	ⓓ
16.	ⓐ	ⓑ	ⓒ	ⓓ	33.	ⓐ	ⓑ	ⓒ	ⓓ	50.	ⓐ	ⓑ	ⓒ	ⓓ
17.	ⓐ	ⓑ	ⓒ	ⓓ	34.	ⓐ	ⓑ	ⓒ	ⓓ					

LEARNINGEXPRESS ANSWER SHEET

Section 5: Biology

1.	ⓐ	ⓑ	ⓒ	ⓓ		18.	ⓐ	ⓑ	ⓒ	ⓓ		35.	ⓐ	ⓑ	ⓒ	ⓓ
2.	ⓐ	ⓑ	ⓒ	ⓓ		19.	ⓐ	ⓑ	ⓒ	ⓓ		36.	ⓐ	ⓑ	ⓒ	ⓓ
3.	ⓐ	ⓑ	ⓒ	ⓓ		20.	ⓐ	ⓑ	ⓒ	ⓓ		37.	ⓐ	ⓑ	ⓒ	ⓓ
4.	ⓐ	ⓑ	ⓒ	ⓓ		21.	ⓐ	ⓑ	ⓒ	ⓓ		38.	ⓐ	ⓑ	ⓒ	ⓓ
5.	ⓐ	ⓑ	ⓒ	ⓓ		22.	ⓐ	ⓑ	ⓒ	ⓓ		39.	ⓐ	ⓑ	ⓒ	ⓓ
6.	ⓐ	ⓑ	ⓒ	ⓓ		23.	ⓐ	ⓑ	ⓒ	ⓓ		40.	ⓐ	ⓑ	ⓒ	ⓓ
7.	ⓐ	ⓑ	ⓒ	ⓓ		24.	ⓐ	ⓑ	ⓒ	ⓓ		41.	ⓐ	ⓑ	ⓒ	ⓓ
8.	ⓐ	ⓑ	ⓒ	ⓓ		25.	ⓐ	ⓑ	ⓒ	ⓓ		42.	ⓐ	ⓑ	ⓒ	ⓓ
9.	ⓐ	ⓑ	ⓒ	ⓓ		26.	ⓐ	ⓑ	ⓒ	ⓓ		43.	ⓐ	ⓑ	ⓒ	ⓓ
10.	ⓐ	ⓑ	ⓒ	ⓓ		27.	ⓐ	ⓑ	ⓒ	ⓓ		44.	ⓐ	ⓑ	ⓒ	ⓓ
11.	ⓐ	ⓑ	ⓒ	ⓓ		28.	ⓐ	ⓑ	ⓒ	ⓓ		45.	ⓐ	ⓑ	ⓒ	ⓓ
12.	ⓐ	ⓑ	ⓒ	ⓓ		29.	ⓐ	ⓑ	ⓒ	ⓓ		46.	ⓐ	ⓑ	ⓒ	ⓓ
13.	ⓐ	ⓑ	ⓒ	ⓓ		30.	ⓐ	ⓑ	ⓒ	ⓓ		47.	ⓐ	ⓑ	ⓒ	ⓓ
14.	ⓐ	ⓑ	ⓒ	ⓓ		31.	ⓐ	ⓑ	ⓒ	ⓓ		48.	ⓐ	ⓑ	ⓒ	ⓓ
15.	ⓐ	ⓑ	ⓒ	ⓓ		32.	ⓐ	ⓑ	ⓒ	ⓓ		49.	ⓐ	ⓑ	ⓒ	ⓓ
16.	ⓐ	ⓑ	ⓒ	ⓓ		33.	ⓐ	ⓑ	ⓒ	ⓓ		50.	ⓐ	ⓑ	ⓒ	ⓓ
17.	ⓐ	ⓑ	ⓒ	ⓓ		34.	ⓐ	ⓑ	ⓒ	ⓓ						

Section 6: Chemistry

1.	ⓐ	ⓑ	ⓒ	ⓓ		18.	ⓐ	ⓑ	ⓒ	ⓓ		35.	ⓐ	ⓑ	ⓒ	ⓓ
2.	ⓐ	ⓑ	ⓒ	ⓓ		19.	ⓐ	ⓑ	ⓒ	ⓓ		36.	ⓐ	ⓑ	ⓒ	ⓓ
3.	ⓐ	ⓑ	ⓒ	ⓓ		20.	ⓐ	ⓑ	ⓒ	ⓓ		37.	ⓐ	ⓑ	ⓒ	ⓓ
4.	ⓐ	ⓑ	ⓒ	ⓓ		21.	ⓐ	ⓑ	ⓒ	ⓓ		38.	ⓐ	ⓑ	ⓒ	ⓓ
5.	ⓐ	ⓑ	ⓒ	ⓓ		22.	ⓐ	ⓑ	ⓒ	ⓓ		39.	ⓐ	ⓑ	ⓒ	ⓓ
6.	ⓐ	ⓑ	ⓒ	ⓓ		23.	ⓐ	ⓑ	ⓒ	ⓓ		40.	ⓐ	ⓑ	ⓒ	ⓓ
7.	ⓐ	ⓑ	ⓒ	ⓓ		24.	ⓐ	ⓑ	ⓒ	ⓓ		41.	ⓐ	ⓑ	ⓒ	ⓓ
8.	ⓐ	ⓑ	ⓒ	ⓓ		25.	ⓐ	ⓑ	ⓒ	ⓓ		42.	ⓐ	ⓑ	ⓒ	ⓓ
9.	ⓐ	ⓑ	ⓒ	ⓓ		26.	ⓐ	ⓑ	ⓒ	ⓓ		43.	ⓐ	ⓑ	ⓒ	ⓓ
10.	ⓐ	ⓑ	ⓒ	ⓓ		27.	ⓐ	ⓑ	ⓒ	ⓓ		44.	ⓐ	ⓑ	ⓒ	ⓓ
11.	ⓐ	ⓑ	ⓒ	ⓓ		28.	ⓐ	ⓑ	ⓒ	ⓓ		45.	ⓐ	ⓑ	ⓒ	ⓓ
12.	ⓐ	ⓑ	ⓒ	ⓓ		29.	ⓐ	ⓑ	ⓒ	ⓓ		46.	ⓐ	ⓑ	ⓒ	ⓓ
13.	ⓐ	ⓑ	ⓒ	ⓓ		30.	ⓐ	ⓑ	ⓒ	ⓓ		47.	ⓐ	ⓑ	ⓒ	ⓓ
14.	ⓐ	ⓑ	ⓒ	ⓓ		31.	ⓐ	ⓑ	ⓒ	ⓓ		48.	ⓐ	ⓑ	ⓒ	ⓓ
15.	ⓐ	ⓑ	ⓒ	ⓓ		32.	ⓐ	ⓑ	ⓒ	ⓓ		49.	ⓐ	ⓑ	ⓒ	ⓓ
16.	ⓐ	ⓑ	ⓒ	ⓓ		33.	ⓐ	ⓑ	ⓒ	ⓓ		50.	ⓐ	ⓑ	ⓒ	ⓓ
17.	ⓐ	ⓑ	ⓒ	ⓓ		34.	ⓐ	ⓑ	ⓒ	ⓓ						

Section 1: Verbal Ability

Find the correctly spelled word in each of the following lists.

1. a. abscessed
   b. absessed
   c. abscesed

2. a. paralel
   b. paralell
   c. parallel

3. a. accidentelly
   b. accidentally
   c. accidently

4. a. tonsillitis
   b. tonsilitis
   c. tonscilitis

5. a. exeled
   b. exceled
   c. excelled

6. a. guardain
   b. guardian
   c. gardain

7. a. accustomed
   b. acustomed
   c. acusstomed

8. a. pastureized
   b. pasteurized
   c. pastuerized

9. a. delirious
   b. delerious
   c. delireous

10. a. disaese
    b. desease
    c. disease

11. a. inundated
    b. innundated
    c. inondatted

12. a. lazyness
    b. lazeness
    c. laziness

13. a. practitoners
    b. practitioners
    c. practishoners

14. a. prosecuted
    b. prossecuted
    c. prosecutted

15. a. counterfiet
    b. counterfit
    c. counterfeit

16. a. symmetrically
    b. symetrically
    c. symmetricully

17. a. dalaying
    b. delaying
    c. deleying

18. a. vacuum
    b. vaccuum
    c. vacum

19. a. acomodate
    b. acommodate
    c. accommodate

20. **a.** coleagues
    b. collegues
    c. colleagues

21. **a.** consceintious
    b. conscientious
    c. consheentious

22. **a.** indescribeable
    b. indiscribable
    c. indescribable

23. **a.** ilegible
    b. illegible
    c. ilegable

24. **a.** penicillen
    b. penicillin
    c. penicillen

25. **a.** adolescense
    b. adolessents
    c. adolescence

26. **a.** preceding
    b. preceeding
    c. preeceding

27. **a.** nusance
    b. nuisance
    c. nuissance

28. **a.** peacable
    b. peaceabel
    c. peaceable

29. **a.** luxurient
    b. luxouriant
    c. luxuriant

30. **a.** gullible
    b. gullable
    c. gullibel

31. **a.** grattitude
    b. gratitude
    c. gratitud

32. **a.** musicaly
    b. musicly
    c. musically

33. **a.** tragedies
    b. tragedys
    c. tragedis

34. **a.** bulletine
    b. bulletin
    c. buletin

35. **a.** embasy
    b. embassie
    c. embassy

36. **a.** nevertheles
    b. nevertheless
    c. neveretheless

37. **a.** questionairre
    b. questionnaire
    c. questionaire

38. **a.** pungent
    b. pungant
    c. pungennt

39. **a.** hygenic
    b. hyginic
    c. hygienic

40.
a. ilegal
b. illegal
c. illegul

41.
a. corosiveness
b. corrosiveness
c. corrossiveness

42.
a. gymnest
b. gymnist
c. gymnast

43.
a. useful
b. usful
c. usefull

44.
a. organising
b. organizing
c. organizeing

45.
a. jewelry
b. jewellry
c. jewelery

46.
a. crazyness
b. crazyiness
c. craziness

47.
a. returnabel
b. returnible
c. returnable

48.
a. chaise
b. chaisse
c. chais

49.
a. extremely
b. extremeley
c. extremly

50.
a. freindly
b. friendly
c. friendlly

Section 2:
Reading Comprehension

Read each passage and answer the questions based on the information in the text. You have 45 minutes to complete this section.

One out of five Americans suffers from an allergic disease, which results from the immune system reacting to a normally innocuous substance such as pollen or dust. Most of these people have allergies that affect nasal passages and sinuses, including allergies to pollen ("hay fever") and allergic reactions in the airways of the lungs that contribute to asthma. Hay fever alone affects some 22 million Americans, who in total see their doctors 9.4 million times a year. Asthma afflicts 10 to 15 million Americans.

An allergic response begins with a process called *sensitization*. When a foreign substance such as pollen (an allergen) first enters the body of an allergic person, cells called *macrophages* engulf the invader, chop it into pieces, and display the pieces on their surfaces. T-helper cells recognize certain allergen fragments and bind to the macrophages. This process causes the T-helper cells to secrete signaling molecules, including interleukin-4 (IL-4). IL-4, in turn, spurs nearby B cells to mature into plasma cells. Plasma cells produce Y-shaped antibody proteins.

One class of antibodies of great importance in allergic diseases and asthma is immunoglobulin E (IgE). The two arms of IgE are tailor-made to specifically attach to the allergen. The stem of the IgE molecule attaches to two classes of immune cells: mast cells, which concentrate in tissues exposed to the outside world, especially the skin, and the linings of the nose, lungs, and gastrointestinal tract; and basophilic cells, which circulate in the blood.

When the same allergen next enters the person's body, it binds to the arms of the IgE molecules protruding from the surfaces of mast cells and basophils. The interaction of an allergen with two IgE molecules triggers enzymes associated with the cell membrane, such as tyrosine kinases. The enzymes start a series of biochemical reactions in the cell, which causes the cell to release chemicals, including histamine, from storage pouches called *granules* in the cell interior.

These chemicals allow fluid to leak from blood vessels, producing symptoms such as redness and swelling in nearby tissues. They also constrict smooth muscles and stimulate mucus production. In addition, the reactions cause such symptoms as a runny nose, sneezing, itching, hives, or abdominal cramps. In severe cases, anaphylactic shock may occur following the release of some chemicals, like histamine, which can constrict the lungs' airways. Also, mast cells secrete chemical messengers that recruit other cells from the bloodstream, including T lymphocytes and eosinophils, into the tissues.

In the tissues, some of the recently arrived cells release substances that can increase and prolong early symptoms and may injure and inflame local tissue. Such responses often occur several hours after the initial encounter with an allergen. Collectively, they are called the *late-phase reaction*. The cells present in late-phase reactions are quite similar to those cells found in the tissues of patients with chronic allergic rhinitis and asthma.

1. Hay fever is an allergy to
   a. dust.
   b. hay.
   c. pollen.
   d. seeds.

2. Cells that surround pollen within the body are known as
   a. T-helper cells.
   b. macrophage cells.
   c. B cells.
   d. plasma cells.

3. The substances that diminish lung capacity
   a. are present during sensitization.
   b. can alleviate skin inflammation.
   c. can trigger the development of plasma cells.
   d. are located inside granules.

4. Which of the following describes the word *concentrate* as it is used in the third paragraph of the passage?
   a. mass
   b. think
   c. reduce
   d. deliberate

5. One result of mast cells' chemical messenger activity is
   a. relief of symptoms such as inflamed tissue.
   b. an allergen connecting to immunoglobulin E.
   c. the development of enzymes such as tyrosine kinases.
   d. an increase in the duration of patients' symptoms.

6. What occurs the second time an allergen enters the body?
   a. Macrophages cut the allergen into pieces.
   b. Mast cells become connected to the allergen.
   c. T-helper cells detect portions of the allergen.
   d. The allergen eliminates tyrosine kinases.

7. How many Americans suffer from either hay fever (allergy to pollen) or asthma?
   a. 32 to 37 million
   b. 22 million
   c. 10 to 15 million
   d. 40 to 80 million

By using tiny probes as neural prostheses, scientists may be able to restore nerve function in quadriplegics and make the blind see or the deaf hear. Thanks to advanced techniques, a single, small, implanted probe can stimulate individual neurons electrically or chemically and then record responses. Preliminary results suggest that the microprobe telemetry systems can be permanently implanted and replace damaged or missing nerves.

The tissue-compatible microprobes represent an advance over the typical aluminum wire electrodes used in studies of the cortex and other brain structures. Researchers accumulate much data using traditional electrodes, but there is a question of how much damage they cause to the nervous system. Microprobes, which are about as thin as a human hair, cause minimal damage and disruption of neurons when inserted into the brain.

In addition to recording nervous system impulses, the microprobes have minuscule channels that open the way for delivery of drugs, cellular growth factors, neurotransmitters, and other neuroactive compounds to a single neuron or to groups of neurons. The probes can have up to four channels, each with its own recording/stimulating electrode.

The probes can be left in place for a fairly long time. In one guinea pig, a probe continued to transmit data from the animal's hearing center for eleven months. The long-term implantability of the probes makes them promising candidates for neural prostheses. Researchers envision the probes being used to affect the motor center of the brain: for example, to stimulate a hand grasp in patients who have lost motor control. They might also be used to create a visual prosthesis, connecting an external miniature video camera to the visual center in the cortex, thereby circumventing damaged eyes and optic nerves.

In quadriplegics and paraplegics, probes might bridge injured areas of the spinal cord and restore nerve connection to the limbs. Additionally, people who lack or produce too little of essential biochemicals or who need drugs could receive minute doses delivered with pinpoint accuracy through permanently implanted probes.

One obstacle to using any electrode as a long-term implant has been the lack of satisfactory connections to the outside world. Wires are bulky, they break easily, and they must be tethered to prevent damage to surrounding tissue. Even with implantable telemetry systems, which have their own power supply and can transmit data via radio waves, leads still must connect the electrodes to the electronic package (a system similar to integrated circuits used on computer chips). To overcome the connection problem, researchers have developed ultra-flexible silicon ribbon cables. The cables are significantly more flexible than a commonly used aluminum wire.

It is easiest to place probes in the brain cortex, compared to deeper structures. Because the probes are so small, implantation must be viewed under the microscope. They can be manually inserted using forceps or affixed to special mounting mechanisms.

8. A major benefit of microprobes is that their wires are
a. strong.
b. thin.
c. stiff.
d. wide.

9. Which of the following is NOT something
with which the author of the passage would
likely agree?
   a. Microprobes are safer to use than traditional electrodes.
   b. There are not any significant concerns
about attaching probes to the brain.
   c. Inadequate connections are a major defect
of electrodes.
   d. The ethics of using probes to cure blind
people needs to be explored more.

10. Who would most likely benefit from permanent implantation of a microprobe telemetry
system?
   a. a patient who is overweight
   b. a patient who has rheumatoid arthritis
   c. a patient who is in a drug-induced coma
   d. a patient who is a quadriplegic

11. The initial function of microprobe channels
is to
   a. create pathways.
   b. disrupt neurons.
   c. replace ribbon cables.
   d. study the brain.

12. The sixth paragraph is chiefly concerned with
the problems with
   a. probes.
   b. implants.
   c. aluminum.
   d. wires.

13. Devising acceptable external telemetry links is
essential to
   a. the implanting of probes with special tools.
   b. the administration of drugs with pinpoint
accuracy.
   c. improvement in the duration of implants.
   d. creation of a usable power supply.

A government report addressing concerns
about the many implications of genetic testing
outlined policy guidelines and legislative
recommendations intended to avoid involuntary and ineffective testing and to protect
confidentiality.

The report identified urgent concerns,
such as quality control measures (including
federal oversight for testing laboratories) and
better genetics training for medical practitioners. It recommended voluntary screening;
urged couples in high-risk populations to
consider carrier screening; and advised caution
in using and interpreting presymptomatic or
predictive tests as certain information could
easily be misused or misinterpreted.

About three in every 100 children are born
with a severe disorder presumed to be genetic or
partially genetic in origin. Genes, often in concert
with environmental factors, are being linked to
the causes of many common adult diseases such
as coronary artery disease, hypertension, various
cancers, diabetes, and Alzheimer's disease. Tests
to determine predisposition to a variety of
conditions are under study, and some are
beginning to be applied.

The report recommended that all
screening, including screening of newborns,
be voluntary. Citing results of two different
voluntary newborn screening programs, the
report said these programs can achieve
compliance rates equal to or better than those
of mandatory programs. State health departments could eventually mandate the offering
of tests for diagnosing treatable conditions in
newborns; however, careful pilot studies for
conditions diagnosable at birth need to be
done first.

Although the report asserted that it would prefer that all screening be voluntary, it did note that if a state requires newborn screening for a particular condition, the state should do so only if there is strong evidence that a newborn would benefit from effective treatment at the earliest possible age. Newborn screening is the most common type of genetic screening today. More than four million newborns are tested annually so that effective treatment can be started in a few hundred infants.

Prenatal testing can pose the most difficult issues. The ability to diagnose genetic disorders in the fetus far exceeds any ability to treat or cure them. Parents must be fully informed about risks and benefits of testing procedures, the nature and variability of the disorders they would disclose, and the options available if test results are positive. Obtaining informed consent—a process that would include educating participants, not just processing documents—would enhance voluntary participation. When offered testing, parents should receive comprehensive counseling, which should be nondirective. Relevant medical advice, however, is recommended for treatable or preventable conditions.

Genetics also can predict whether certain diseases might develop later in life. For single-gene diseases, population screening should only be considered for treatable or preventable conditions of relatively high frequency. Children should be tested only for disorders for which effective treatments or preventive measures could be applied early in life.

14. As it is used in the passage, the word *predisposition* most nearly means
    a. willingness.
    b. susceptibility.
    c. impartiality.
    d. composure.

15. The author stresses the need for caution in the use and interpretation of
    a. predictive tests.
    b. newborn screening.
    c. informed consent.
    d. pilot studies.

16. According to the report, most screenings should not be
    a. optional.
    b. insured.
    c. mandatory.
    d. complementary.

17. One intention of the policy guidelines was to
    a. implement compulsory testing.
    b. minimize concerns about quality control.
    c. endorse the expansion of screening programs.
    d. preserve privacy in testing.

18. When discussing prenatal testing in the sixth paragraph, the author's tone could best be described as
    a. jovial.
    b. anxious.
    c. assured.
    d. difficult.

TYPES OF SCREENINGS		
NAME	**DETECTS**	**ACCURACY**
First trimester combined screen	Down syndrome	83%
	Trisomy 18	75%
Second trimester quad screen	Spina bifida	80%
	Down syndrome	75%
	Trisomy 18	98%
Cell free fetal DNA screen	Down syndrome	99%
	Trisomy 18	98%

19. Which of the following is true based on the above table?

a. Getting screened during the third trimester will yield the most accurate results.

b. The most accurate screening for Down syndrome is performed in the first trimester.

c. Spina bifida cannot be tested accurately with a prenatal screening.

d. The most accurate screening for trisomy 18 is performed in the second trimester.

Scientists have developed an innovative procedure that reveals details of tissues and organs that are difficult to see by conventional magnetic resonance imaging (MRI). By using "hyperpolarized" gases, scientists have taken the first clear MRI pictures of human lungs and airways. Researchers hope the new technique will aid the diagnosis and treatment of lung disorders, and perhaps lead to improved visualization of blood flow.

The air spaces of the lungs have been notoriously difficult for clinicians to visualize. Chest X-rays can detect tumors or inflamed regions in the lungs but provide poor soft-tissue contrast and no clear view of air passages. Computed tomography, a cross sectional X-ray scan, can provide high resolution images of the walls of the lungs and its airways but gives no measure of function. Conventional MRI, because it images water protons, provides poor images of the lungs, which are filled with air, not water.

The new MRI technique detects not water but inert gases whose nuclei have been strongly aligned, or hyperpolarized, by laser light. Initially this technique seemed to have no practical application, but exhaustive research has proven its potential. Scientists plan to further refine this technology with animal and human studies, in part because they have yet to produce a viable 3-D image of human lungs.

By 1995 researchers had produced the first 3-D MRI pictures of a living animal's lungs. In the first human test, a member of the research team inhaled hyperpolarized helium-3. His lungs were then imaged using a standard MRI scanner that had been adjusted to detect helium. The results were impressive, considering that the system had yet to be optimized and there was only a relatively small volume of gas with which to work.

When a standard MRI is taken, the patient enters a large magnet. Many of the body's hydrogen atoms (primarily the hydrogen atoms in water) align with the magnetic field like tiny bar magnets, and the nucleus at the center of each atom spins constantly about its north-south axis. Inside the MRI scanner, a radio pulse temporarily knocks the spinning nuclei out of position, and as their axes gradually realign within the magnetic field, they emit faint radio signals. Computers convert these faint signals into an image.

The new gas-based MRI is built around similar principles. But circularly polarized light, rather than a magnet, is used to align spinning nuclei, and the inert gases helium-3 or xenon-129 (rather than hydrogen) provide the nuclei that emit the image-producing signals. The laser light polarizes the gases through a technique known as *spin exchange*. Helium-3 and xenon-129 are ideal for gas-based MRI because they take hours to lose their polarization. Most other gases readily lose their alignment. The clarity of an MRI picture depends in part on the volume of aligned nuclei.

20. The MRI innovation is different from the standard MRI in that it
   a. distinguishes gases rather than water.
   b. uses magnets rather than light.
   c. has a range of useful applications.
   d. provides better images of blood circulation.

21. Chest X-rays have the most difficulty photographing
   a. tumors.
   b. inflammations.
   c. lungs.
   d. air passages.

22. Standard MRI scanners detect radio signals emitted
   a. before nuclei rotate on an axis.
   b. before atoms align with magnets.
   c. after nuclei are aligned by magnetism.
   d. after signals are transformed into pictures.

23. The word that can best be interchanged with *hyperpolarization* in the passage is
   a. visualization.
   b. alignment.
   c. emission.
   d. tomography.

24. Use of which of the following is substituted for use of a magnet in one of the MRI techniques?
   a. light
   b. hydrogen
   c. helium-3
   d. X-rays

25. An image lacking in clarity is likely to be the result of
   a. a high number of aligned nuclei.
   b. hydrogen being replaced with xenon.
   c. an abbreviated period of alignment.
   d. nuclei regaining their aligned position.

Once people wore garlic around their necks to ward off disease. Today, most Americans would scoff at the idea of wearing a necklace of garlic cloves to enhance their well-being. However, you might find a number of Americans willing to ingest capsules of pulverized garlic or other herbal supplements in the name of health.

Complementary and alternative medicine (CAM), which includes a range of practices outside of conventional medicine such as herbs, homeopathy, massage, yoga, and acupuncture, holds increasing appeal for Americans. In fact, according to one estimate, 42% of Americans have used alternative therapies. A Harvard Medical School survey found that young adults (those born between 1965 and 1979) are the most likely to use alternative treatments, whereas people born before 1945 are the least likely to use these therapies. Nonetheless, in all age groups, the use of unconventional healthcare practices has steadily increased since the 1950s, and the trend is likely to continue.

CAM has become a big business as Americans dip into their wallets to pay for alternative treatments. A 1997 American Medical Association study estimated that the public spent $21.2 billion for alternative medicine therapies in that year, more than half of which were "out-of-pocket" expenditures, meaning they were not covered by health insurance. Indeed, Americans made more out-of-pocket expenditures for alternative services than they did for out-of-pocket payments for hospital stays in 1997. In addition, the number of total visits to alternative medicine providers (about 629 million) exceeded the tally of visits to primary care physicians (386 million) in that year.

However, the public has not abandoned conventional medicine for alternative healthcare. Most Americans seek out alternative therapies as a complement to their conventional healthcare whereas only a small percentage of Americans rely primarily on alternative care. Why have so many patients turned to alternative therapies? Frustrated by the time constraints of managed care and alienated by conventional medicine's focus on technology, some feel that a holistic approach to healthcare better reflects their beliefs and values. Others seek therapies that will relieve symptoms associated with chronic disease, symptoms that mainstream medicine cannot treat.

Some alternative therapies have crossed the line into mainstream medicine as scientific investigation has confirmed their safety and efficacy. For example, today physicians may prescribe acupuncture for pain management or to control the nausea associated with chemotherapy. Most U.S. medical schools teach courses in alternative therapies and many health insurance companies offer some alternative medicine benefits. Yet, despite their gaining acceptance, the majority of alternative therapies have not been researched in controlled studies. New research efforts aim at testing alternative methods and providing the public with information about which ones are safe and effective and which ones are a waste of money, or possibly dangerous.

So what about those who swear by the health benefits of the "smelly rose," garlic?

Observational studies that track disease incidence in different populations suggest that garlic use in the diet may act as a cancer-fighting agent, particularly for prostate and stomach cancer. However, these findings have not been confirmed in clinical studies. And yes, reported side effects include garlic odor.

26. The author describes wearing garlic as an example of
    a. an arcane practice considered odd and superstitious today.
    b. the ludicrous nature of complementary and alternative medicine.
    c. a scientifically tested medical practice.
    d. a socially unacceptable style of jewelry.

27. As it is used in the second paragraph, the word *conventional* most nearly means
    a. appropriate.
    b. established.
    c. formal.
    d. moralistic.

28. According to the Harvard Medical School survey cited in the passage, the people most likely to use alternative treatments were
    a. people born between 1921 and 1946.
    b. people born between 1948 and 1960.
    c. people born between 1965 and 1979.
    d. people born between 1980 and 2007.

29. The statistic in the third paragraph comparing total visits to alternative medicine practitioners with those to primary care physicians is used to illustrate the
    a. popularity of alternative medicine.
    b. public's distrust of conventional healthcare.
    c. accessibility of alternative medicine.
    d. affordability of alternative therapies.

30. In paragraph four, *complement* most nearly means
    a. tribute.
    b. commendation.
    c. replacement.
    d. addition.

31. CAM may have disadvantages that are
    a. medical.
    b. ethical.
    c. conventional.
    d. financial.

In space flight, there are the obvious hazards of meteors, debris, and radiation; however, astronauts must also deal with two vexing physiological foes—muscle atrophy and bone loss. Space shuttle astronauts, because they spend only about a week in space, undergo minimal wasting of bone and muscle. But when longer stays in microgravity or zero gravity are contemplated, as in the space station or a two-year round-trip voyage to Mars, these problems are of particular concern because they could become acute.

Some studies show that muscle atrophy can be kept largely at bay with appropriate exercise, but bone loss caused by reduced gravity cannot. Scientists can measure certain flight-related hormonal changes and can obtain animal bone biopsies immediately after flights, but they do not completely understand how gravity affects the bones or what happens at the cellular level.

Even pounding the bones or wearing a suspender-like pressure device does nothing to avert loss of calcium from bones. Researchers say that after a three-month or longer stay in space, much of the profound bone loss may be irreversible. Some argue that protracted missions should be curtailed. They are conducting a search for the molecular mechanisms behind bone loss, and they hope these studies will help develop a prevention strategy to control tissue loss associated not only with weightlessness but also with prolonged bed rest.

Doctors simulate bone-depleting microgravity conditions by putting volunteers to bed for long time periods. The bed support of the supine body decreases the load on it significantly, thus simulating reduced gravity. One study involves administering either *alendronate*, a drug that blocks the breakdown of bone, or a placebo, a look-alike substance without medical effects, to volunteers for two weeks prior to and then during a three-week bed rest.

Prior to bed rest, alendronate-treated volunteers excreted only about one-third as much calcium as did the persons receiving the placebo. Bed rest increased urinary calcium excretion in both groups, but in alendronate-treated persons the urinary calcium levels were even lower than those in the placebo group before bed rest. Blood levels of parathyroid hormone and vitamin D, which are involved in regulation of bone metabolism, were also significantly elevated in drug recipients.

Although these results suggest that alendronate inhibits bone loss and averts high urinary calcium concentrations that can cause kidney stones, they do not point to the precise molecular mechanisms at work. Thus, plans are to initiate a more prolonged bed rest project over the next several years.

32. One factor that has a negative affect on bones in space is
    a. radiation.
    b. calcium.
    c. microgravity.
    d. hormones.

33. Compared to volunteers who received a placebo, volunteers who received alendronate experienced
   a. lower levels of parathyroid hormone.
   b. lower levels of hormonal changes.
   c. higher levels of vitamin D.
   d. higher levels of calcium excretion.

34. Specialized equipment for astronauts in weightless conditions
   a. reduces the amount of calcium in their bones.
   b. makes lengthy space flights more feasible.
   c. enables scientists to better comprehend molecular mechanisms.
   d. has a negligible impact on bone loss.

35. The passage suggests that the bone-loss studies may yield information that could aid the treatment of
   a. kidney stones.
   b. muscular atrophy.
   c. thyroid disease.
   d. urinary infections.

36. Doctors simulated bone-depleting micro-gravity conditions by
   a. having volunteers work out on treadmills for an hour.
   b. having volunteers stay in bed for three weeks.
   c. having volunteers run in a marathon.
   d. having volunteers stay in bed for three months.

About three million Americans have open-angle glaucoma, the most common form of glaucoma in the United States. For unknown reasons, small changes within the eye gradually interfere with the normal flow of fluids that feed tissues in the front of the eye. If these fluids do not drain properly, the resulting higher pressure inside the eye can damage the optic nerve and narrow the field of vision. This change happens so slowly that many people are not diagnosed with glaucoma until they have significant loss of vision.

Laser therapy is a safe and effective alternative to eyedrops as a first-line treatment for patients with newly diagnosed primary open-angle glaucoma. This finding comes from a follow-up study undertaken to learn if early laser treatment is safe and whether it offers any medical advantages over eyedrops for newly diagnosed open-angle glaucoma. A total of 271 patients were enrolled in the initial study. Each patient had laser treatment in one eye and medication in the other eye. Over 200 patients were followed for an average of seven years after treatment.

Post-study analysis revealed that all measures used to evaluate the two treatments showed that the "laser-first" eyes and the "medication-first" eyes had a similar status on all measures used to evaluate the two treatments. Researchers assessed changes in the patient's visual field, visual acuity, intraocular pressure, and optic nerve. The results suggested that initial treatment with laser surgery is at least as effective as initial treatment with eyedrops. However, researchers cautioned that neither treatment method is a "magic bullet" for long-term control of glaucoma. They noted that two years after the start of treatment, 56% of "laser-first" eyes and 70% of "medication-first" eyes needed new or extra medications to control pressure inside the eye.

Researchers noted that both treatments caused side effects. However, the side effects of laser treatment were temporary or made no apparent difference in the long run, whereas the side effects of eyedrops were troublesome for some patients for as long as the drops were used. Eyedrops used for glaucoma treatment can cause discomfort in the eye, blurry vision, headaches, and fast or slow heartbeat.

In 34% of "laser-first" eyes, the laser treatment caused a temporary jump in intraocular pressure for the first few days after treatment. Also, some 30% of the "laser-first" eyes developed *peripheral anterior synechiae*—adhesions that form when the iris sticks to part of the cornea.

37. Over half the patients in the study discussed in the passage required supplemental treatment for
    a. optic nerve damage.
    b. intraocular pressure.
    c. visual field weakness.
    d. lack of visual acuity.

38. The fourth paragraph is chiefly concerned with
    a. eyedrops.
    b. headaches.
    c. research.
    d. side effects.

39. Greater pressure within the eye results from
    a. a disruption of fluid concentration.
    b. the rapid accumulation of fluids.
    c. a gradual broadening of the field of vision.
    d. initial treatment with eyedrops.

40. The study concluded that, compared with medication, laser therapy is
    a. slightly more effective.
    b. significantly more effective.
    c. just as effective.
    d. less effective.

41. The study was conducted on patients who were
    a. in the initial stages of open-angle glaucoma.
    b. experiencing a rare form of glaucoma.
    c. given eyedrop medication in both eyes.
    d. in the late stages of open-angle glaucoma.

Almost 50% of American teens are not vigorously active on a regular basis, contributing to a trend of sluggishness among Americans of all ages, according the U.S. Centers for Disease Control (CDC). Adolescent female students are particularly inactive—29% are inactive compared with 15% of male students. Unfortunately, the sedentary habits of young "couch potatoes" often continue into adulthood. According to the Surgeon General's Report on Physical Activity and Health, Americans become increasingly less active with each year of age. Inactivity can be a serious health risk factor, setting the stage for obesity and associated chronic illnesses like heart disease or diabetes. The benefits of exercise include building bone, muscle, and joints, controlling weight, and preventing the development of high blood pressure.

Some studies suggest that physical activity may have other benefits as well. One CDC study found that high school students who take part in team sports or are physically active outside of school are less likely to engage in risky behaviors, like using drugs or smoking. Physical activity does not need to be strenuous to be beneficial. The CDC recommends moderate, daily physical activity for people of all ages, such as brisk walking for 30 minutes or 15–20 minutes of more intense exercise. A survey conducted by the National Association for Sport and Physical Education questioned teens about their attitudes toward exercise and about what it would take to get them moving. Teens chose friends (56%) as their most likely motivators for becoming more active, followed by parents (18%) and professional athletes (11%).

42. The author defines smoking as behavior that is
   a. deadly.
   b. unhygienic.
   c. risky.
   d. chronic.

43. In the first paragraph, *sedentary* most nearly means
   a. slothful.
   b. apathetic.
   c. stationary.
   d. stabilized.

BENEFITS OF EXERCISE— REPORTED BY TEENS

BENEFIT	PERCENTAGE THAT REPORTED BENEFIT
Good self-image	53%
Good mood	40%
Less stressed	32%

44. Which of the following is true based on the table?
   a. Exercise is an essential component of self-esteem.
   b. Exercise is a key tactic for lowering stress.
   c. Exercise has more dramatic effects on adults than teens.
   d. Exercise can have emotional benefits for certain teens.

45. The primary purpose of the passage is to
   a. refute an argument.
   b. make a prediction.
   c. praise an outcome.
   d. promote a change.

Section 3: Math

Choose the correct answer for each problem. You have 45 minutes to complete this section.

1. How many inches are there in $3\frac{1}{3}$ yards?
   a. 120
   b. 126
   c. 160
   d. 168

2. Lori ran 45 miles over the last three weeks. Paola ran $\frac{2}{3}$ the number of miles that Lori ran over the same time period. How many miles did Paola run?
   a. 20 miles
   b. 90 miles
   c. 30 miles
   d. 15 miles

3. A patient started a particular test at 7:15 A.M. After two hours, he had a break for 15 minutes. The rest of the test took three hours 10 minutes. What time did the patient finish the test?
   a. 12:40 P.M.
   b. 9:30 A.M.
   c. 12:30 P.M.
   d. 11:40 A.M.

4. In a triangle, angle *A* is 70° and angle *B* is 30°. What is the measure of angle *C*?
   a. 90°
   b. 70°
   c. 80°
   d. 100°

5. 6^3 is equal to
   a. 36.
   b. 1,296.
   c. 18.
   d. 216.

6. Dr. Drake charges $36.00 for an office visit, which is $\frac{3}{4}$ of what Dr. Jean charges. How much does Dr. Jean charge?
   a. $48.00
   b. $27.00
   c. $38.00
   d. $57.00

7. The nursing assistants give baths to the patients every morning at 7:00. Tasha gives Ms. Rogers her bath in 20 minutes. Lou gives Mr. Taft his bath in 17 minutes, and Marie gives Ms. Johnson her bath in 14 minutes. What is the average time for the three baths?
   a. 20 minutes
   b. 17 minutes
   c. 14 minutes
   d. 12 minutes

8. What percentage of 50 is 12?
   a. 4%
   b. 14%
   c. 24%
   d. 34%

9. A hospital waiting room is 8 feet wide and 10 feet long. What is the area of the waiting room?
   a. 18 square feet
   b. 40 square feet
   c. 60 square feet
   d. 80 square feet

10. Mr. Beard's temperature is 98° Fahrenheit. What is his temperature in degrees Centigrade? $C = \frac{5}{9}(F - 32)$
   a. 35.8°
   b. 36.7°
   c. 37.6°
   d. 31.1°

11. $6(3^3 - 7) + 50 \div 2$ is equal to
   a. 85.
   b. 145.
   c. 31.
   d. 28.

12. Order the numbers from least to greatest.
   $\frac{3}{8}, 0.7, 0.44, \frac{5}{7}, 0.35$
   a. $\frac{5}{7}, 0.35, \frac{3}{8}, 0.44, 0.7$
   b. $0.35, \frac{3}{8}, 0.44, 0.7, \frac{5}{7}$
   c. $0.35, 0.44, 0.7, \frac{5}{7}, \frac{3}{8}$
   d. $\frac{5}{7}, \frac{3}{8}, 0.7, 0.44, 0.35$

13. Which of the following is 14% of 232?
   a. 3.248
   b. 32.48
   c. 16.57
   d. 165.7

14. One side of a square bandage is 4 inches long. What is the perimeter of the bandage?
   a. 4 inches
   b. 8 inches
   c. 12 inches
   d. 16 inches

15. $12(9 \times 4)$ is equal to
   a. 432.
   b. 72.
   c. 108.
   d. 336.

16. 33 is 12% of which of the following numbers?
   a. 3,960
   b. 396
   c. 275
   d. 2,750

17. 945.6 ÷ 24 is equal to
    a. 3,940.
    b. 394.
    c. 39.4.
    d. 3.946.

18. A medical assistant makes $14.25 an hour. He receives a 10% raise. What is his hourly pay after he receives the raise?
    a. $1.43
    b. $16.25
    c. $17.10
    d. $15.68

19. The radius of a circle is 13. What is the approximate area of the circle?
    a. 81.64
    b. 1,666.27
    c. 530.66
    d. 169

20. $\frac{7}{8} - \frac{3}{5}$ is equal to
    a. $\frac{11}{40}$.
    b. $1\frac{1}{3}$.
    c. $\frac{1}{10}$.
    d. $1\frac{19}{40}$.

21. All the rooms on the orthopedic ward are rectangular with 8-foot ceilings. One room is 9 feet wide by 11 feet long. What is the combined area of the four walls, including doors and windows?
    a. 99 square feet
    b. 160 square feet
    c. 320 square feet
    d. 72 square feet

22. What is the value of 195.6 divided by 7.2, rounded to the nearest hundredth?
    a. 271.67
    b. 27.17
    c. 27.16
    d. 2.717

23. What is the correct way to write the number 65.19?
    a. sixty-five and nine tenths
    b. sixty-five and nineteen thousandths
    c. sixty-five and nineteen hundredths
    d. sixty-five and nine hundredths

24. $\frac{5}{8} \div 3$ is equal to
    a. $\frac{5}{24}$.
    b. $\frac{3}{8}$.
    c. $1\frac{7}{8}$.
    d. $\frac{3}{24}$.

25. On the cardiac ward, there are seven nursing assistants. Emily has eight patients; Luis has five patients; Keisha has nine patients; Ray has ten patients; Dawn has ten patients; James has 14 patients, and Sheela has seven patients. What is the average number of patients per nursing assistant?
    a. 7
    b. 8
    c. 9
    d. 10

26. $(25 + 17)(64 - 49)$ is equal to
    a. 57.
    b. 630.
    c. 570.
    d. 63.

27. What percentage of 18,000 is 234?
    a. 1,300%
    b. 130%
    c. 13%
    d. 1.3%

28. How many minutes are in $7\frac{1}{6}$ hours?
    a. 430 minutes
    b. 2,580 minutes
    c. 4,300 minutes
    d. 258 minutes

29. 72.687 + 145.29 is equal to
    a. 87.216.
    b. 217.977.
    c. 217.877.
    d. 882.16.

30. $12(84 - 5) - (3 \times 54)$ is equal to
    a. 54,000.
    b. 841.
    c. 796.
    d. 786.

31. The perimeter of an equilateral triangle is 22.5 centimeters. What is the length of one side of the triangle?
    a. 11.25 centimeters
    b. 7.5 centimeters
    c. 7 centimeters
    d. 9 centimeters

32. 6.35×5 is equal to
    a. 31.75.
    b. 30.75.
    c. 3.175.
    d. 317.5.

33. $2,273 \times 4$ is equal to
    a. 9,092.
    b. 8,982.
    c. 8,892.
    d. 8,882.

34. The floor of an operating room has a length of 11 yards and a width of 9 yards. The flooring for the room costs $12.25 per square yard. How much does the flooring of the operating room cost?
    a. $140.25
    b. $1,212.75
    c. $490.00
    d. $1,245.25

35. 703×365 is equal to
    a. 67,595.
    b. 255,695.
    c. 256,595.
    d. 263,595.

36. $4\frac{1}{5} + 1\frac{2}{5} + 3\frac{3}{10}$ is equal to
    a. $9\frac{1}{10}$.
    b. $8\frac{9}{10}$.
    c. $8\frac{4}{5}$.
    d. $8\frac{6}{15}$.

37. A store puts its pens on sale by 25%. Kathy buys a pen with a sale price of $22.50. What was the amount of her discount?
    a. $7.50
    b. $5.50
    c. $37.50
    d. $30.00

38. $76\frac{1}{2} + 11\frac{5}{6}$ is equal to
    a. $87\frac{1}{2}$.
    b. $88\frac{1}{3}$.
    c. $88\frac{5}{6}$.
    d. $89\frac{1}{6}$.

39. Juan makes a special window for the waiting room of a clinic. The window has a width of 4 feet 3 inches and a length of 3 feet 5 inches. Juan needs to put trim around the window. How much trim does he need?
- **a.** 8 feet 6 inches
- **b.** 13 feet 3 inches
- **c.** 6 feet 10 inches
- **d.** 15 feet 4 inches

40. $30 \div 2\frac{1}{2}$ is equal to
- **a.** $\frac{1}{15}$.
- **b.** 12.
- **c.** 15.
- **d.** 75.

41. 172×0.56 is equal to
- **a.** 9.632.
- **b.** 96.32.
- **c.** 963.2.
- **d.** 0.9632.

42. $7,400 \div 74$ is equal to
- **a.** 1.
- **b.** 10.
- **c.** 100.
- **d.** 1,000.

43. $\left(-\frac{3}{10}\right) \div \left(-\frac{1}{5}\right)$ is equal to
- **a.** $1\frac{1}{2}$.
- **b.** $-\frac{2}{3}$.
- **c.** $-\frac{3}{50}$.
- **d.** $\frac{3}{50}$.

44. 35% of what number is equal to 14?
- **a.** 4
- **b.** 40
- **c.** 49
- **d.** 400

45. A piece of gauze 3 feet 4 inches long was divided into 5 equal parts. How long was each part?
- **a.** 1 foot 2 inches
- **b.** 10 inches
- **c.** 8 inches
- **d.** 6 inches

46. What is 0.716 rounded to the nearest tenth?
- **a.** 0.7
- **b.** 0.8
- **c.** 0.72
- **d.** 1.0

47. Which of these has a 9 in the thousandths place?
- **a.** 3.0095
- **b.** 3.0905
- **c.** 3.9005
- **d.** 3.0059

48. Out of 100 shoppers polled, 80 said they buy fresh fruit every week. How many shoppers out of 30,000 could be expected to buy fresh fruit every week?
- **a.** 2,400
- **b.** 6,000
- **c.** 22,000
- **d.** 24,000

49. Which of the following means $5n + 7 = 17$?
- **a.** seven more than five times a number is 17.
- **b.** five more than seven times a number is 17.
- **c.** seven less than five times a number is 17.
- **d.** 12 times a number is 17.

50. What is the value of y when $x = 3$ and $y = 5 + 4x$?
- **a.** 6
- **b.** 9
- **c.** 12
- **d.** 17

Section 4: General Science

There are 50 questions in this section. You have 45 minutes to complete this section.

1. Earth's core is
   a. divided into two parts.
   b. also called the mantle.
   c. largely composed of lead.
   d. located 400 miles beneath the surface.

2. When did Earth form?
   a. 4.6 billion years ago
   b. 3.5 billion years ago
   c. 4.6 hundred million years ago
   d. 3.5 hundred million years ago

3. The lithosphere is
   a. relatively buoyant and deep in the Earth.
   b. relatively buoyant and on the Earth's surface.
   c. relatively dense and deep in the Earth.
   d. relatively dense and on the Earth's surface.

4. Most weather phenomena occur in the
   a. lithosphere.
   b. troposphere.
   c. thermosphere.
   d. stratosphere.

5. Which of the following is the primary driving force behind ocean tides?
   a. the Moon
   b. the Sun
   c. wind
   d. Coriolis effect

6. Earth's mantle
   a. is between the crust and the core.
   b. is under the core and the crust.
   c. is heavier than the core.
   d. contains both crust and core.

7. Most of the rock at Earth's surface is
   a. sedimentary.
   b. metamorphic.
   c. igneous.
   d. bedrock.

8. Which of the following is the metric (SI) unit for mass?
   a. newton
   b. ounce
   c. pound
   d. gram

9. The four planets known as the gas giants are Jupiter, Saturn, Neptune, and
   a. Mars.
   b. Uranus.
   c. Pluto.
   d. Venus.

10. What kind of rock is obsidian?
   a. sedimentary
   b. igneous
   c. metamorphic
   d. mantle

11. In which century did the world see the biggest increase in its population?
   a. thirteenth
   b. twentieth
   c. nineteenth
   d. seventeenth

12. How long does it take the global atmosphere to circulate?
   a. one day
   b. one year
   c. one decade
   d. one century

13. What ultimately drives the circulation of the atmosphere and ocean?
a. biosphere
b. the Sun
c. volcanism
d. lithosphere

14. Which of the following correctly places the four layers of Earth's atmosphere in order beginning at the surface of Earth and increasing in altitude toward space?
a. stratosphere, thermosphere, troposphere, mesosphere
b. troposphere, stratosphere, mesosphere, thermosphere
c. thermosphere, mesosphere, stratosphere, troposphere
d. mesosphere, troposphere, thermosphere, stratosphere

15. The timescale for the entire ocean to mix is about
a. one year.
b. one decade.
c. one thousand years.
d. one hundred thousand years.

16. Why do oceans have waves, but small ponds do not?
a. Ponds do not have enough depth for waves to develop.
b. The surface area of a pond is not large enough for wind to create waves.
c. Oceans experience much greater, steadier wind duration than ponds.
d. Wind velocities are much greater over the open ocean than small ponds.

17. Soil is thickest, generally, where
a. vegetation is densest.
b. climate is coldest.
c. vegetation is hardiest.
d. climate is wettest.

18. Today, we have classified about 310,000 species of vascular plants. Which of these groups has an even larger number of species already described?
a. insects
b. fungi
c. viruses
d. mollusks

19. A tropical entomologist wants to know how many species of insects still remain to be discovered, especially in the tropical rain forests. The entomologist observes that 100 species of insects are specialized to just the canopy of a particular species of tropical tree. Half the species of insects that are specialized to this tree species live in the canopy, and half live underground in and around the roots of that species. How many total species of insects are specialized to that species of tree?
a. 50
b. 100
c. 200
d. 400

20. Which biome has the thickest soils that are hugely abundant in organic matter, because decomposition is so slow?
a. tropical rain forests
b. tundra
c. tropical dry forests
d. chaparral

21. In which biome are the solar collecting organs of the net primary producers particularly tough with the chemical called lignin?
a. tundra
b. tropical dry forest
c. deciduous forest
d. boreal forest

22. Which of the following is true in biological classification?
   a. Family is equal to genus.
   b. A genus has many families.
   c. Genus is equal to species.
   d. A genus has many species.

23. Uranus and Neptune are composed mainly of
   a. rocks.
   b. metals.
   c. various ices.
   d. hydrogen.

24. High-temperature magma behaves much like
   a. running water.
   b. rubber.
   c. thick oil.
   d. a sponge.

25. The special type of cell division that creates sex cells with half the number of chromosomes (and thus genes) from an individual male or female in a sexual species is called
   a. mitosis.
   b. symbiosis.
   c. parthenogenesis.
   d. meiosis.

26. The Northern spotted owl is protected because it requires the old growth forests of the Pacific northwest. It therefore is an example of a(n)
   a. umbrella species.
   b. invasive species.
   c. keystone species.
   d. extinct species.

27. What is an invasive species?
   a. a nonnative species that is introduced from elsewhere and spreads
   b. a native species that suddenly booms in population, threatening the other native species
   c. an endemic species that suddenly booms in population, threatening the native species
   d. an endemic species that is introduced from elsewhere and spreads

28. The loudness of a sound wave depends on its
   a. pitch.
   b. amplitude.
   c. frequency.
   d. wavelength.

29. The functional role that bacteria play in the recycling of elements in the ocean is the equivalent to the role played on land by
   a. leaf litter.
   b. worms.
   c. root nodules.
   d. soil bacteria.

30. Dolly the sheep was involved in what scientific achievement?
   a. the first genetically modified animal
   b. the first animal-to-human organ transplant
   c. the first cloned mammal
   d. the first animal-human hybrid

31. The limit to a population of a species in a community, determined by environmental conditions or species interactions, is called the
   a. ultimate yield.
   b. maximum sustainable yield.
   c. carrying capacity.
   d. deadlock number.

32. A steady influx of nutrients makes which of these regions of the ocean among the most productive fishing grounds?
   a. hydrothermal vents
   b. transition zones
   c. upwelling zones
   d. deep layers

33. In the carbon cycle, photosynthesis removes carbon (in the form of CO_2) from the atmosphere, while which process returns it back to the atmosphere?
   a. burial
   b. respiration
   c. dissolution
   d. sequestration

34. Two gases that contain carbon and are released by bacteria are
   a. sulfuric acid and methane.
   b. carbon dioxide and methane.
   c. sulfuric acid and water.
   d. water and carbon dioxide.

35. Bacteria that live in nodules attached to the roots of certain plants perform the chemical transformation called
   a. denitrification.
   b. ammoniafication.
   c. nitrification.
   d. nitrogen fixation.

36. Negative population growth in some countries is due to
   a. sub-replacement fertility rates.
   b. overpopulation.
   c. high fertility rates.
   d. medical technology.

37. The main supply of phosphorus to the ocean (and thus to marine life in the ocean) is as phosphate ions, via
   a. wind.
   b. undersea volcanoes.
   c. rain.
   d. rivers.

38. From most to least, in terms of mass, the four most abundant elements in the human body are
   a. H, C, Fe, P.
   b. H, C, P, Fe.
   c. C, H, P, Fe.
   d. C, P, Fe, H.

39. Which is NOT a macronutrient?
   a. copper
   b. magnesium
   c. nitrogen
   d. sulfur

40. During the hunting and gathering stage of human history, prior to agriculture, the global population was about
   a. 10 thousand.
   b. 10 billion.
   c. 100 thousand.
   d. 10 million.

41. Although coal is a relatively abundant energy resource, many environmentalists oppose the construction of new coal power plants because these plants release which of the following into the atmosphere?
   a. ammonia, sucrose, calcium carbonate
   b. carbon dioxide, volatile organic compounds, radiation
   c. sulfur dioxide, carbon monoxide, nitrogen oxide
   d. radon, lead, asbestos

42. Toxicology is the study of
   a. viruses.
   b. transportation.
   c. poisons.
   d. cancers.

43. The remaining land that can be converted to agriculture might not be as good as the land already employed for agriculture, because
   a. erosion from irrigation has already taken a toll.
   b. its soils are less rich.
   c. it is closer to the poles.
   d. it would be reclaimed from former urbanized land.

44. The urbanized area of the world is
   a. about 1%.
   b. shrinking as people move to dense cities.
   c. about equal to the tundra biome.
   d. about 10%.

45. What is removed from water in the process of desalination?
   a. salt
   b. lead
   c. electrolytes
   d. pollution

46. The burning of a fossil fuel does not create
   a. greenhouse gases.
   b. stratospheric ozone.
   c. carbon dioxide.
   d. acid rain.

47. Methane in Earth's atmosphere, like CO_2, is a greenhouse gas. A greenhouse gas
   a. absorbs shortwave radiation and is transparent to long-wave radiation.
   b. absorbs shortwave radiation and reflects long-wave radiation.
   c. absorbs long-wave radiation and is transparent to shortwave radiation.
   d. absorbs long-wave radiation and reflects shortwave radiation.

48. One would expect acid rainfall to be worst downwind of a
   a. coal power plant.
   b. nuclear power plant.
   c. wind farm.
   d. wastewater treatment plant.

49. Nitrates and sulfates in Earth's atmosphere create
   a. polar melting.
   b. acid rain.
   c. a greenhouse effect.
   d. equilibrium clouds.

50. Which of the following is the term for a mathematical system that attempts to simulate a natural phenomenon?
   a. calculation
   b. variable
   c. statistic
   d. model

Section 5: Biology

There are 50 questions in this section. You have 45 minutes to complete this section.

1. Which of the following vitamins prevents scurvy, aids in the production of collagen, and may boost the immune system?
   a. vitamin K
   b. vitamin C
   c. vitamin A
   d. vitamin D

2. Which of the following is a viral disease?
   a. botulism
   b. syphilis
   c. tuberculosis
   d. polio

3. Which of the following actions is controlled by smooth muscles?
   a. running
   b. heart beat
   c. peristalsis
   d. movement of bones and joints

4. The resting potential of a neuron is
   a. −70 mV.
   b. +70 mV.
   c. −50 mV.
   d. 0 mV.

5. An important function of a plant's root system is to
   a. produce glucose through photosysnthesis.
   b. break down organic compounds.
   c. release carbon dioxide.
   d. absorb minerals and water from the soil.

6. Carbohydrates are much better foods for quick energy than fats because they
   a. are digested more easily and absorbed more quickly.
   b. supply essential amino acids, which provide energy.
   c. are high in both protein and iron.
   d. carry oxygen to the blood.

7. Which of the following systems contains sebaceous glands?
   a. integumentary system
   b. digestive system
   c. circulatory system
   d. respiratory system

8. The process that yields four gametes, each containing half the chromosome number of the parent cell, is
   a. morphogenesis.
   b. mitosis.
   c. metamorphosis.
   d. meiosis.

9. What are the two kinds of chambers of the heart, and how are they different from one another?
   a. A superior vena cava pumps blood to areas above the heart, and an inferior vena cava pumps blood to the lower body.
   b. A superior vena cava pumps blood to the lower body, and an inferior vena cava pumps blood to areas above the heart.
   c. An atrium pumps blood away from the heart, and a ventricle receives blood coming from the heart.
   d. An atrium receives blood coming into the heart, and a ventricle pumps blood away from the heart.

10. An aneurysm is best described as a
   a. weak spot that swells in a main artery.
   b. coronary heart attack.
   c. buildup of fatty deposits.
   d. calcium deposit in the wall of an artery.

11. Which of the following groups of organisms produce flowers?
   a. angiosperms
   b. mosses
   c. gymnosperms
   d. fungi

12. Which of the following is NOT an effect of the hormone adrenaline?
   a. enhancement of the effects of sympathetic nerves
   b. decrease in blood sugar
   c. increase in the heartbeat rate
   d. inhibition of movement of smooth muscles in the stomach and intestines

13. Which organ is made up of nephrons?
   a. heart
   b. kidney
   c. liver
   d. pancreas

14. Which of the following structures is present in both eukaryotic and prokaryotic cells?
   a. nucleus
   b. chloroplast
   c. chromosome
   d. mitochondrion

15. All of the following bones are found in a human leg EXCEPT the
   a. fibula.
   b. ulna.
   c. patella.
   d. femur.

16. Which of the following parts of the brain controls breathing rates?
   a. the medulla oblongata
   b. the cerebellum
   c. the thalamus
   d. the temporal lobe

17. For the DNA segment 5'-AAT-GAC-TGG-3', what mRNA segment will be generated by transcription?
   a. 5'-TTA-CTG-ACC-3'
   b. 5'-UUA-CUG-ACC-3'
   c. 5'-CCA-GUC-AUU-3'
   d. 5'-CCA-GTC-ATT-3'

18. In what organelle does most protein synthesis occur?
   a. the nucleus
   b. the ribosome
   c. the cytoplasm
   d. the lysosome

19. Which of the following best defines an antigen?
   a. a chemical that prevents blood clotting
   b. a chemical extracted from a living microbe
   c. an antibody that attaches itself to a toxin and makes the toxin harmless
   d. a substance that stimulates the production of antibodies

20. Cell membranes generally have which of the following structures?
   a. phospholipid bilayer
   b. amino acid monolayer
   c. aminopeptide bilayer
   d. phosphopeptide monolayer

21. Which of the following is a vertebrate?
   a. a sponge
   b. a starfish
   c. an octopus
   d. a snake

22. In genetics, what kind of diagram indicates all of the possible genotypes in the F_2 generation of a Mendelian cross?
    a. Punnett square
    b. flow chart
    c. periodic table
    d. test square

23. Which of the following is the function of a ligament?
    a. to connect bones together
    b. to connect muscles together
    c. to attach muscle to bone
    d. to serve as a cushion between vertebrae

24. Which of the following plants lacks a vascular system?
    a. a moss
    b. a fern
    c. a fir tree
    d. a peanut plant

25. An energy-rich molecule found in cells is
    a. adrenaline.
    b. adenosine triphosphate.
    c. acetylcholine.
    d. amino acids.

26. In humans, wet earwax (W) is dominant to dry earwax (w). What is the chance that two heterozygous parents (Ww) will have an offspring that has the homozygous dominant genotype (WW)?
    a. 0%
    b. 25%
    c. 50%
    d. 100%

27. Which organ is affected by meningitis?
    a. brain
    b. liver
    c. lungs
    d. spleen

28. Which of the following causes a seed's first stem to grow upward?
    a. gravitropism
    b. phototropsim
    c. hydrotropism
    d. thermotropism

29. A group of individuals that belong to the same species and inhabit a particular geographic area is called
    a. a community.
    b. an ecosystem.
    c. a population.
    d. a kingdom.

30. Which of the following types of substances is lipase?
    a. vitamin
    b. lipid
    c. enzyme
    d. steroid

31. What molecule is the terminal source of electrons during photosynthesis?
    a. H_2O
    b. O_2
    c. CO_2
    d. $C_6H_{12}O_6$

32. The transition between the G1 and S phases of the cell cycle that prevents abnormal cells from dividing is called the
    a. interphase boundary.
    b. mitotic boundary.
    c. resting phase.
    d. restriction point.

33. An osteocyte is a
   a. muscle cell.
   b. blood cell.
   c. nerve cell.
   d. bone cell.

34. Bat wings and bird wings are an example of
   a. homologous structures.
   b. vestigial structures.
   c. analogous structures.
   d. divergent structures.

35. In the scientific name for the emperor penguin, *Aptenodytes forsteri*, the word *Aptenodytes* indicates the
   a. phylum.
   b. genus.
   c. species.
   d. order.

36. Which category of living things creates the energy that all organisms need to survive?
   a. consumers
   b. producers
   c. decomposers
   d. herbivores

37. The human appendix and the coccyx are examples of
   a. homologous structures.
   b. vestigial structures.
   c. analogous structures.
   d. convergent structures.

38. A chemical signal emitted by one animal to stimulate a specific response in another animal of the same species is called
   a. a hormone.
   b. a pheromone.
   c. an antigen.
   d. a receptor.

39. In messenger RNA, a codon contains how many nucleotides?
   a. one
   b. two
   c. three
   d. four

40. Which of the following is another word for the digits in the hands and feet of vertebrates?
   a. carpals
   b. tarsals
   c. phalanges
   d. metacarpals

41. During protein synthesis, the process of synthesizing RNA from DNA is known as
   a. translation.
   b. transcription.
   c. elongation.
   d. initiation.

42. What are the blood vessels that carry blood toward the heart?
   a. arteries
   b. veins
   c. capillaries
   d. arterioles

43. A human embryo will be female if the
   a. mother's egg contributes an X chromosome.
   b. mother's egg contributes a Y chromosome.
   c. father's sperm contributes an X chromosome.
   d. father's sperm contributes a Y chromosome.

44. What is the term for the skeleton of soft-bodied animals such as mollusks and annelid worms?
   a. internal skeleton
   b. hydrostatic skeleton
   c. exoskeleton
   d. external skeleton

45. In warm-blooded animals, shivering is an aspect of
   a. thermoregulation.
   b. freezing.
   c. osmoregulation.
   d. hibernation.

46. Which of the following is the region between two nerve cells across which electronic impulses are transmitted?
   a. neuron
   b. myelin sheath
   c. synapse
   d. axon

47. When egg cells are produced and grow in an animal ovary, the process is called
   a. oogenesis.
   b. oocyte.
   c. oogonia.
   d. ova.

48. A genetic disorder caused by a mutation on the X chromosome
   a. will affect only men.
   b. will affect only women.
   c. is more likely to affect men.
   d. is more likely to affect women.

49. In humans, the ossicles, utricle, and cochlea are all part of which organ?
   a. the stomach
   b. the heart
   c. the ear
   d. the brain

50. An embryo first develops three germ layers (endoderm, mesoderm, and ectoderm) during which stage of development?
   a. cleavage
   b. gastrulation
   c. fertilization
   d. organogenesis

Section 6: Chemistry

There are 50 questions in this section. Use the periodic table on page 365 when necessary to help you answer the questions. You have 45 minutes to complete this section.

1. Give the number of protons, neutrons, and electrons of this isotope of oxygen: $^{17}_{8}O$
   a. 8 protons, 8 neutrons, 17 electrons
   b. 8 protons, 8 neutrons, 9 electrons
   c. 8 protons, 9 neutrons, 8 electrons
   d. 8 protons, 17 neutrons, 8 electrons

2. What are the spectator ions in the following equation?
$Ca(NO_3)_2$ (aq) + $2KCl$ (aq) → $CaCl_2$ (sol) + $2KNO_3$ (aq)
   a. Ca^{2+} (aq), $2NO_3^-$ (aq), $2K^+$(aq), $2Cl^-$(aq)
   b. Ca^{2+} (aq), $2NO_3^-$ (aq)
   c. Ca^{2+} (aq), $2K^+$ (aq), $2Cl^-$ (aq)
   d. $2NO_3^-$ (aq), $2K^+$ (aq)

3. What are the products of the following equation? sodium chloride (aq) + lead(II) nitrate (aq) →
   a. sodium nitrate + lead(II) chloride
   b. sodium + chloride
   c. sodium + chloride + lead(II) + nitrate
   d. sodium(II) nitrate + lead chloride

4. What is the net ionic equation of the following transformations?
$Ca(NO_3)_2$ (aq) + $2KCl$ (aq) → $CaCl_2$ (sol) + $2KNO_3$ (aq)
   a. $2NO_3^-$ (aq) + $2K^+$ (aq) → $2KNO_3$ (aq)
   b. Ca^{2+} (aq) + $2Cl^-$ (aq) → $CaCl_2$ (sol)
   c. Ca^{2+} (aq) + $2NO_3^-$ (aq) + $2K^+$ (aq) + $2Cl^-$ (aq) → $CaCl_2$ (sol) + $2K^+$ (aq) + $2NO_3^-$ (aq)
   d. Ca^{2+} (aq) +$2NO_3^-$ (aq) + $2K^+$ (aq)+$2Cl^-$ (aq) → Ca^{2+} (aq)+$2Cl^-$ (aq)+$2K^+$ (aq)+$2NO_3^-$ (aq)

1 IA																		18 VIIIA
1 **H** 1.00794	2 IIA												13 IIIA	14 IVA	15 VA	16 VIA	17 VIIA	2 **He** 4.002602
3 **Li** 6.941	4 **Be** 9.012182												5 **B** 10.811	6 **C** 12.0107	7 **N** 14.00674	8 **O** 15.9994	9 **F** 8.9984032	10 **Ne** 20.1797
11 **Na** 22.989770	12 **Mg** 24.3050	3 IIIB	4 IVB	5 VB	6 VIB	7 VIIB	8	9 VIIIB	10	11 IB	12 IIB		13 **Al** 26.981538	14 **Si** 28.0855	15 **P** 30.973761	16 **S** 32.066	17 **Cl** 35.4527	18 **Ar** 39.948
19 **K** 39.0983	20 **Ca** 40.078	21 **Sc** 44.955910	22 **Ti** 47.867	23 **V** 50.9415	24 **Cr** 51.9961	25 **Mn** 54.938049	26 **Fe** 55.845	27 **Co** 58.933200	28 **Ni** 58.6934	29 **Cu** 63.546	30 **Zn** 65.39		31 **Ga** 69.723	32 **Ge** 72.61	33 **As** 74.92160	34 **Se** 78.96	35 **Br** 79.904	36 **Kr** 83.80
37 **Rb** 85.4678	38 **Sr** 87.62	39 **Y** 88.90585	40 **Zr** 91.224	41 **Nb** 92.90638	42 **Mo** 95.94	43 **Tc** (98)	44 **Ru** 101.07	45 **Rh** 102.90550	46 **Pd** 106.42	47 **Ag** 107.8682	48 **Cd** 112.411		49 **In** 114.818	50 **Sn** 118.710	51 **Sb** 121.760	52 **Te** 127.60	53 **I** 126.90447	54 **Xe** 131.29
55 **Cs** 132.90545	56 **Ba** 137.327	57 **La*** 138.9055	72 **Hf** 178.49	73 **Ta** 180.9479	74 **W** 183.84	75 **Re** 186.207	76 **Os** 190.23	77 **Ir** 192.217	78 **Pt** 195.078	79 **Au** 196.96655	80 **Hg** 200.59		81 **Tl** 204.3833	82 **Pb** 207.2	83 **Bi** 208.98038	84 **Po** (209)	85 **At** (210)	86 **Rn** (222)
87 **Fr** (223)	88 **Ra** (226)	89 **Ac**** (227)	104 **Rf** (265)	105 **Db** (268)	106 **Sg** (271)	107 **Bh** (270)	108 **Hs** (277)	109 **Mt** (276)	110 **Ds** (281)	111 **Rg** (280)	112 **Cn** (285)		113 **Nh** (286)	114 **Fl** (289)	115 **Mc** (289)	116 **Lv** (293)	117 **Ts** (294)	118 **Og** (294)

*Lanthanide series	58 **Ce** 140.116	59 **Pr** 140.90765	60 **Nd** 144.24	61 **Pm** (145)	62 **Sm** 150.36	63 **Eu** 151.964	64 **Gd** 157.25	65 **Tb** 158.92534	66 **Dy** 162.50	67 **Ho** 164.93032	68 **Er** 167.26	69 **Tm** 168.93421	70 **Yb** 173.04	71 **Lu** 174.967

**Actinide series	90 **Th** 232.0381	91 **Pa** 231.03588	92 **U** 238.0289	93 **Np** (237)	94 **Pu** (244)	95 **Am** (243)	96 **Cm** (247)	97 **Bk** (247)	98 **Cf** (251)	99 **Es** (252)	100 **Fm** (257)	101 **Md** (258)	102 **No** (259)	103 **Lr** (262)

5. Complete the following precipitation reaction knowing that nitrate ions remain in solution:
$Hg_2(NO_3)_2$ (aq) + 2KI (aq) → _____ + _____

a. Hg_2I_2 (s) + $2K^+$ (aq) + $2(NO_3)^-$ (aq)

b. Hg_2I_2 (s) + $2KNO_3$ (s)

c. Hg_2^{2+} (aq) + $2(NO_3)^-$ (aq) + $2K^+$ (aq) + $2(NO_3)^-$ (aq)

d. Hg_2I_2 (aq) + $2K^+$ (aq) + $2(NO_3)^-$ (aq)

6. What is the product when an acid and a base are combined?

a. water and a salt

b. hydrogen and a salt

c. an oxidant and a reductant

d. no reaction occurs

7. Identify the oxidizing agent and the reducing agent in the following reaction:
$8H^+$ (aq) + $6Cl^-$ (aq) + Sn (s) + $4NO_3^-$ (aq) → $SnCl_6^{2-}$ (aq) + $4NO_2$ (g) + $4H_2O$ (l)

a. oxidizing agent: $8H^+$(aq), reducing agent: Sn (s)

b. oxidizing agent: $4NO_3^-$(aq), reducing agent: Sn (s) (g)

c. oxidizing agent: $4NO_3^-$(aq), reducing agent: $4NO_2$ (g)

d. oxidizing agent: $4NO_3^-$(aq), reducing agent: $8H^+$(aq)

8. Which two atoms would form a covalent bond?

a. sodium and chloride

b. iron and oxygen

c. nitrogen and oxygen

d. magnesium and sulfur

9. Classify the following reaction as combination, decomposition, or single or double displacement reaction:

$Cr(NO_3)_3$ (aq) + Al (s) → $Al(NO_3)_3$ (aq) + Cr (s)

a. decomposition

b. combination

c. double displacement

d. single displacement

10. Classify the following reaction as combination, decomposition, or single or double displacement reaction:

PF_3 (g) + F_2 (g) → PF_5 (g)

a. combination

b. decomposition

c. simple displacement

d. double displacement

11. Balance the following equation:

$Ba(OH)_2$ (aq) + HNO_3 (aq) → $Ba(NO_3)_2$ (aq) + H_2O(l)

a. $Ba(OH)_2$ (aq) + $2HNO_3$ (aq) → $Ba(NO_3)_2$ (aq) + $2H_2O$ (l)

b. $Ba(OH)_2$ (aq) + $2HNO_3$ (aq) → $Ba(NO_3)_2$ (aq) + $4H_2O$ (l)

c. $Ba(OH)_2$ (aq) + $2HNO_3$ (aq) → $Ba(NO_3)_2$ (aq) + H_2O (l)

d. $Ba(OH)_2$ (aq) + HNO_3 (aq) → $Ba(NO_3)_2$ (aq) + H_2O (l)

12. The chemical formula for the polyatomic ion nitrite is

a. N_2O^-.

b. NO^{2-}.

c. NO_2^-.

d. NO_3^-.

13. Which reactant is oxidized and which is reduced in the following reacton?

C_2H_4 (g) + $3O_2$ (g) → $2CO_2$ (g) + $2H_2O$ (g)

a. oxidized: C_2H_4 (g), reduced: $3O_2$ (g)

b. oxidized: C_2H_4 (g), reduced: $2H_2O$ (g)

c. oxidized: C_2H_4 (g), reduced: $2CO_2$ (g)

d. oxidized: $2CO_2$ (g), reduced: C_2H_4 (g)

14. Which one of the following compounds is a nonelectrolyte when dissolved in water?

a. KOH

b. NH_3

c. NaBr

d. $CaCl_2$

15. Which of the following solutions will have the highest electrical conductivity?

a. 0.1M $AlCl_3$

b. 0.15M $SrBr_2$

c. 0.2M NaBr

d. 0.25M $Mg(NO_3)_2$

16. A precipitate will form when an aqueous solution of $Ba(NO_3)_2$ is added to an aqueous solution of Na_2SO_4. How many moles of sodium sulfate are required to produce 10.0 g of the precipitate?

a. 1 mole

b. 10.0 mole

c. 0.04 mole

d. 0.4 mole

17. A 1.0 L sample of gas with a pressure of 2.0 atm is placed in an expandable container at 25°C. If the temperature remains constant, to what volume does the container need to be expanded for the pressure to be lowered to 1.8 atm?

a. 0.9 L

b. 1.1 L

c. 1.8 L

d. 3.6 L

18. When vinegar (acetic acid, CH_3COOH) is combined with baking soda (sodium bicarbonate, $NaHCO_3$), a gas is released. What is the identity of the gas?
a. O_2
b. H_2
c. CO_2
d. CO

19. What ions form NaCl?
a. Na and Cl
b. Na^+ and Cl^+
c. Na^+ and Cl^-
d. Na^- and Cl^+

20. The density of acetic acid is 1.05 g/mL. What is the volume of 275 g of acetic acid?
a. 275 mL
b. ~262 mL
c. ~100 mL
d. 22.4 L

21. The correct formula for converting Fahrenheit to Centigrade is given by: $°C = \frac{5}{9}(°F - 32)$. Convert 72°F into temperature in Centigrade.
a. 72°C
b. 40°C
c. 25°C
d. 22.2°C

22. Which of the following compounds is held together by ionic bonds?
a. $CaCl_2$
b. CCl_4
c. SiO_4
d. H_2O

23. A chemical reaction has an enthalpy change of −285 kJ. Which of the following can be determined from this?
a. The reaction is exothermic.
b. The reaction is endothermic.
c. The reaction involved oxidation.
d. The reaction involved reduction.

24. What is the concentration of ions when 47.6 g magnesium chloride is dissolved in 2 L water?
a. 0.250
b. 0.500
c. 0.750
d. 1.50

25. Find all the enantiomeric pairs (i.e., mirror image) among the following sets of stereoisomers (a, b, c, d, e, f, g, h) on page 368.
a. a, b, c, e, h
b. b, c, d, h
c. a, c, f
d. d, e, g

26. Find all the diastereomeric pairs among the sets of stereoisomers shown on page 368.
a. b, d, g
b. b, d
c. g
d. h

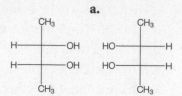

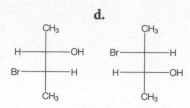

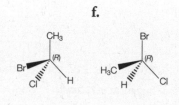

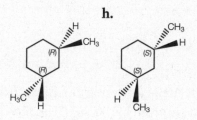

27. Choose the correct answer (correct number of significant figures) for the following calculation: $3.33 \times 10^{-5} + 8.13 \times 10^{-7}$

a. 3.41×10^{-5}

b. 11.46×10^{-7}

c. 11.46×10^{-5}

d. 11.46×10^{-12}

28. Express 0.05620 in exponential notation.

a. 0.057×10^{-3}

b. 57×10^{-3}

c. 563×10^{-4}

d. 5.620×10^{-2}

29. Which pairs of stereoisomers represent diastereomers?

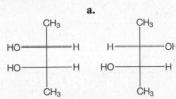

a.

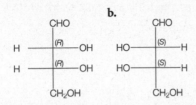

b.

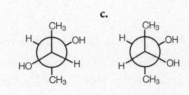

c.

d.

a. a, b
b. a, c
c. a, d
d. a

30. Which of the following describes a Bronsted base?
a. a proton donor
b. a proton acceptor
c. an electron donor
d. an electron acceptor

31. What volume of a 0.5 M solution of NaOH is required to fully neutralize a 100 mL solution of 1 M H_2SO_4?
a. 50 mL
b. 100 mL
c. 200 mL
d. 400 mL

32. How many significant figures are there in the value 0.00250?
a. 2
b. 3
c. 5
d. 6

33. Identify the following as an oxidation, a reduction, a decomposition, or a dismutation reaction.
$Cl_2 + 2e^- \rightarrow 2Cl^-$
a. a reduction
b. an oxidation
c. a decomposition
d. a dismutation

34. What is the $[OH^-]$ of a solution that has a pH of 3?
a. 1×10^{-3}
b. 1×10^{-4}
c. 1×10^{-6}
d. 1×10^{-11}

35. When linoleic acid, an unsaturated fatty acid, reacts with hydrogen, it forms a saturated fatty acid.

$$C_{18}H_{32}O_2 + 2H_2 \rightarrow C_{18}H_{36}O_2$$

How many moles of hydrogen H_2 are required to hydrogenate 5.0 g of unsaturated linoleic acid?

a. 1 mol

b. 10 mol

c. 0.20 mol

d. 0.36 mol

36. Valence electrons are those in the outermost shell of an atom. Indicate the number of valence electrons for Sc (Scandium).

a. 1

b. 2

c. 4

d. 3

37. Based on its position in the periodic table, which element is most likely to be a semiconductor?

a. potassium

b. chromium

c. oxygen

d. germanium

38. In an atom, how many orbitals have a principal quantum number, n, of 2?

a. one

b. two

c. three

d. four

39. Elements in the same period of the periodic table have the same number of

a. protons.

b. neutrons.

c. electron shells.

d. valence electrons.

40. Which of the following is the formula for the simplest alkene?

a. CH_4

b. C_2H_4

c. C_2H_2

d. CH_3OH

41. When a chemical reaction occurs between two atoms, their valence electrons are reorganized so that an attractive force, called a *chemical bond*, occurs between atoms. Name the type of bond that is formed when electrons are transferred from one atom to another.

a. molecular bond

b. covalent bond

c. ionic bond

d. transfer bond

42. When CO_2 is processed by plants during photosynthesis, what happens to the carbon?

a. It is oxidized.

b. It is reduced.

c. It undergoes α-decay.

d. It is expelled as waste.

43. What is the equilibrium constant (K_a) for the dissociation of the weak acid H_2CO_3 (carbonic acid)? $H_2CO_{3(aq)} \rightleftharpoons H^+_{(aq)} + HCO^-_{3(aq)}$

a. $K_a = \dfrac{[H^+][HCO_3^-]}{[H_2CO_3]}$

b. $K_a = \dfrac{[H^+][H_2CO_3]}{[HCO_3^-]}$

c. $K_a = \dfrac{[H_2CO_3]}{[H^+][HCO_3^-]}$

d. $K_a = [H^+][HCO_3^-]$

44. Methane (CH_4) has four hydrogen atoms bonded to a carbon atom. Based on the VSEPR model, what shape is a methane molecule?
a. tetrahedral
b. trigonal pyramidal
c. trigonal planar
d. linear

45. Give the number of valence electrons for boron (B).
a. 5
b. 3
c. 2
d. 13

46. What is the maximum number of electrons that can be described by a principal quantum number of 3 and an orbital quantum number of 2?
a. 1
b. 2
c. 5
d. 10

47. Which of the following molecules is nonpolar?
a. NH_3
b. H_2O
c. PCl_3
d. N_2

48. Write the Lewis electron dot structures for kitchen salt (NaCl).
a. Na:C̈l:
b. Na:Cl
c. :N̈a:C̈l:
d. Na-Cl

49. In a storage area where the temperature has reached 55° C, the pressure of oxygen gas in a 15.0 L steel cylinder is 965 torr. To what temperature would the gas have to be cooled to reduce the pressure to 850 torr?
a. 40° C
b. 30° C
c. 15° C
d. 50° C

50. What is the volume of 64.0 g of oxygen gas (O_2) at the standard temperature and pressure (STP) conditions?
a. 4 L
b. 2 L
c. 22.4 L
d. 44.8 L

Answers

Section 1: Verbal Ability

1. **a.** abscessed
2. **c.** parallel
3. **b.** accidentally
4. **a.** tonsillitis
5. **c.** excelled
6. **b.** guardian
7. **a.** accustomed
8. **b.** pasteurized
9. **a.** delirious
10. **c.** disease
11. **a.** inundated
12. **c.** laziness
13. **b.** practitioners
14. **a.** prosecuted
15. **c.** counterfeit
16. **a.** symmetrically
17. **b.** delaying
18. **a.** vacuum
19. **c.** accommodate
20. **c.** colleagues
21. **b.** conscientious
22. **c.** indescribable
23. **b.** illegible
24. **b.** penicillin
25. **c.** adolescence
26. **a.** preceding
27. **b.** nuisance
28. **c.** peaceable
29. **c.** luxuriant
30. **a.** gullible
31. **b.** gratitude
32. **c.** musically
33. **a.** tragedies
34. **b.** bulletin
35. **c.** embassy
36. **b.** nevertheless
37. **b.** questionnaire
38. **a.** pungent
39. **c.** hygienic
40. **b.** illegal
41. **b.** corrosiveness
42. **c.** gymnast
43. **a.** useful
44. **b.** organizing
45. **a.** jewelry
46. **c.** craziness
47. **c.** returnable
48. **a.** chaise
49. **a.** extremely
50. **b.** friendly

Section 2: Reading Comprehension

1. **c.** The answer to this question is in the first paragraph of the passage, which defines allergies to pollen as *hay fever*.
2. **b.** See the second paragraph: *Cells called macrophages engulf the invader* (i.e., pollen).
3. **d.** The fourth paragraph states that histamines (chemicals) are stored in and released from granules. The fifth paragraph says that histamines can constrict the lungs' airways.
4. **a.** Each answer choice is a synonym for *concentrate*, but only mass explains how the word is used in the context of the third paragraph, which explains how cells mass together in tissues.
5. **d.** The fifth paragraph says that *mast cells secrete chemical messengers that recruit other cells* into the tissues. As a result (according to the sixth paragraph), *some of the recently arrived cells release substances that can increase and prolong early symptoms.*
6. **b.** See the fourth paragraph, which states, *When the same allergen next enters the person's body, it binds to the arms of the IgE molecules protruding from the surfaces of mast cells and basophils.* Macrophages cut the allergen the first time it enters the body. The same is true for T-helper cells detecting fragments of the allergen.

7. a. The first paragraph gives the facts that hay fever affects 22 million Americans and asthma affects 10 to 15 million, so in tandem, the two conditions affect 32 to 37 million people.

8. b. Unlike traditional electrodes, which have relatively wide and stiff wires of aluminum, the silicon wires of microprobes are as *thin as a human hair*, which helps them to *cause minimal damage and disruption of neurons when inserted into the brain*, according to the second paragraph of the passage.

9. d. The author only writes of probes in positive terms, and even uses the word *thanks* to imply gratitude for the use of probes in repairing nerve damage in the first paragraph. Therefore, it is most likely that the author would not think there are ethical issues with using probes to cure anyone.

10. d. According to the first paragraph, the tiny probes may restore nerve function in quadriplegics.

11. a. The first sentence of the third paragraph says that microprobes have channels that *open the way for delivery of drugs*.

12. d. The sixth paragraph is mainly about how bulky wires cause problems when using electrodes in surgical procedures.

13. c. See the sixth paragraph, in which it is understood that long-term implantation has to rely on *satisfactory connections to the outside world*.

14. b. *Susceptible* means being *liable to be affected by something*. According to the third paragraph, some patients are genetically predisposed, or susceptible, to some diseases.

15. a. The last sentence of the second paragraph indicates that the report *advised caution in using . . . predictive tests*.

16. c. The answer to this question can be found in the fourth paragraph. The paragraph begins with the statement *The report recommended that all screening, including screening of newborns, be voluntary* and states that they should only be mandatory in the case of *diagnosing treatable conditions in newborns*.

17. d. The first paragraph says that the report addressed concerns *to protect confidentiality*.

18. c. Although the paragraph discusses the potentially anxiety-inducing topic of the difficulties of prenatal testing and the importance of performing them, the tone does not alter significantly. The sixth paragraph is as professional and assured as the rest of the passage.

19. d. According to the table, the first trimester combined screen for trisomy 18 are not as accurate as the second trimester quad screens are. Choice **a** is incorrect because the third trimester is not mentioned in the table at all.

20. a. According to the first sentence of the third paragraph, the new MRI *detects not water but inert gases*.

21. d. The answer to this question can be found in the second paragraph, which states that *chest X-rays can detect tumors or inflamed regions in the lungs but provide poor soft-tissue contrast and no clear view of air passages*.

22. c. See the fifth paragraph: Radio signals knock nuclei out of position, but as they are realigned, they transmit faint radio signals.

23. b. The first sentence of the third paragraph states the equivalency: Nuclei are *aligned, or hyperpolarized*.

24. a. The last paragraph says that light, rather than a magnet, is used to align nuclei, suggesting that the two serve equivalent purposes in the two MRI processes.

25. c. See the last sentence of the passage. Since lesser gases lose their alignment more quickly, a shorter period of alignment would lead to poorer clarity. A higher number of aligned nuclei would theoretically lead to a better image.

26. a. The author contrasts the public's dismissal of the arcane practice of wearing garlic with its increasing acceptance of herbal remedies.

27. b. In this context, *conventional* refers to the established system of Western medicine or biomedicine.

28. c. The second paragraph states that the survey found those born between 1965 and 1979 most likely to use alternative treatments.

29. a. The statistic illustrates the popularity of alternative therapies without giving any specific information as to why.

30. d. The author states that Americans are not replacing conventional healthcare but are adding to or supplementing it with alternative care.

31. d. According to the third paragraph of the passage, nearly half of CAM expenses had to be paid out of pocket because they were not covered by medical insurance. Therefore, it is reasonable to infer that CAM has financial disadvantages.

32. c. The answer to this question can be found in the first paragraph of the passage. The paragraph suggests that *longer stays in microgravity* can have an *acute* effect on bone loss.

33. c. According to the fifth paragraph, levels of vitamin D were elevated in drug recipients.

34. d. The third paragraph states that a pressure device *does nothing to avert loss of calcium*.

35. a. The last paragraph states that high urinary calcium concentrations can cause kidney stones. Treatment that inhibits urinary discharge of calcium, such as use of alendronate, could therefore help in the treatment of kidney stones.

36. b. The last sentence of the fourth paragraph states that volunteers took a three-week bed rest.

37. b. The last sentence of the third paragraph states that 56% of "laser-first" and 70% of "medication-first" patients (over half) needed new or extra medications *to control pressure inside the eye*.

38. d. The fourth paragraph is chiefly about the side effects of both laser surgery and medication such as eyedrops.

39. a. See the second and third sentences of the first paragraph.

40. c. The third sentence of the third paragraph states that *initial treatment with laser surgery is at least as effective as initial treatment with eyedrops*.

41. a. The second paragraph says that the patients were *newly diagnosed*.

42. c. In the second paragraph, the author states that exercise can help teens to avoid *risky behaviors* and uses smoking as an example of such behavior.

43. c. One meaning of *sedentary* is settled; another meaning is doing or requiring much sitting. *Stationary,* defined as fixed in a course or mode, is closest in meaning.

44. d. The chart shows that roughly half of the teens surveyed enjoyed emotional benefits from exercising. This is not a very dramatic percentage, but it does support choice **d** as the best answer. Choices **a** and **b** imply emotional benefits more dramatic than this survey indicates, so they are not the best answers.

45. d. The passage promotes change in teenagers' exercise habits by emphasizing the benefits of exercise, the moderate amount of exercise needed to achieve benefits, and some factors that may encourage teenagers to exercise.

Section 3: Math

1. a. To solve this problem, you must first convert yards to inches. There are 36 inches in a yard. $36 \times 3\frac{1}{3} = 120$.

2. c. Multiply $\frac{2}{3}$ by 45 and cancel common factors: $\frac{2}{3} \times \frac{45}{1} = \frac{2}{3} \times \frac{\overset{15}{\cancel{45}}}{1} = 30$. Paola ran 30 miles.

3. a. The test starts at 7:15 A.M. Two hours later is 9:15 A.M. Add 15 minutes to get a time of 9:30 A.M. Three hours later is 12:30 P.M. Add 10 more minutes to get a time of 12:40 P.M., which is the time the patient finished the test.

4. c. The sum of the measure of the angles in a triangle is 180°; 70° + 30° = 100°; 180° − 100° = 80°. Therefore, angle C measures 80°.

5. d. 6^3 is equal to $6 \times 6 \times 6$, or 216.

6. a. The ratio of Drake's charge to Jean's charge is 3 to 4, or $\frac{3}{4}$. To find what Jean charges, you must use the proportion $\frac{3}{4} = \frac{36}{x}$, or $3x = 4 \times 36$; $4 \times 36 = 144$, which is then divided by 3 to arrive at $x = 48$.

7. b. To find the average time for the three baths, you must add the times for all the baths and divide by the number of baths: 20 + 17 + 14 = 51; 51 ÷ 3 = 17.

8. c. A percentage is a portion of 100, or $\frac{x}{100}$. The proportion here is $\frac{x}{100} = \frac{12}{50}$, or $12 \times 100 = 50x$. Divide both sides by 50 to get $x = 24\%$.

9. d. The area is the width times the length—in this case, 10 × 8, or 80 square feet.

10. b. Use the formula beginning with the operation in parentheses: 98 − 32 = 66. After that, multiply 66 by $\frac{5}{9}$, first multiplying 66 by 5 to get 330; 330 divded by 9 is $36.\overline{6}$, which is rounded up to 36.7.

11. b. Simplify the parentheses first: $6(3^3 − 7) + 50 ÷ 2 = 6(27 − 7) + 50 ÷ 2 = 6(20) + 50 ÷ 2$. Then do the multiplication or division from left to right: $6(20) + 50 ÷ 2 = 120 + 25$. Then add or subtract: 120 + 125 = 145.

12. b. First, convert the fractions to decimals: $\frac{3}{8} = 0.375$ and $\frac{5}{7} = 0.72$. Then the order from least to greatest is: $0.35, \frac{3}{8}, 0.44, 0.7, \frac{5}{7}$.

13. b. Convert the percentage to a decimal: 232 × 0.14 = 32.48.

14. d. The perimeter is the total length of all sides. In a square, all four sides are of equal length, so the perimeter is 4 + 4 + 4 + 4, or 16.

15. a. Perform the operation in parentheses first: 9 × 4 = 36; 36 × 12 = 432.

16. c. The proportion is $\frac{12}{100} = \frac{33}{x}$, or $100 \times 33 = 12x$; $3,300 ÷ 12 = 275$; therefore, $x = 275$.

17. c. It is important to keep the decimal values aligned. Divide as usual, and then bring the decimal point straight up into the answer in order to get 39.4.

18. d. 10% of $14.25 is 0.10 × 14.25 = $1.43. Then add $14.25 and $1.43 to get $15.68 as the new hourly wage.

19. c. The formula for finding the area of a circle is $A = \pi r^2$. First, square the radius: 13 × 13 = 169. Then, multiply by the approximate value of π, 3.14, to get 530.66.

20. a. In order to subtract fractions, you must first find the least common denominator, in this case, 40. The problem is then $\frac{35}{40} − \frac{24}{40}$, or $\frac{11}{40}$.

21. c. Each 9-foot wall has an area of 9 × 8 or 72 square feet. There are two such walls, so those two walls combined have an area of 72 × 2 or 144 square feet. Each 11-foot wall has an area of 11 × 8 or 88 square feet, and again, there are two such walls: 88 × 2 = 176. Finally, add 144 and 176 to get 320 square feet.

22. b. 195.6 ÷ 7.2 yields a repeating decimal, 27.1666666 . . . , which rounded up to the nearest hundredth is 27.17.

23. c. 65.19 is read as *sixty-five and nineteen hundredths*. Choice **a** is 65.9. Choice **b** is 65.019. Choice **d** is 65.09.

24. a. The first step is to convert 3 to a fraction, which is $\frac{3}{1}$. Divide by inverting the second fraction, making it $\frac{1}{3}$, and multiplying: $\frac{5}{8} \times \frac{1}{3} = \frac{5}{24}$.

25. **c.** To find the average, first find the total number of patients: $8 + 5 + 9 + 10 + 10 + 14 + 7 = 63$. Then, divide the number of patients by the number of nursing assistants: $63 \div 7 = 9$.

26. **b.** Perform the operations within the parentheses first: $25 + 17 = 42$; $64 - 49 = 15$; $42 \times 15 = 630$.

27. **d.** A percentage is a portion of 100, or $\frac{x}{100}$. The equation here is $\frac{x}{100} = \frac{234}{18,000}$, or $234 \times 100 = 18,000x$; $23,400 \div 18,000 = 1.3$.

28. **a.** There are 60 minutes in an hour. Multiply $60 \times 7\frac{1}{6}$ by multiplying $60 \times 7 = 420$ and $60 \times \frac{1}{6} = 10$. Then add $420 + 10$ to get 430 minutes.

29. **b.** Think of 145.29 as 145.290, and then line up the decimal points and add the numbers to get the correct answer, 217.977.

30. **d.** Perform the operations in parentheses first, left to right: $84 - 5 = 79$. Now, multiply $12(79) = 948$. Next, do the other parenthetical operation: $3 \times 54 = 162$. Now, do the final operation: $948 - 162 = 786$.

31. **b.** The sides of an equilateral triangle are of equal length. Divide 22.5 by 3 to get the length of each side: $22.5 \div 3 = 7.5$ centimeters.

32. **a.** The correct answer is 31.75. Not lining up the decimal points when multiplying is the most common error in this type of problem.

33. **a.** This is a simple multiplication problem. The correct answer is 9,092.

34. **b.** The area of the operating room is $11 \times 9 = 99$ square yards. The cost of the flooring is $99 \times 12.25 = \$1,212.75$.

35. **c.** The correct answer is 256,595. When multiplying three-digit numbers, be careful in computation and in aligning numbers.

36. **b.** The correct answer is $8\frac{9}{10}$. Incorrect answers could result from adding both the numerator and the denominator or not converting fifths to tenths properly.

37. **a.** $22.50 is 75% of the original price. To find x, solve the equation $22.50 = 0.75x$. Divide both sides by 0.75. The original price is $30. The amount of the discount is $30 - \$22.50 = \$7.50$.

38. **b.** The correct answer is $88\frac{1}{3}$. To work the problem, you must first convert $\frac{1}{2}$ to $\frac{3}{6}$.

39. **d.** Find the perimeter of the window: 4 feet 3 inches + 4 feet 3 inches + 3 feet 5 inches + 3 feet 5 inches = 14 feet 16 inches = 15 feet 4 inches. Juan needs 15 feet 4 inches of trim.

40. **b.** To do division with mixed numbers, you must first rewrite the mixed numbers as improper fractions: $30 \div 2\frac{1}{2} = 30 \div \frac{5}{2}$. Then, in order to perform the division, use the reciprocal of the second fraction and turn the problem into multiplication: $30 \div \frac{5}{2} = 30 \times \frac{2}{5} = \frac{60}{5} = 12$.

41. **b.** The correct answer has only two decimal places: 96.32.

42. **c.** The number 74 goes into 7,400 one hundred times.

43. **a.** Remember that two negatives multiplied yield a positive. Invert the second fraction and multiply: $-\frac{3}{10} \times (-5) = \frac{3}{2} = 1\frac{1}{2}$.

44. **b.** To find the answer, divide 14 by 0.35 to get 40.

45. **c.** Three feet 4 inches equals 40 inches; 40 divided by 5 is 8.

46. **a.** Choice **b** is rounded up instead of down; choice **c** is rounded to the nearest hundredth; choice **d** is rounded to the nearest whole number.

47. **a.** In choice **b**, the 9 is in the hundredths place; in choice **c**, it is in the tenths place; and in choice **d**, it is in the ten thousandths place.

48. **d.** Eighty out of 100 is 80%. Eighty percent of 30,000 is 24,000.

49. **a.** The expression $5n$ means 5 times n. The addition sign before the 7 indicates the phrase *more than*.

50. **d.** Substitute 3 for x in the expression $5 + 4x$ to determine that $y = 17$.

Section 4: General Science

1. a. Earth's core is divided into two parts: the solid inner core and the liquid outer core.

2. a. It was 4.6 billion years ago, which we know from radioactive dating of meteorites, which all come in about that age.

3. b. The lithosphere has a low density and "floats" on the more dense layers of Earth that are below.

4. b. The troposphere is the lowest portion of Earth's atmosphere, and it is where most weather phenomena take place. The word comes from the Greek *tropos*, meaning "turning or mixing," since the troposphere's structure and behavior are caused by mixing.

5. a. The gravitational pull of the Moon is the primary force creating ocean tides. The Sun's gravitational force also influences tides, but because of the great distance between Earth and the Sun, it influences tides with about half the force as the Moon.

6. a. The mantle is the thick zone beneath Earth's crust but not as deep as the inner core.

7. a. Most of Earth's surface is sedimentary rock, or rock formed from the breakdown of other rocks.

8. d. The metric (SI) unit for mass is the gram. The newton is the unit for weight, which is the force exerted on an object by gravity. While in common language weight and mass are interchangeable, they are not the same in scientific terms.

9. b. Uranus is the fourth planet known as a gas giant—a large planet not composed primarily of rock or solid matter.

10. b. Obsidian is igneous rock, formed from lava that has cooled rapidly.

11. b. The twentieth century had the world's largest population increase. This was due to medical advances and agricultural technology.

12. b. In about one year, the entire atmosphere mixes, even between the northern and southern hemispheres.

13. b. The energy of the Sun that falls upon the land and ocean creates difference in temperature, which drives the circulation of atmosphere and ocean.

14. b. The troposphere is the atmospheric layer where weather occurs. Next is the stratosphere, where temperature actually increases with altitude because energy from the Sun is absorbed by ozone here. Next is the mesosphere, where temperatures drop. Last is the thermosphere, where the air is very thin.

15. c. The mixing time for the entire world's oceans is about one thousand years.

16. b. Although depth, surface area, wind duration, and wind velocity all influence wave generation and behavior, it is the limited surface area, or "fetch," of ponds that keeps waves from forming. Even sustained hurricane-force winds would create no more than ripples on a small pond because the wind does not have a large enough surface area over which to generate waves.

17. b. Temperature is the main determinant of bacterial activity in the soil, which decomposes organic matter. Where it is cold, bacterial activity is low, and that explains the famously thick soils of the arctic tundra, often called peat. Moisture comes into play as well, but temperature is influence number one.

18. a. Insects are the most species-rich type of creature on Earth. Most of the estimated millions of species yet to be discovered and classified are insects.

19. c. If 100 species live in the canopy, and those are only half of the total that are specialized for that species of tree (because the other half live underground in and around the roots), then twice the number from the canopy must be the total for the tree. Twice 100 is 200.

20. b. Paradoxically, though tundra has a low amount of plants because of the cold, lack of sunlight, and short growing season, it has a huge amount of organic matter in its soil.

21. d. Boreal forests, with their evergreens of fir and pine, sport tough needles with lots of lignin to give them strength to endure the winds and freezing of winter in the very high latitudes.

22. d. A genus consists of many species (usually, in rare cases, a genus might only have one living species, but would have had more in the past). A family consists of many genera.

23. c. Uranus and Neptune are mostly composed of ammonia, water, and methane frozen into ices, and are often referred to as "ice giants."

24. c. Magma is a high-temperature fluid substance, and it behaves like thick oil.

25. d. Meiosis is the process in which parent sex cells from males and females create four gametes (eggs or sperm in the case of animals) with half the genes and chromosomes of the parents.

26. a. Preserving the owl means preserving the old growth forests and thereby all other species that require the old growth forests. Preserving the owl acts like an umbrella for many other species, protecting them all from extinction as a group.

27. a. A nonnative species introduced from elsewhere and that spreads is called an invasive species (also called an *introduced* or *alien* species). *Endemic* means extremely native (occurring nowhere else), so **c** makes no sense. Choice **b** is not the definition of an invasive species, and choice **d** makes no sense, since an endemic species cannot, by definition, be introduced from elsewhere.

28. b. The loudness of a sound wave depends on its amplitude, or height of its wave crests. The pitch depends on its frequency.

29. d. Both in the ocean and in the soil, bacteria recycle nutrients from their organic forms into their inorganic forms.

30. c. In 1996, Dolly became the first mammal to be cloned using a process called nuclear transfer.

31. c. The carrying capacity is the limit asked for in the question. Words with "yield" usually refer to the human harvesting of creatures, such as fish.

32. c. Areas of upwelling bring cool, nutrient-rich waters from ocean depths to the surface, allowing for plankton blooms, which in turn attract large fish. By weight, over 50% of ocean fish are fed by upwelling zones, making these regions productive grounds for fishing.

33. b. When organisms use respiration to convert carbon-based sugars into energy, they release CO_2 back into the atmosphere. The other processes listed all take carbon out of the atmosphere and lock it into the land or oceans.

34. b. Bacteria (different kinds) make the gases carbon dioxide and methane as wastes from their metabolisms.

35. d. Bacteria in root nodules are nitrogen fixers.

36. a. Negative population growth in some countries is due to sub-replacement fertility rates (less than 2.1 children per woman in developed countries).

37. d. Rivers carry the most phosphorus to the sea. There is some phosphorus in the dust carried by wind, which is less than the phosphorus in rivers. Regardless, the phosphorus in dust is not in the dissolved ion form, which was asked for.

38. c. Although you wouldn't be expected to memorize numbers, it should be noted that carbon is the most abundant and iron is a micronutrient. In between these two, hydrogen is in all organic molecules, while phosphorus has specialized uses in cells. Therefore, it is logical that carbon is first, followed by hydrogen, then phosphorus, then iron.

39. a. Copper is needed by cells in only trace amounts; it is therefore not a macronutrient but a micronutrient.

40. d. Estimates place the preagricultural population at about ten million. The other answers are either definitely too little or too big.

41. c. Old coal-fired power plants release many pollutants into the atmosphere; the most dominant of these are sulfur dioxide, carbon monoxide, and nitrogen oxide. Efforts are taken to "scrub" or remove some of these harmful byproducts before they are released into the atmosphere. "Clean coal" technology is expensive and impractical economically on a large scale. Not a single "clean coal" plant has yet opened in the United States.

42. c. Toxicology is the study of poisons and the adverse effects of chemicals on living organisms. It comes from the Greek *toxicos*, which means "poisonous."

43. b. Land already used for agriculture tends to be prime land that was formerly grasslands and prairies in Europe, the United States, Russia, and China. Remaining land still convertible to agriculture includes land in the Amazon with thin soils and land in Africa with workable but still less than ideal soils.

44. a. The urbanized land use is about 1% of the world's land.

45. a. Desalination is the process of removing salt from water. It is done to convert saltwater into freshwater that is suitable for human use.

46. b. The burning creates all those items except stratospheric ozone. Natural processes high in Earth's atmosphere create that kind of ozone.

47. c. Solar radiation is primarily shortwave radiation, which greenhouse gases are transparent to. Greenhouse gases do absorb long-wave radiation, so the concentration of these gases is very important in determining how much energy the atmosphere absorbs.

48. a. A major source of acid rain is the sulfur dioxide produced by the combustion of fossil fuels for energy, the main source of which are coal power plants.

49. b. Acid rain forms when nitrates and sulfates in clouds fall to Earth as nitric and sulfuric acids in rainwater.

50. d. A model is a complex mathematical or conceptual system that tries to explain a natural phenomenon. The other choices can all be part of a model but are too simple to be models on their own.

Section 5: Biology

1. b. Vitamin K is important in the clotting of blood, vitamin A is important in vision, and vitamin D is important in the formation of bone.

2. d. Polio, or poliomyelitis, is a viral disease. Botulism, syphilis, and tuberculosis are all bacterial diseases.

3. c. The other actions are controlled by skeletal muscles (choices **a** and **d**) or cardiac muscles (choice **b**).

4. a. The resting potential of a neuron is –70 millivolts (mV).

5. d. Glucose production (glycolysis) is done primarily in the leaf chloroplasts, breakdown of organic compounds is primarily done in the mitochondria, and roots do not release carbon dioxide.

6. a. Carbohydrates are digested more easily and absorbed more quickly than fats. Choice **b** is incorrect because amino acids are the building blocks of proteins. Choices **c** and **d** are not true of carbohydrates.

7. a. Sebaceous glands, or oil glands, are glands in the skin that secrete oil to lubricate the skin and to kill bacteria on the skin. The sebaceous glands are part of the integumentary system.

8. d. Meiosis results in four reproductive cells, each with half the number of chromosomes found in the parent cell. This is often confused with mitosis, the result of which is two daughter cells with the same number of chromosomes as the parent cell.

9. **d.** Choices **a** and **b** are incorrect because the superior and inferior vena cava are not chambers of the heart. Choice **c** is incorrect because the functions of the atrium and ventricle are reversed.

10. **a.** A weak spot in a main artery, such as the aorta, causes an aneurysm, or swelling.

11. **a.** Gymnosperms produce pine cones with seeds, not flowers; mosses are not vascular plants and do not produce flowers; fungi are not plants and produce spores from fruiting bodies, not flowers.

12. **b.** Adrenaline causes an increase in blood sugar by releasing stored carbohydrates. Choice **d** is incorrect because adrenaline does inhibit these muscles, even though it stimulates muscles in the spleen, hair follicles, and eyes.

13. **b.** Nephrons are processing units that filter blood and form urine. Each kidney contains over one million nephrons.

14. **c** Both eukaryotic and prokaryotic cells contain chromosomes, which make up the genetic material of an organism. Prokaryotic cells do not contain any membrane-bound organelles, so they do not have any of the other choices, while eukaryotic cells can have all of them.

15. **b.** The ulna is a bone in the lower arm.

16. **a.** The medulla oblongata controls many involuntary responses including heart and breathing rates.

17. **c.** DNA is transcribed to mRNA by pairing A→U, T→A, G→C, and C→G. The 5' end of DNA aligns with the 3' end of RNA, so the mRNA sequence is the complement of the DNA sequence when it is read from 3' to 5'.

18. **b.** The ribosome is the site of protein synthesis within the cell. The nucleus houses the genetic material; the cytoplasm is the fluid inside the cell membrane, and the lysosome manages waste.

19. **d.** Antigens are chemicals recognized as foreign by the immune system. Viruses and bacteria are typically antigenic because of their structure.

20. **a.** Cell membranes are generally composed of phospholipids—molecules arranged in two layers with the phosphate ends pointing in toward the cell's center in one layer and to the outside environment in the other layer; the lipid ends of the molecules are sandwiched in the middle of the membrane.

21. **d.** The snake is the only vertebrate—that is, it is the only one of the four animals that has a backbone.

22. **a.** The Punnett square is a grid that represents all of the possible genotypic combinations in the F_2 generation produced by a male (gametes listed horizontally) and a female (gametes listed vertically).

23. **a.** Ligaments are the dense parallel bundles of collagen fibers that hold bones together at a joint.

24. **a.** Mosses are bryophytes, which are characterized by their lack of a vascular system.

25. **b.** Adrenaline is a hormone, acetylcholine is a neurotransmitter, and amino acids are the building block molecules of proteins.

26. **b.** Each heterozygous parent will provide one dominant (W) and one recessive allele (w), so there is a 25% chance that they will have a homozygous dominant offspring, a 25% chance for a homozygous recessive offspring, and a 50% chance for a heterozygous offspring.

27. **a.** The meninges are connective tissue membranes in the brain. Meningitis is a bacterial or viral disease that involves inflammation of the meninges.

28. **a.** Gravitropism refers to a growth response based on gravity, which causes a seed's first root to grow downward and its first stem to grow upward.

29. c. Choice **a** is incorrect because a community includes the protists, plants, and animals living in a particular area. Choice **b** is incorrect because an ecosystem includes all the organisms in a particular area plus the abiotic factors with which they interact. Choice **d** is incorrect because a kingdom is a much broader classification than a species.

30. c. Enzymes are substances that act as catalysts for chemical reactions. The enzyme lipase acts as a catalyst in the reactions that break down lipid molecules.

31. a. Photosynthesis oxidizes water into O_2 and protons (with electrons released during the reaction). These electrons and protons are ultimately used to reduce CO_2 into more complex molecules.

32. d. Abnormal cells are stopped from dividing at the restriction point between the G1 and S phases of the cell cycle. A cell must have a large enough size and energy reserves, as well as undamaged DNA, to pass the restriction point and begin replicating its DNA.

33. d. Osteocytes are living cells within the minerals of bone. *Osteo* is the combining form for *bone*.

34. c. Analogous structures describe two unrelated species separately evolving similar traits. The closest common ancestor of birds and bats did not have wings, yet each evolved them.

35. b. In binomial nomenclature, the genus name (*Aptenodytes*) precedes the species name (*forsteri*).

36. b. Producers are living things that use sunlight to produce food and are mainly plants. Producers create the food all living things need to survive.

37. b. Vestigial structures are structures within an organism that have lost their original function through evolution. The appendix was part of the digestive system of a human ancestor, and the coccyx is a remnant of a tail.

38. b. Pheromones are chemical signals that may be released either in a secretion or as an odor.

39. c. A codon is a triplet of nucleotides that, during protein synthesis, usually represents a genetic code for an amino acid.

40. c. Vertebrate digits are also referred to as phalanges.

41. b. Protein synthesis involves two stages: transcription and translation. Transcription involves synthesizing RNA from DNA. This is followed by translation, which is where proteins are synthesized from the RNA.

42. b. Veins carry blood in the direction of the heart.

43. c. In humans, an embryo's sex is always determined by the sperm. The egg always contributes an X chromosome, while the sperm contributes either an X (for a female) or a Y (for a male).

44. b. The hydrostatic skeleton works by muscles pressing against a fluid-filled area to produce movement. Humans have internal skeletons. Insects have exoskeletons, otherwise known as external skeletons.

45. a. In a cold environment, warm-blooded animals may shiver involuntarily in order to thermoregulate or raise their body temperature. Choice **c**, osmoregulation, is an organism's way of keeping a constant internal water level.

46. c. The junction of two nerve cells is called a synapse.

47. a. Oogenesis is the name of the process in which the ova (egg cells) are produced and grow in the ovary. Special ovarian cells called oogonia divide repeatedly to make large numbers of prospective eggs called oocytes.

48. c. Men are more likely to be affected by an X-linked disorder, as they possess only one copy of the gene, whereas women possess two copies. Therefore, X-linked recessive disorders are often inherited through the mother—who is a carrier and shows no symptoms as she has a second, functional allele.

49. c. The ossicles, utricle, and cochlea are all components of the human ear.

50. b. The embryo first develops into the three germ layers during gastrulation, after it has implanted in the uterus. Organogenesis (formation of organs) occurs later. Fertilization and cleavage occur earlier, when the embryo is still a zygote.

Section 6: Chemistry

1. c. # electrons = # protons for atomic neutrality, # neutrons = mass number – # protons.

2. d. Spectator ions (in bold in the following equation) stay in solution (i.e., aqueous) before and after the reaction.
Ca^{2+} (aq) + **$2NO_3^-$ (aq)** + **$2K^+$ (aq)** + $2Cl^-$ (aq) → $CaCl_2$ (sol) + **$2K^+$ (aq)** + **$2NO_3^-$ (aq)**

3. a. Sodium nitrate + lead(II) chloride. A double displacement reaction: $A^+B^- + C^+D^- → A^+D^- + B^-C^+$.

4. b. A precipitation reaction produces solid $CaCl_2$ from Ca^{2+} and $2Cl^-$ ions.

5. a. Nitrate ions recombine with potassium ions, which both remain in solution, while mercury[II] ions and iodide ions form the precipitate in this double displacement reaction.
Hg_2^{2+} (aq) + $2(NO_3)^-$ (aq) + $2K^+$ (aq) + $2I^-$ (aq) → Hg_2I_2 (s) + $2K^+$ (aq) + $2(NO_3)^-$ (aq)

6. a. Acids and bases neutralize each other, creating water and a salt ($HA + BOH → H_2O + AB$).

7. b. Oxidation: increase of the oxidation # of Sn from Sn [0] to $SnCl_6^{2-}$ [+4]. Oxidizing agent: $4NO_3^-$ (aq), while Sn (s) is the reducing agent (it is oxidized).

8. c. A covalent bond is one where electrons are shared between atoms. Nitrogen and oxygen would form a covalent bond. Sodium and chloride, iron and oxygen, and magnesium and sulfur would all form ionic bonds.

9. d. Cr in $Cr(NO_3)_3$ is displaced by Al.

10. a. Combination of PF_3 (g) and F_2 (g).

11. a. $Ba(OH)_2$ (aq) + $2HNO_3$ (aq) → $Ba(NO_3)_2$ (aq) + $2H_2O$ (l)
The left side of the equation must equal the right side of the equation for all atoms:
1 Ba [in $Ba(OH)_2$] for 1 Ba [in $Ba(NO_3)_2$],
2 N (in $2HNO_3$) for 2 N [in $Ba(NO_3)_2$],
8 O [2 in $Ba(OH)_2$ and 6 in $2HNO_3$] for 8 O [6 in $Ba(NO_3)_2$ and 2 in $2H_2O$]
4 H [2 in $Ba(OH)_2$ and 2 in $2HNO_3$] for 4 H [4 in $2H_2O$]

12. c. The formula for nitrite is NO_2^- and nitrate is NO_3^-.

13. a. C_2H_4 (g) + $3O_2$ (g) → $2CO_2$ (g) + $2H_2O$ (g)
Oxidation: increase of the oxidation # of C from [–2] in C_2H_4 (g) to [+4] in CO_2 (g) and reduction: decrease of the oxidation # of O from [0] in O_2 (g) to [–2] in CO_2 (g).

14. b. Only NH_3 is not ionic and cannot be broken into ions.

15. d. 3 ions: $2 NO_3^-$ and $1 Mg^{2+}$: $3 × 0.25 M = 0.75 M$, which is greater than 0.4 M (Al^{3+} and $3 Cl^-$), 0.45 M (Sr^{2+} and $2 Br^-$), and 0.4 M (Na^+ and Br^-).

16. c. In the equation $Ba(NO_3)_2 + Na_2SO_4 →$ $BaSO_4$ (s) + $2NaNO_3$, 1 mole of sodium sulfate produces 1 mole of the precipitate barium sulfate [137.3 (Ba) + 32 (S) + 4 × 16 (4O) = 233.3 g]. So, to produce 10.0 g of barium sulfate, only $(\frac{10.0}{233.3}) × 1$ mol = 0.04 mol of sodium sulfate is required.

17. b. At constant T, $P_1V_1 = P_2V_2$, so $V_2 = \frac{P_1V_1}{P_2}$
$= \frac{(2.0 \text{ atm})(1.0 \text{ L})}{1.8 \text{ L}} = 1.1 \text{ L}$.

18. c. $CH_3COOH + NaHCO_3 → NaCH_3COO + H_2CO_3$ is an acid-base reaction. Carbonic acid decomposes to H_2O and CO_2, which is released as a gas.

19. c. Na^+ and Cl^- form NaCl.

20. b. $d = \frac{m}{v}$ implies that $v = \frac{m}{d} = \frac{275 \text{ g}}{1.05 \text{ g/mL}}$ ~ 262 mL.

21. d. $\frac{5}{9}(72 - 32) = \frac{5}{9} × 40 = 22.2°C$

22. a. Ionic complexes are formed from combinations of metals and nonmetals. All other choices contain only nonmetals, which form covalent bonds with each other.

23. a. The enthalpy change of a chemical reaction indicates whether the reaction is exothermic or endothermic. A reaction with a negative enthalpy change is exothermic, while a reaction with a positive enthalpy change is endothermic.

24. c. 47.6 g $MgCl_2$ is equivalent to 0.500 mol. 0.500 mol ÷ 2.00 L = 0.250 M $MgCl_2$. In solution, $MgCl_2$ dissociates into three ions (1 Mg^{2+} and 2 Cl^-), so the total concentration of ions is 0.750 M.

25. b. Mirror images are two structures that are not superposable (upon rotation/flipping of the structure or not). In (a), (e), and (f), we have the same structure: On rotating the *second* structure (in plane strictly for (a) and (c) since these are Fischer projections and out of plane for (f)) by 180°, we obtain the *first* structure: (a), (e) and (f) are not pairs of enantiomers or mirror images. Set (g) is labeled (R),(S) for one and (R),(R) for the other structure and cannot therefore constitute a set of enantiomers (in which absolute configuration shouldn't be the same for same chiral carbons of the structures). Choices (b), (c), (d), (h) are sets of enantiomers or mirror images, with (h) showing (R),(R) and (S),(S) (opposite configurations) for the same chiral carbons that is characteristic of enantiomeric pairs.

383

26. c. Since (g) is labeled (R),(S) for one and (R),(R) for the other structure and cannot therefore constitute a set of enantiomers, it's a set of diastereomers.

27. a. $3.33 \times 10^{-5} + 8.13 \times (10^{-5} \times 10^{-2}) = (3.33 + 8.13 \times 10^{-2}) \times 10^{-5} = 3.41 \times 10^{-5}$ (2 decimal digits as in 3.33 and 8.13)

28. d. $0.05620 = 0.5620 \times 10^{-1} = 5.620 \times 10^{-2}$

29. b. By assigning the absolute configurations, set (a) is (R),(S) and (S),(S) and therefore clearly a pair of diastereomers and set (c) shows groups that are not symmetrical by a mirror located between the two Newman projections.

30. b. Bronsted theory defines acids as proton donors and bases as proton acceptors. Lewis theory defines acids as electron acceptors and bases as electron donors.

31. d. The acid concentration of H_2SO_4 is 2 M (2 H^+ per H_2SO_4). The acid is neutralized when it has been reacted with an equimolar amount of base. Using $M_1V_1 = M_2V_2$: $(2\ M)(0.1\ L) = (0.5\ M)(x\ L) \rightarrow x = 0.4\ L$ (400 mL).

32. b. Significant figures include all nonzero digits and trailing zeros in a number that contains a decimal point. In the number 0.00250, the bolded digits are significant.

33. a. This is a reduction reaction because it reduces the oxidation number of Cl from [0] in Cl_2 to [−1] in Cl.

34. d. $[H^+] = 1 \times 10^{-pH} = 1 \times 10^{-3}$
$[H^+][OH^-] = 1 \times 10^{-14}$
$[OH+] = \frac{1 \times 10^{-14}}{[H^+]} = \frac{1 \times 10^{-14}}{1 \times 10^{-3}} = 1 \times 10^{-11}$

35. d. 2 mol of H_2 react with 1 mol (280 g) of linoleic acid. To form 5.0 g of linoleic acid, the required amount of H_2 is $\left(\frac{5.0}{280}\right) \times 2$ mol $= \frac{1}{28}$ mol.

36. d. Sc has 3 valence electrons ($3d^1 4s^2$) and is therefore in group IIIB (group 3, or transition metals).

37. d. A metalloid is an element with properties between those of metals and nonmetals. One of the common properties of metalloids is that they are semiconductors. Germanium, silicon, and arsenic are all metalloids.

38. d. For a principal quantum number of 2, there are four orbitals: $2s$, $2p_x$, $2p_y$, and $2p_z$.

39. c. Elements in the same period, or row, of the periodic table have the same number of electron shells, or levels. In other words, these elements all have the same principal quantum number.

40. b. An alkene is an organic compound made up of carbon and hydrogen atoms, where the carbon atoms are joined by a double bond. The simplest alkene is ethene, which is made up of two double-bonded carbon atoms and four hydrogen atoms.

41. c. An ionic bond forms when electrons are transferred from one atom (now a positively charged cation) to another (which becomes a negatively charged anion).

42. b. In CO_2, carbon has a +4 oxidation state. During photosynthesis, it is reduced to a lower oxidation state as it is converted into carbohydrates that are used as fuel.

43. a. For the dissociation of a weak acid, $HA \rightleftharpoons H^+ + A^-$, the equilibrium constant K_a (also known as the acid dissociation constant), is $K_a = \frac{[H^+][A^-]}{[HA]}$. As with any equilibrium constant, K_a is the product of the concentration of the products over the product of the concentration of the reactants. So for carbonic acid, $K_a = \frac{[H^+][HCO_3^-]}{[H_2CO_3]}$.

44. a. The VSEPR model describes the shape of molecules based on the number of bonds and the number of unbonded electron pairs. The carbon atom of methane has four bonds and no unbonded pairs, so its shape is tetrahedral.

45. b. Boron is in group IIIA (group 13), so it has 3 valence electrons.

46. d. An orbital quantum number of 2 corresponds to a d orbital. There are five d orbitals, each of which can hold two electrons, for a total of 10 electrons that can have these quantum numbers.

47. d. $N \equiv N$

N_2 is nonpolar since both N atoms are identical in nature and physical properties.

48. a. Na:$\overset{\cdot\cdot}{\underset{\cdot\cdot}{Cl}}$: displays 8 dots (a complete octet) around Cl and 2 dots around Na (the particular "He" octet for group IA/group 1 atoms is 2 electrons). In NaCl, Na has transfered its lone valence electron to Cl (which has added it to its original 7 to make a complete octet).

49. c. At constant V, $\frac{P_i}{T_i} = \frac{P_f}{T_f}$ implies that, in Kelvins $T_f = P_f \frac{T_i}{P_i} = \left(\frac{850}{965}\right) \times 328 \text{ K} = 288.64 \text{ K} = 15° \text{ C}$.

50. d. At STP conditions, the molar volume of 1 mole (i.e., 32 g) of O_2 is 22.4 L. Thus, 64.0 g (2 moles) of O_2 gas will occupy $2 \times 22.4 \text{ L} = 44.8$ L volume.

Scoring

Your scores on the six sections of the exam and on the test as a whole will be reported both as scaled scores and as percentiles. A scaled score is a way of converting the number you got right on this test to a number that can be compared with the number other people got right on other forms of the test, which may have been harder or easier. A percentile is a comparison of your scaled score with the scaled scores of other test takers. If your percentile score is 60, you scored higher than 60% of all test takers; if your percentile score is 84, you scored higher than 84% of all test takers.

There is no "passing" scale or percentile score. Individual schools set their own standards, and it's worth your while to find out what scores the schools you want to apply to will accept.

The testing agency uses complicated formulas to come up with scaled and percentile scores. A more meaningful way for you to look at your performance on this practice test is to convert your scores to percentages so that you will be able to compare how you did on the six sections of the test. A *percentage* is not the same as the *percentile* that will appear on your score report. The percentage is simply the number you would have gotten right if there had been 100 questions in the section; it will enable you to compare your scores among the various sections. The *percentile* compares your score with that of other candidates.

In order to find your percentage scores, first add up the number you got right in each section and write it in the following blanks. Questions you didn't answer or got wrong don't count; only count the ones you got right. Then add up the total number of questions you got right.

Section 1: _____ of 50 questions right
Section 2: _____ of 45 questions right
Section 3: _____ of 50 questions right
Section 4: _____ of 50 questions right
Section 5: _____ of 50 questions right
Section 6: _____ of 50 questions right

To figure the percentages for each section and for your total, divide your raw score by the number of questions, and then move the decimal point two places to the right to arrive at a percentage.

Now that you know what percentage of the questions on each section you got right, you can diagnose your strengths and weaknesses. The sections on which you got the lowest percentages are the ones you should plan on studying hardest. Sections on which you got higher percentages may not need as much of your time. However, unless you scored over 90% on a given section, you can't afford to skip studying that section altogether. After all, you want the highest score you can manage in the time left before the exam.

Having taken this practice exam is one important step toward that high score. Simply knowing what to expect is a big help in taking a standardized exam. You are now familiar with the format and content of the exam—an advantage many test takers don't have. Make the most of this advantage by using your scores to help you focus your additional study.

ADDITIONAL ONLINE PRACTICE

Using the codes below, you'll be able to log in and access additional online practice materials!

Your free online practice access codes are:

FVEU034UMN2C2ULBLX2I

FVEFW3S7K17NJEEBH847

FVEGK756BF4H6Q7XG1E3

FVE0K744MI2TWP1WB6KF

FVE8EOA5MS3I5747VOAV

FVEB537QGGS50N74Q72D

Follow these simple steps to redeem your code:

- Go to **www.learningexpresshub.com/affiliate** and have your access code handy.

If you're a new user:

- Click the **New user? Register here** button and complete the registration form to create your account and access your products.
- Be sure to enter your unique access code only once. If you have multiple access codes, you can enter them all—just use a comma to separate each code.
- The next time you visit, simply click the **Returning user? Sign in** button and enter your username and password.
- Do not re-enter previously redeemed access codes. Any products you previously accessed are saved in the **My Account** section on the site. Entering a previously redeemed access code will result in an error message.

If you're a returning user:

- Click the **Returning user? Sign in** button, enter your username and password, and click **Sign In**.
- You will automatically be brought to the **My Account** page to access your products.
- Do not re-enter previously redeemed access codes. Any products you previously accessed are saved in the **My Account** section on the site. Entering a previously redeemed access code will result in an error message.

If you're a returning user with a new access code:

- Click the **Returning user? Sign in** button, enter your username, password, and new access code, and click **Sign In**.
- If you have multiple access codes, you can enter them all—just use a comma to separate each code.
- Do not re-enter previously redeemed access codes. Any products you previously accessed are saved in the **My Account** section on the site. Entering a previously redeemed access code will result in an error message.

If you have any questions, please contact Customer Support at Support@ebsco.com. All inquiries will be responded to within a 24-hour period during our normal business hours: 9:00 A.M.–5:00 P.M. Eastern Time. Thank you!

NOTES

NOTES